Female Pelvic Medicine

Kathleen C. Kobashi • Steven D. Wexner
Editors

Female Pelvic Medicine

Challenging Cases with Expert Commentary

Springer

Editors
Kathleen C. Kobashi, MD, FACS
Department of Urology
Virginia Mason Medical Center
Seattle, WA
USA

Steven D. Wexner, MD, PhD (Hon), FACS, FRCS (Eng), FRCS (Ed), FRCSI (Hon), Hon FRCS (Glasg)
Cleveland Clinic Florida
Weston, FL
USA

ISBN 978-3-030-54838-4 ISBN 978-3-030-54839-1 (eBook)
https://doi.org/10.1007/978-3-030-54839-1

This Springer imprint is published by the registered company Springer Nature Switzerland AG
The registered company address is: Gewerbestrasse 11, 6330 Cham, Switzerland

I dedicate this book to my parents, Luis and Hiroko Kobashi, for their guidance and faith in me from day one and to my husband, Christopher Porter, for his tireless support of me each and every day of my life.

Kathleen C. Kobashi

I thank Dr. Kathleen C. Kobashi for inviting me to co-edit this unique and much needed textbook and Elektra McDermott for her invaluable editorial assistance. I dedicate this book to my sons Wesley and Trevor Wexner for several decades of patience and love as I pursued my clinical and academic endeavors and to my partner in life Mariana Berho for her wisdom, guidance, and love. Lastly, I dedicate this book to my father and mother who encouraged, inspired, and supported me to achieve my goals.

Steven D. Wexner

Foreword

Over the past two decades, the field of Female Pelvic Medicine and Reconstructive Surgery has evolved and since 2013 has been recognized as an official domain of medicine by the American Board of Medical Specialties. During that same period of time, I have had the honor and privilege of working with Kathleen Kobashi on numerous projects related to the specialty that we call our own. She brings unique insights and an unbridled passion to the care of her patients and the advancement of the art and science of the field. Her vision for this book is to provide its readers with advanced knowledge of the more complex challenges encountered by a group of experienced experts. In this era in which the field of Pelvic Floor Medicine has appropriately evolved toward a more truly multidisciplinary approach to our patients, Dr. Kobashi has partnered with Dr. Steven Wexner, a world-renowned colorectal surgeon, to include experts in colorectal surgery to provide their important input.

Drawing from both the experiences of the authors and the practical use of the evidence-based data and information available, Dr. Kobashi and Dr. Wexner have created a resource that focuses on the thought-leader's approach to complex FPMRS problems and scenarios. Hence its uniqueness—a book that provides its readers with evidence-based, experience-based, and case-based learning. I believe that the type and style of learning provided in this text is exactly what is needed for the ultimate benefit of our patients as the specialty of FPMRS continues to grow and evolve in the decades to come.

Los Angeles, CA, USA — Victor W. Nitti

Preface

Female Pelvic Medicine and Reconstructive Surgery (FPMRS) has recently become recognized as an official domain of medicine by the American Board of Medical Specialties. As such, attention to this subspecialty that intersects urology, gynecology, and colorectal surgery has significantly increased during the past decade. Indeed, FPMRS has become an integral part of the core curriculum of urology residencies, and with more individuals achieving advanced training in the field, a notable evolution of the entire discipline has been realized. Importantly, with more clinicians being trained, more patients are being treated, and new challenges are continually arising. It must also be emphasized that with this evolution, the close anatomical and functional relationships of the lower genitourinary and colorectal systems have come to the forefront of thinking, underscoring the importance of a multidisciplinary approach to the pelvic floor as a global entity.

This book offers a resource that focuses on advanced scenarios in pelvic floor medicine. While there are many textbooks in urology, urogynecology, gynecology, and colorectal surgery that discuss pelvic floor disorders (PFD), this book is exclusively dedicated to comprehensive strategies to address the clinical challenges in PFD. The issues presented in this textbook are essential to all practitioners of pelvic floor surgery.

In a general sense, the book is organized by PFD, including the evaluation and treatment of urinary incontinence, fecal incontinence, and pelvic organ prolapse. In order to offer a logical perspective, the initial chapters in each part review the fundamentals of a proper comprehensive assessment of patients with PFDs of any complexity and the treatment options that are available for each. However, the overarching theme of this book is a focus on more complex and challenging situations that are becoming more frequently encountered as more clinicians enter this field. As the sheer number of patients treated each year rises and the length of follow-up continues to increase, new scenarios have arisen that require a shift in approach from that of the treatment-naïve patients.

In order to maintain clinical relevance and applicability for the reader, each chapter is written based on clinical scenarios. The book is designed to impart to the reader the reflections and opinions of numerous internationally renowned experts who have been in the field as it has evolved. The format is unique in that it presents the material in a practical manner that can be applied to daily practice. Our hope is that the reader will learn how to approach the most challenging of multidisciplinary clinical situations with confidence.

Seattle, WA, USA Kathleen C. Kobashi
Weston, FL, USA Steven D. Wexner

Acknowledgments

We would like to thank the following authors for their contribution to the Commentary section in all the chapters.

Chapter 1: Eric S. Rovner
Chapter 2: Kathleen C. Kobashi
Chapter 3: J. Marcio N. Jorge
Chapter 4: Ann C. Lowry
Chapter 5: Polina Reyblat
Chapter 6: Jason Kim
Chapter 7: John P. Lavelle
Chapter 8: Marcio A. Averbeck
Chapter 9: E. Ann Gormley
Chapter 10: David E. Rapp
Chapter 11: Tracy L. Hull
Chapter 12: Massarat Zutshi
Chapter 13: Donato F. Altomare
Chapter 14: Tracy L. Hull
Chapter 15: Benjamin M. Brucker
Chapter 16: Howard B. Goldman
Chapter 17: Una Lee
Chapter 18: Alexander Gomelsky
Chapter 19: W. Stuart Reynolds
Chapter 20: Amanda S. J. Chung
Chapter 21: Jaspreet S. Sandhu

Contents

Contributors

Donato F. Altomare, MD Azienda Ospedaliero Universitaria Policlinico Bari, Department of Emergency and Organ Transplantation, University Aldo Moro of Bari, Bari, Italy

Jennifer T. Anger, MD, MPH Cedars-Sinai Medical Center, Department of Surgery, Division of Urology, Los Angeles, CA, USA

Marcio A. Averbeck, MD, MSc, PhD Neuro-urology, Video-urodynamics Unit, Moinhos De Vento Hospital, Department of Urology, Porto Allegre, Brazil

Rachel C. Barratt, BMedSci, BMBS, FRCS(Urol) University College London Hospitals and University College London, Department of Urology, UCLH@Westmoreland Street Hospital, London, UK

Marylise Boutros, MDCM, FRCSC Jewish General Hospital, Division of Colon and Rectal Surgery, Montreal, QC, Canada

Amallia Brair, MBBD, CABOG Birmingham Women's and Children's NHS Foundation Trust, Department of Pelvic Floor Medicine, Birmingham, UK

Benjamin M. Brucker, MD Division of Female Pelvic Medicine and Reconstructive Surgery and Neurourology, New York University Langone Health, Department of Urology and Obstetrics and Gynecology, New York, NY, USA

Claire S. Burton, MD University of California – Los Angeles, Department of Urology, Los Angeles, CA, USA

Amanda S. J. Chung, BSc(Med)/MBBS, MS, FRACS The University of Sydney, Sydney, NSW, Australia

Royal North Shore Hospital, St Leonards, NSW, Australia

Concord Repatriation General Hospital, Concord, NSW, Australia

Macquarie University Hospital, Department of Urology, Sydney, NSW, Australia

Craig V. Comiter, MD Stanford University, Department of Urology, Stanford, CA, USA

Giovanna da Silva, MD Department of Colorectal Surgery, Cleveland Clinic Florida, Weston, FL, USA

Sophia D. Delpe, MD Vanderbilt University Medical Center, Department of Urology, Nashville, TN, USA

Samir Derisavifard, MD Cleveland Clinic, Glickman Urological and Kidney Institute, Cleveland, OH, USA

Roger R. Dmochowski, MD, MMHC, FACS Vanderbilt University Medical Center, Department of Urology, Nashville, TN, USA

Amy D. Dobberfuhl, MD Stanford University, Department of Urology, Stanford, CA, USA

Ekene A. Enemchukwu, MD, MPH Stanford University, Department of Urology, Stanford, CA, USA

Dee E. Fenner, MD University of Michigan, Department of Obstetrics and Gynecology, Ann Arbor, MI, USA

David Alan Ginsberg, MD Keck School of Medicine USC, Department of Urology, Los Angeles, CA, USA

Howard B. Goldman, MD Cleveland Clinic, Glickman Urologic and Kidney Institute, Cleveland, OH, USA

Alexander Gomelsky, MD, FACS LSU Health – Shreveport, Department of Urology, Shreveport, LA, USA

E. Ann Gormley, MD Geisel School of Medicine at Dartmouth, Hanover, NH, USA

Dartmouth-Hitchcock Medical Center, Section of Urology, Department of Surgery, Lebanon, NH, USA

Tamsin J. Greenwell, MBChB, MD, FRCS (Urol) University College London Hospitals and University College London, Department of Urology, UCLH@Westmoreland Street Hospital, London, UK

Deborah S. Hess, MD, MS Wilmington Health, Department of Urology, Wilmington, NC, USA

Christine Jeanne Horton, MD MSCR Keck School of Medicine USC, Department of Urology, Los Angeles, CA, USA

Vanessa W. Hui, MD University of Miami, Department of General Surgery, Division of Colorectal Surgery, Miami, FL, USA

Tracy L. Hull, MD Cleveland Clinic, Department of Colon and Rectal Surgery, Cleveland, OH, USA

J. Marcio N. Jorge, MD, PhD Hospital das Clinicas, University of Sao Paulo, Department of Gastroenterology – Colorectal Division, Sao Paulo, Brazil

Jason Kim, MD Women's Pelvic Health and Continence Center, Stony Brook University Hospital, Department of Urology, Stony Brook, NY, USA

Kathleen C. Kobashi, MD, FACS Virginia Mason Medical Center, Department of Urology and Renal Transplantation, Seattle, WA, USA

Madeline Rovira Koerner, MD, MBA Louisiana State University Health Sciences Center, Department of Urology, New Orleans, LA, USA

Casey G. Kowalik, MD University of Kansas Health System, Department of Urology, Kansas City, KS, USA

Victoria Valinluck Lao, MD, PhD Memorial Hospital West, Division of Colon and Rectal Surgery, Pembroke Pines, FL, USA

John P. Lavelle, MB, FRCSI Veterans Affairs Palo Alto Health Care System, Department of Surgical Service, Urology Section, Palo Alto, CA, USA

Chun Hin Angus Lee, MD Cleveland Clinic, Department of Colorectal Surgery, Digestive Disease and Surgery Institute, Cleveland, OH, USA

Una Lee, MD Virginia Mason Medical Center, Department of Urology, Seattle, WA, USA

Gary E. Lemack, MD University of Texas Southwestern Medical Center, Department of Urology, Dallas, TX, USA

Ann C. Lowry, MD University of Minnesota, Department of Colon and Rectal Surgery, Minneapolis, MN, USA

Alvaro Lucioni, MD Virginia Mason Medical Center, Department of Urology, Seattle, WA, USA

Dena Moskowitz, MD Virginia Mason Medical Center, Department of Urology, Seattle, WA, USA

Victor W. Nitti, MD Department of Urology Georgetown University, Female Pelvic Medicine and Reconstructive Surgery, New York University, Department of Urology, New York, NY, USA

Lucia Camara Castro Oliveira, MD, PhD, FASCRS Anorectal Physiology Department, CEPEMED, Rio de Janeiro, Brazil

Allison Pang, MD, MSc, FRCSC Jewish General Hospital, Division of Colon and Rectal Surgery, Montreal, QC, Canada

David E. Rapp, MD, FPMRS University of Virginia, Department of Urology, Charlottesville, VA, USA

Charles R. Rardin, MD Woman and Infants Hospital, Department of Obstetrics and Gynecology, Providence, RI, USA

Polina Reyblat, MD Kaiser Permanente, Los Angeles Medical Center, Department of Urology, Los Angeles, CA, USA

W. Stuart Reynolds, MD, MPH Vanderbilt University Medical Center, Department of Urology, Nashville, TN, USA

Eric S. Rovner, MD Medical University of South Carolina, Department of Urology, Charleston, SC, USA

Jessica J. Rueb, MD Cleveland Clinic, Glickman Urological and Kidney Institute, Cleveland, OH, USA

Jaspreet S. Sandhu, MD Memorial Sloan-Kettering Cancer Center, Department of Surgery, Urology Service, New York, NY, USA

Dana R. Sands, MD Cleveland Clinic Florida, Department of Colorectal Surgery, Weston, FL, USA

Payton Schmidt, MD University of Michigan, Department of Obstetrics and Gynecology, Ann Arbor, MI, USA

Karen L. Sherman, MD, MS Duke University Hospital, Department of Surgery, Raleigh, NC, USA

Ariana L. Smith, MD, FPMRS Pelvic Medicine & Reconstructive Surgery, University of Pennsylvania Health System, Philadelphia, PA, USA

Lauren E. Stewart, MD Female Pelvic Medicine and Reconstructive Surgery, Departments of Urology and Obstetrics and Gynecology, NYU Grossman School of Medicine/NYU Langone Health, New York, NY, USA

Rachael D. Sussman, MD Department of Urology Georgetown University, Female Pelvic Medicine and Reconstructive Surgery, New York University, Department of Urology, New York, NY, USA

Raveen Syan, MD Stanford University, Department of Urology, Stanford, CA, USA

Philip Toozs-Hobson, MD, FRCOG Birmingham Women's and Children's NHS Foundation Trust, Department of Urogynecology, Birmingham, UK

Megan C. Turner, MD, MHS Department of Surgery, Duke University Medical Center, Durham, NC, USA

Philip E. V. Van Kerrebroeck, MD, PhD, MMSc Maastricht University Medical Center, Department of Urology, Maastricht, The Netherlands

Julie Ann Van Koughnett, MD, MEd, FRSCS, FACS London Health Sciences Centre – University Hospital, Departments of Surgery and Oncology, London, ON, Canada

Sandip Vasavada, MD Cleveland Clinic, Department of Urology, Cleveland, OH, USA

Steven J. Weissbart, MD Stony Brook University Hospital, Department of Urology, Stony Brook, NY, USA

Steven D. Wexner, MD, PhD (Hon), FACS, FRCS (Eng), FRCS (Ed), FRCSI (Hon), Hon FRCS (Glasg) Department of Colorectal Surgery, Cleveland Clinic Florida, Weston, FL, USA

Cleveland Clinic Lerner College of Medicine of Case Western Reserve University, Cleveland, OH, USA

Charles E. Schmidt College of Medicine, Florida Atlantic University, Boca Raton, FL, USA

Herbert Wertheim College of Medicine, Florida International University, Miami, FL, USA

Ohio State University Wexner College of Medicine, Cleveland, OH, USA

Department of Surgery, University of South Florida Morsani College of Medicine, Tampa, FL, USA

Division of Surgery and Interventional Science, Department of Targeted Intervention, University College London, London, UK

J. Christian Winters, MD, FACS Louisiana State University Health Sciences Center, Department of Urology, New Orleans, LA, USA

Massarat Zutshi, MD Cleveland Clinic, Department of Colorectal Surgery, Digestive Disease and Surgery Institute, Cleveland, OH, USA

Part I

Evaluation

1 Basic Evaluation of the Patient with Pelvic Floor Dysfunction (General Review)

Raveen Syan, Ekene A. Enemchukwu, Amy D. Dobberfuhl, and Craig V. Comiter

Abbreviations

AUA	American Urological Association
FI	Fecal incontinence
MMSE	Mini-mental status exam
MUI	Mixed urinary incontinence
OAB	Overactive bladder
PFD	Pelvic floor dysfunction
PFMT	Pelvic floor muscle training
POP	Pelvic organ prolapse
POP-Q	Pelvic Organ Prolapse Quantification system
PVR	Post-void residual
SUFU	Society of Urodynamics, Female Pelvic Medicine and Urogenital Reconstruction
SUI	Stress urinary incontinence
UTI	Urinary tract infection
UI	Urge incontinence

Commentary by Eric S. Rovner, Medical University of South Carolina, Department of Urology, Charleston, SC, USA

R. Syan (✉) · E. A. Enemchukwu · A. D. Dobberfuhl
C. V. Comiter
Stanford University, Department of Urology, Stanford, CA, USA
e-mail: rsyan@stanford.edu

Case Scenarios

Case Scenario 1

A 45-year-old woman presents with stress urinary incontinence. She denies any storage/overactive bladder or prolapse symptoms. Physical examination reveals a positive supine cough stress test and urethral hypermobility with no evidence of prolapse.

Case Scenario 2

A 62-year-old female presents with bothersome symptoms of urinary urgency and frequency, nocturia, and urge incontinence. She denies stress incontinence. She has never been treated with medical or surgical therapy.

Case Scenario 3

A 58-year-old G3P3 woman presents with a bothersome vaginal bulge and constipation. This is associated with a sensation of incomplete bladder emptying with mild urinary frequency. She has a prior history of stress urinary incontinence that spontaneously resolved 2 years ago. On pelvic examination, the patient has a grade 3 cystocele, a grade 2 rectocele, and a negative empty

K. C. Kobashi, S. D. Wexner (eds.), *Female Pelvic Medicine*,
https://doi.org/10.1007/978-3-030-54839-1_1

supine cough stress test with or without the cystocele reduced.

Introduction

Pelvic floor dysfunction (PFD) is a condition that may manifest as multiple complaints, such as urinary incontinence, fecal incontinence, and pelvic organ prolapse. PFD is highly prevalent and increases with advancing age. Twenty-five percent of women in the United States report symptoms related to one or more of these complaints [1–3]. It is commonly associated with obstetric injury following childbirth; however, there are many contributing causes of PFD that include neurologic disorders, prior surgeries, trauma, or unknown causes [1].

While PFD-related symptomatology often varies from patient to patient, the effect on individual quality of life and the burden of disease on the healthcare system can be significant. Hu et al. performed a cost-of-illness analysis in the United States and found that the total cost of urinary incontinence (UI) was \$19.5 billion dollars and overactive bladder (OAB) was \$12.6 billion dollars in the year 2000 [4]. With an aging population in the United States, the prevalence of these disorders is expected to rise. Therefore, understanding the diagnosis and treatment of these disorders is of great importance.

Essentials in History and Physical Exam Including Urinary and Fecal Incontinence Scores

Symptoms of PFD such as urinary symptoms, defecatory symptoms, or prolapse symptoms can occur alone or in combination. As a result, a thorough history is essential. An assessment of the impact each symptom has on a patient's quality of life is also important, as this can guide the clinician regarding goals of care. Several validated questionnaires are available for quality-of-life assessment, which allows the patient and physician to treat the most bothersome symptom first. Finally, a careful physical exam plays an important role in elucidating the pathophysiology of the patient's symptoms.

Terminology

Lower urinary tract symptoms typically lead the patient to seek care. Symptoms can be variable and include both storage and voiding complaints. The International Continence Society published a report that standardized terminology for many of the lower urinary tract symptoms in 2002 [5] and a recent updated terminology report on PFD in 2017 [6]. Examples of lower urinary tract symptoms are summarized in Table 1.1, along with the underlying anatomical changes and

Table 1.1 Terminology used for lower urinary symptoms

Term	Symptom	Common pathophysiology
Stress urinary incontinence (SUI)	Complaint of involuntary urinary loss with physical exertion, sneezing/coughing, or other activities raising intra-abdominal pressure	Weak urinary sphincter
Urinary urgency	Complaint of sudden compelling desire to urinate that is difficult to defer	Detrusor overactivity
Urinary frequency	Complaint of voiding too often by day	Detrusor overactivity
Urge incontinence (UI)	Complaint of involuntary urinary loss associated with sensation of urgency	Detrusor overactivity
Mixed urinary incontinence (MUI)	Complaint of involuntary urinary loss associated with physical exertion/rise in intra-abdominal pressure and also with urgency	Detrusor overactivity and weak urinary sphincter
Overactive bladder (OAB)	Complaint of urinary urgency, with or without urge incontinence, typically with frequency and nocturia	Detrusor overactivity
Fecal incontinence (FI)	Complaint of involuntary loss of feces, with or without urgency	Weak anal sphincter

Adapted from "The standardisation of terminology of lower urinary tract function: report from the Standardisation Subcommittee of the International Continence Society," 2002 and updated in 2017 [5, 6]

pathophysiology most commonly associated with these symptoms.

Patient History

A thorough patient history, including exacerbating and alleviating factors, can help to identify the specific cause of the patient's pelvic floor symptoms. Once the chief complaint is established, it is important to determine any contributing medical conditions. For instance, disease processes such as diabetes can lead to high volumes of urine production and present as urinary frequency or nocturia. Neurologic conditions such as Parkinson's disease or stroke can be associated with urinary storage dysfunction [7, 8].

A detailed history of surgical procedures is important, especially prior abdominal and vaginal surgeries, as these can have adverse consequences on the pelvic floor. Prior vaginal surgery can result in surgical disruption of the normal pelvic floor support, alter bladder anatomy and neurologic function, and in some cases result in changes in the caliber of the vaginal canal, contributing to subsequent PFD. For example, a history of hysterectomy for an indication other than prolapse repair has been shown to be a risk factor for subsequent prolapse [9].

A careful gynecologic history can be especially important in the setting of pelvic organ prolapse. This history should include parity, vaginal versus cesarean route of delivery, infant birth weight, use of forceps versus vacuum assistance, and associated obstetric lacerations to the vagina and rectum, as these are all known to be associated with pelvic organ prolapse [10]. Current menopausal status is important to ascertain, as vaginal atrophy related to menopause is associated with voiding and sexual dysfunction. Hormone replacement therapy has been shown to be effective and may be indicated [11]. Treatment should be individualized based on patient history and symptoms, with oral therapy, topical therapy, or a combined approach. Any history of abnormal vaginal bleeding or discharge should also be elicited to determine if procedures such as pelvic ultrasound or Papanicolaou smear are needed prior to intervention.

The clinician should always review the patient's medication list, as many medications have side effects that can result in voiding dysfunction, constipation, and dry mouth. For example, sympathomimetics can result in increased tone of the urinary sphincter and therefore an obstructive pattern of voiding. Anticholinergics can weaken detrusor contractions and cause incomplete bladder emptying or, in some cases, urinary retention [12]. Diuretics and antihypertensives increase urine production that can cause urinary frequency and nocturia [13].

Studies suggest that there is a genetic component to the development of both pelvic organ prolapse and urinary incontinence [14–16]. Therefore, obtaining a family history can help determine a patient's likelihood of developing these disorders and may help predict eventual severity of disease [17].

Urinary, fecal, and pelvic symptoms can be complex, and evaluation should be directed toward understanding the degree of bother. For example, when a patient presents with urinary incontinence, it is important to differentiate urge from stress. Clinicians should determine the frequency of incontinence, the exacerbating behaviors, the presence of urgency symptoms, the volume of leakage, and the sensory awareness of the incontinence. It is helpful to distinguish between daytime and nighttime incontinence to help understand diurnal variations in functional bladder capacity and urine production. Obstructive voiding symptoms should be evaluated. These include hesitancy, intermittency, straining to void, and feelings of incomplete bladder emptying. A post-void residual can be obtained to identify incomplete emptying or urinary retention. A timeline detailing the onset of symptoms and associated events such as pregnancies or surgical interventions should be established.

Bothersome pelvic organ prolapse (POP) is often associated with a bulge sensation or pressure-like sensation in the vaginal canal. Patients should be asked if they must "splint" or manually reduce the vaginal bulge in order to urinate or defecate. Obstructive patterns of urination or defecation should raise index of suspicion for POP-Q stage 3 or greater prolapse.

Finally, an assessment of patient's physical activity can be useful when it is used to identify the exacerbating maneuvers, adverse impairment of patient's mobility, prevention of physical activity, and the impact each of these may have on a patient's quality of life.

Pad Tests, Voiding Diaries, and Questionnaires

Given the complex relationship among PFD symptoms, questionnaires are useful tools for quantifying the severity and degree of bother associated with each symptom. There are many questionnaires available for the assessment of PFD. The most commonly used questionnaires are summarized in Table 1.2 [18–29].

Pad weight tests are commonly used to quantify volume of incontinence. Pads are counted and weighed over a 24-hour period to assess urinary leakage. These pads are weighed, and patients are categorized as having mild, moderate, or severe incontinence based on pad weight [30]. However, this can be burdensome to perform for both patients and clinicians, and Nitti et al. demonstrated that patient report of pad number and subjective description of pad saturation is as effective as a pad weight test [31]. Pad tests are especially useful in clinical trials where they provide objective measurements of incontinence. However, they are less commonly used in clinical practice and have been mostly replaced by patient self-report of pad use.

Voiding diaries are completed by patients and document the number of voids, the number of incontinence episodes, the presence of urgency or stress-related episodes, and a detailed report of fluid intake. This allows the clinician to better understand the type of incontinence as well as the severity of the symptoms. There is no consensus on the ideal duration of the voiding diary; however, 2- to 7-day voiding diaries have been shown to be reliable [32]. Schick et al. found that a 4-day diary was as effective as a 7-day diary [33]. Voiding diaries also help clinicians identify areas

Table 1.2 Commonly used questionnaires for evaluating pelvic floor dysfunction

Questionnaire	Utility
Fecal incontinence	
Fecal Incontinence Quality of Life (FIQL) [18]	Assessment of symptoms of fecal incontinence and impact on quality of life
Fecal Incontinence Severity Index (FISI) (from the American Society of Colon and Rectal Surgeons) [19]	Assessment of the severity of symptoms of fecal incontinence and can be used to evaluate change following treatment
Cleveland Clinic Florida- Fecal Incontinence Score (CCF-FIS) [20]	Assessment of degree and frequency of incontinence and quality of life assessment
Pelvic organ prolapse	
Pelvic Floor Distress Inventory (PFDI) [21]	Assessment of pelvic organ prolapse symptoms
Pelvic Floor Impact Questionnaire (PFIQ) [21]	Assessment of the impact of pelvic organ prolapse symptoms on quality of life
Urinary incontinence	
Bristol Female Urinary Tract Symptoms Questionnaire (BFLUTS) [22]	Assessment of urinary symptoms and impact on quality of life and can be used to evaluate change following treatment
International Consultation on Incontinence Modular Questionnaire Short Form (ICIQ-UI-SF) [23]	Assessment of urinary incontinence
Incontinence Impact Questionnaire – Short Form (IIQ-SF) [24]	Assessment of the impact of urinary incontinence on quality of life
Incontinence Quality of Life Questionnaire (IQOL) [25]	Assessment of the impact of urinary incontinence on quality of life
Overactive Bladder Questionnaire – Short Form (OABq-SF) [26]	Assessment of symptoms of overactive bladder and the impact on quality of life
Overactive Bladder Symptom Score (OAB-SS) [27]	Often used as a screening questionnaire evaluating for overactive bladder symptoms
Questionnaire for Urinary Incontinence Diagnosis (QUID) [28]	Often used as a screening questionnaire evaluating for overactive bladder and/or stress incontinence symptoms
Urogenital Distress Inventory – Short Form (UDI-6) [24]	Assessment of degree of bother due to urinary tract symptoms
Urinary Incontinence Severity Score (UISS) [29]	Assessment of severity of symptoms and impact on quality of life

that may benefit from behavioral modification, such as limiting fluids at night, limiting bladder irritants such as caffeine, and avoiding excessive fluid intake.

Physical Exam

Abdominal and Bimanual Exam

A basic examination of the abdomen should be routinely performed in all patients. Suprapubic fullness may indicate incomplete bladder emptying. Abdominal exam should include evaluation of surgical scars, which may help identify operations known to contribute to the development of PFD. Scars from laparoscopic, suprapubic, groin, laparotomy, and Pfannenstiel incisions should be documented and compared to the patient's surgical history. If surgical intervention is warranted, the site, number, and location of surgical scars may impact surgical approach.

The bimanual exam should also include evaluation of the uterus and the adnexa for masses, as this may lead to deferment of elective interventions until a malignant workup is complete. Pelvic floor strength, the presence of vaginal atrophy, and fascial integrity are also key aspects of the pelvic exam in PFD.

Neurologic Exam

An overall picture of neurologic and cognitive health of a patient should be elicited while taking the patient's history. Additional information can be obtained by evaluating a patients' gait and ability to transfer their body weight from the chair to the table for the physical exam. If cognitive deficits that raise concern for prior stroke or other neurologic disease are observed, a mini-mental state exam (MMSE) should be performed (Table 1.3). A score less than 24 is suggestive of cognitive impairment [34].

Table 1.3 Mini-mental status examination

Question	Score
Orientation	
What is the year/season/date/day/month?	5
Where are we (state/country/town/hospital/floor)?	5
Registration	
The examiner names three unrelated objects and asks the patient to repeat all three. The examiner repeats them until the patient learns them, if possible. The number of trials is documented	3
Attention and calculation	
Serial 7s: 1 point for each correct answer, and stop after 5 answersCan also ask the patient to spell "world" backward	5
Recall	
Ask the patient to repeat the three objects previously given. 1 point is given for each correct answer	3
Language	
Name a pencil and a watch	2
Repeat the following: "No ifs, ands, or buts"	1
Follow a three-stage command ("Take a paper, fold it, place on floor")	3
Reach and obey the following: CLOSE YOUR EYES	1
Write a sentence	1
Copy a design shown (typically interlocking pentagons)	1
Total	30

Adapted from "The Mini-Mental State Examination in general medical practice: clinical utility and acceptance" by Tangalos et al. [34]

A basic neurologic exam should be performed during every pelvic examination to assess motor and sensory response. The first assessment that should be performed is visually, by asking the patient to perform a pelvic floor Kegel contraction, and assessing visually for a symmetric contraction of the perineum, pelvic floor, vagina, and anus. Tactile response should be assessed next, with an assessment of laterality and sensory discrimination.

Following these tests, the most commonly used neurologic reflex test of afferent and efferent function is the anal wink or perineal reflex test. This is performed by gently touching the skin around the anus. The test is positive (or normal) if a symmetric contraction is elicited from the anal sphincter.

Following vaginal exam, the clinician should assess anal sphincter tone, sensation, as well as volitional anal sphincter contractility. If normal, then the clinician can assume that sacral innervation is present.

Evaluation for Stress Urinary Incontinence

According to the American Urological Association (AUA) guidelines on female stress urinary incontinence (SUI), it is important to objectively demonstrate SUI in patients who complain of incontinence with activity [35]. During the pelvic exam, a cough stress test should be performed, during which the patient should be asked to cough. If the patient has already voided, an empty supine cough stress test may be performed. During the pelvic exam, urethral hypermobility should be visually assessed using the Q-tip test (see Fig. 1.1). A lubricated sterile cotton swab is placed in the urethra, and the patient is asked to perform a Valsalva maneuver. The maximal urethral deflection from the horizon is noted. Having a greater than 30-degree deflection from the horizon is consistent with urethral hypermobility. If incontinence and hypermobility are identified, then Marshall's test may be performed to elevate the vaginal fornices and assess for cessation of leakage [36]. If this results in continence during a cough or stress maneuver, this may indicate symptom success with a retropubic sling.

If the patient has a cystocele, the tip of the half speculum, a vaginal packing, or pessary should be used to reduce the cystocele and assess for stress incontinence with and without the prolapse reduced. This is especially useful in patients who do not complain of SUI and are considering treatment of the cystocele, either surgically or with a pessary. If occult SUI is unmasked, the patient should be counseled regarding the risk of bothersome SUI. As part of this discussion, the clinician should manage expectations while discussing the role of SUI procedures.

Speculum Exam and Evaluation for Prolapse

A standard speculum exam should be performed on all females with symptoms of PFD. The clinician should evaluate the external genitalia for abnormal masses and perform a general examination of the vaginal walls and cervix.

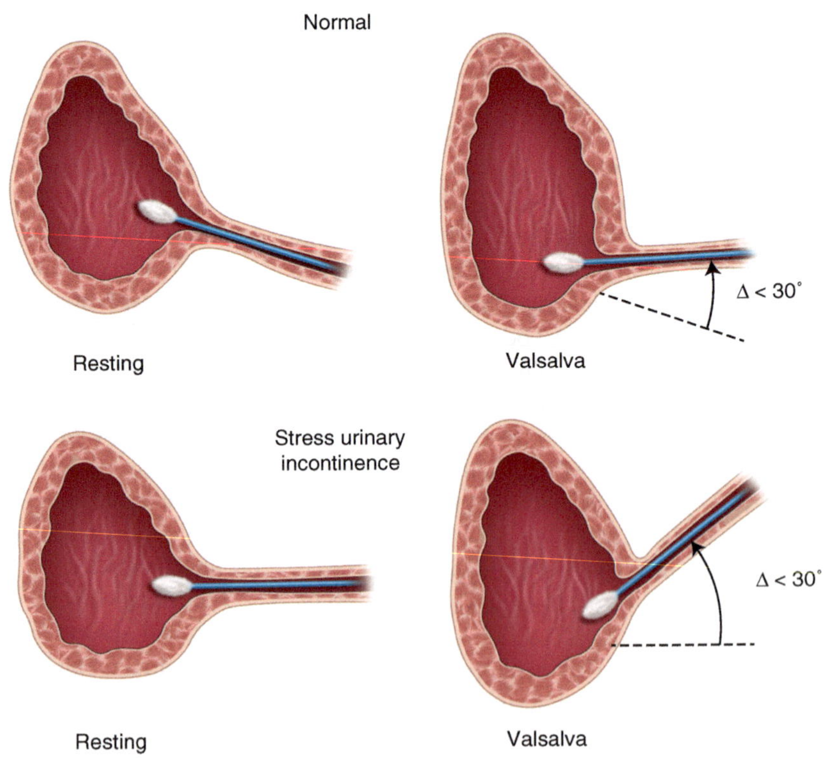

Fig. 1.1 Q-tip test for stress incontinence: with a sterile cotton tip within the urethra, a greater than 30° deflection from the horizon with cough or strain is indicative of urethral hypermobility

The Pelvic Organ Prolapse Quantification (POP-Q) system exam is a standardized system used for quantifying the degree of POP. A complete POP-Q exam is performed using a measuring stick and a vaginal speculum. The exam entails assessment of vaginal length with the full speculum. A general appearance of the vaginal walls can be evaluated at this time. Half of the speculum is then used to retract the posterior wall for evaluation of the anterior wall and then subsequently to retract the anterior wall for posterior wall evaluation. The degree of descent with straining is quantified using the measuring stick during the speculum exam, and staging is quantified using the POP-Q staging system (see Fig. 1.2). The degree of descent of the apex can be evaluated during both anterior and posterior wall examinations, though this can be difficult to assess in some patients. Alternatively, the apex can also be assessed by placing a finger against the cervix and evaluating degree of descent down the vaginal canal during Valsalva maneuver. A limited POP-Q exam can also be performed using just a half speculum and should be combined with a bimanual exam.

Pelvic Floor Exam

The caliber of the vagina is assessed visually and by placing one or two fingers in the vagina. During this evaluation, the patient should be asked to contract her pelvic floor (Kegel exercise) to determine if the patient is able to appropriately recruit the pelvic floor muscles. Patients with incontinence, prolapse symptoms, and poor contraction effort may benefit from pelvic floor muscle training (PFMT) and biofeedback focused on strengthening the pelvic floor muscles, with or without the assistance of a formal pelvic floor physical therapist [37, 38].

Pelvic floor muscle tone, tenderness, and spasticity should be evaluated to assess both pelvic floor strength and excessive tightness of the pelvic floor muscles. High-tone pelvic floor can cause obstructive urinary symptoms, constipation, pelvic pain, and dyspareunia. In this setting, pelvic floor physical therapy is targeted toward relaxation of the pelvic floor during voiding, defecation, and sexual intercourse. Assessment of pelvic floor tone is critical to directing the patient to the correct therapy, as a high-tone pelvic floor is best treated with pelvic floor down-training and biofeedback. The goal of therapy is to help patients identify strategies to isolate the pelvic floor musculature and relax the pelvic floor, in concert with a coordinated detrusor contraction if voiding complaints predominate, or Valsalva for defecatory dysfunction [39].

Perineal and Rectal Exam

An evaluation of the perineum and rectum in patients with defecatory dysfunction or a rectocele is important. A rectal exam assesses anal sphincter tone and helps evaluate for the common causes of fecal incontinence. With a finger in the rectum, the posterior vaginal wall should be evaluated to assess for presence and degree of rectocele. The perineum is often attenuated in women with obstetric injuries; thus, the clinician must assess for the presence of an intact perineal body. Finally, rectal prolapse is often associated with pelvic organ prolapse and can often be treated concomitantly with pelvic organ prolapse repair. Thus, the clinician should visually assess for rectal prolapse as the patient is asked to bear down. If present, patients should be referred to a colorectal surgeon for consideration of surgical management.

Adjunct Studies in the Straightforward Patient

Post-void Residual

When a patient enters a urologic and gynecologic clinic, a urine sample is often obtained for a screening urinalysis for the evaluation of lower urinary tract symptoms. At this point, an assessment of a patient's ability to empty her bladder can be easily performed using clean intermittent catheterization or an ultrasound bladder scanner to measure the patient's post-void residual (PVR). The American Urological Association and the Society of Urodynamics, Female Pelvic Medicine

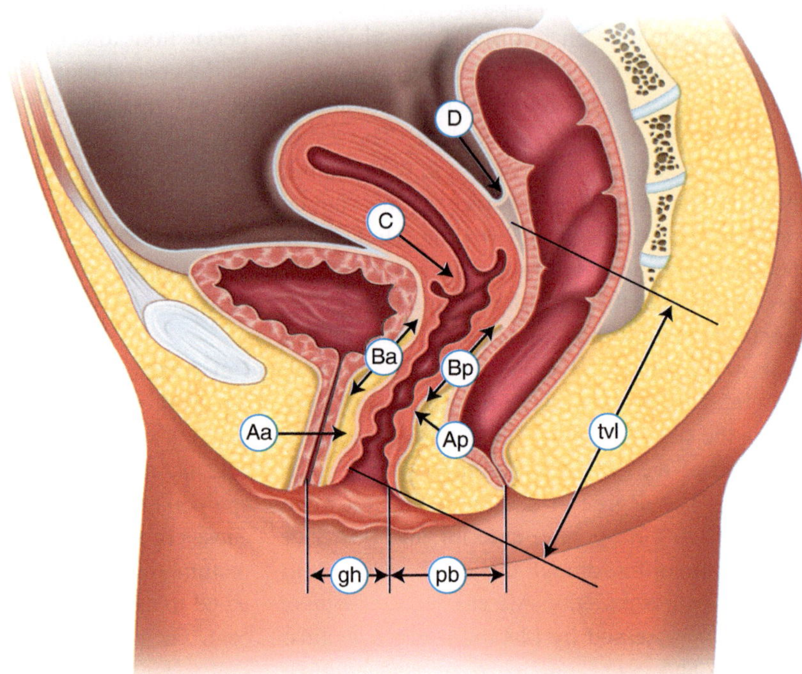

Fig. 1.2 The Pelvic Organ Prolapse Quantification (POP-Q) system and the points that are measured

Point	Description	Range of valves
Aa	Anterior vaginal wall 3 cm proximal to the hymen	-3 cm to +3 cm
Ba	Most distal position of remaining upper anterior vaginal wall	-3 cm to +tvl
C	Most distal edge of cervix or vaginal cuff scar	-
D	Posterior fornix (N/A if post-hysterectomy)	-
Ap	Posterior vaginal wall 3 cm proximal to the hymen	-3 cm to +3 cm
Bp	Most distal position of remaining upper posterior vaginal wall	-3 cm to +tvl
gh (genital hiatus)	Measured from middle of external urethral meatus to posterior midline hymen	-
pb (perineal body)	Measured from posterior margin of gh to middle of anal opening	-
tvl (total vaginal length)	Depth of vagina when point D or C is reduced to normal position	-

and Urogenital Reconstruction (AUA/SUFU) guidelines on OAB recommend a PVR be obtained on all patients, as an elevated PVR can be associated with increased risk of voiding dysfunction following surgical intervention [40, 41].

Uroflowmetry is often available in the outpatient clinical setting. Using a noninvasive machine, it measures the voided volume, the maximum rate of flow, the average rate of flow, and the pattern of flow. This is especially useful in patients with obstructive urinary symptoms or incomplete bladder emptying.

Laboratory Testing

Routine laboratory testing is typically unnecessary for the initial evaluation. A urinalysis with or without urine culture may be obtained in symptomatic patients to rule out urinary tract infection (UTI) and quantify the presence or absence of microscopic hematuria. In a patient with three or greater red blood cells per high-power field, in the absence of a UTI, a hematuria workup should be considered [42]. Otherwise, laboratory testing in the uncomplicated patient is reserved for preoperative testing and may include a urinalysis with reflex urine culture when indicated, a complete blood count (CBC), and blood type and screen. Additional testing is based on an individual patient's comorbidities and surgical risk.

Evaluation of the Complex Patient

Patients often present with multiple symptoms of PFD or a complex history that may trigger additional intervention. Additional testing is recommended according to the AUA stress urinary incontinence guidelines when the diagnosis is unclear or if there is mixed incontinence, obstructive urinary symptoms, urinary retention, a history of prior pelvic surgery, suspicion for neurogenic bladder, a negative stress test despite patient complaint of SUI, an elevated PVR, advanced POP, or other dysfunctional voiding [35].

Physical Exam in the Complex Patient

Patients may complain of SUI; however, some patients may not demonstrate this on routine examination. Clinicians may be hesitant to perform a procedure without objective demonstration of SUI. A simple maneuver is to place a sterile catheter and fill the bladder with water or saline, remove the catheter, and ask the patient to cough. For patients who report SUI with specific maneuvers such as standing from a seated position or during exercise, a pad can be placed on the floor and the patient asked to squat and jump to see if SUI is demonstrated. Urodynamic studies can also be utilized to assess for SUI by asking the patient to perform provocative maneuvers.

A fistula should be suspected in patients with complaints of continuous or unaware fecal or urinary incontinence. The clinician should have a high index of suspicion in those who have a history of either a severe obstetric injury or prior pelvic surgery. Fistulas can be challenging to diagnose, as they are often not visible to the naked eye. The double-dye tampon test can be performed for suspicion of a vesicovaginal or ureterovaginal fistula. A patient is given a phenazopyridine pill that changes the urine color to orange. At the same time, the bladder is filled via a catheter with dilute methylene blue. A clean dry tampon is placed in the vagina. The patient is allowed to resume normal activity for approximately 1 hour. The tampon is removed. The presence of orange staining in the tip of the tampon indicates a likely ureterovaginal fistula, while the presence of blue along the middle of the tampon indicates a vesicovaginal fistula. If blue is present on the distal edge of the tampon, it can be difficult to discern between incontinence and a distal vesicovaginal fistula. The use of fluoroscopy during the filling and voiding phase of the urodynamic studies can also be helpful in diagnosing a fistula.

Urodynamics

Urodynamic testing is used to evaluate bladder storage and voiding function. This test is especially useful in cases of mixed urinary incontinence, where the predominant type of incontinence can be evaluated and aid in counseling patient on effective interventions. Patients in whom neurogenic bladder is suspected should undergo urodynamics to evaluate bladder function and importantly bladder compliance, as poor compliance places patients at risk for renal dysfunction. The AUA and SUFU have published guidelines on when to perform urodynamics in adults and recommend testing in patients with signs or symptoms of obstructive urination, suspected neurogenic voiding dysfunction, mixed incontinence, and high-grade POP and patients with prior pelvic surgery [43].

Cystoscopy and Imaging Studies

Routine cystoscopy is often unnecessary for the evaluation of PFD. However, in patients with symptoms of a urinary tract malignancy such as hematuria, cystoscopy should be performed prior to intervention for elective procedures.

Patients with a history of pelvic mesh placement, intermittent hematuria, recurrent UTI, dysuria, bladder calculi, and urethral and pelvic pain should have cystoscopy performed in order to rule out mesh erosion. If it is suspected that prior mesh may be contributing to symptoms of PFD, patients may benefit from mesh removal. However, patients rarely know the details of their mesh surgery, including mesh type, surgical approach (e.g., suprapubic versus transobturator), or location, and it may not be obvious on exam. Prior to surgical intervention, the clinician must obtain operative records to aid in surgical planning. If records are not available, transvaginal ultrasound may be helpful. Staack et al. reported that a transvaginal ultrasound in the hands of a skilled operator may help identify the location of mesh preoperatively [44].

For patients with symptoms of POP where an examination is difficult or inconclusive, a dynamic pelvic MRI may be considered. MRI has been shown to be particularly useful in evaluation of a posterior compartment prolapse and distinguishing between a rectocele and an enterocele [45], though it may have a more limited role in evaluating apical prolapse [46].

Discussion of Case Scenarios

A. A 45-year-old woman presents with stress urinary incontinence. She denies any storage/overactive bladder or prolapse symptoms. Physical examination reveals a positive supine cough stress test and urethral hypermobility with no evidence of prolapse.

This case represents the index case described in the AUA/SUFU guidelines of SUI. The patient has symptoms consistent with SUI with no other competing PFD symptoms and has objective demonstration of SUI. No additional testing is needed, and the patient may be counseled on interventions to treat SUI. Chapter 7 outlines treatment options for SUI.

B. A 62-year-old female presents with bothersome symptoms of urinary urgency and frequency, nocturia, and urge incontinence. She denies stress incontinence. She has never been treated with medical or surgical therapy.

This patient represents the index case described in the AUA/SUFU guidelines on OAB. No additional workup is needed. The patient can be counseled on the various treatment options available to patients with OAB. Treatment approaches for OAB are discussed in Chapters. 7 and 10.

C. A 58-year-old G3P3 woman presents with a bothersome vaginal bulge and constipation. This is associated with a sensation of incomplete bladder emptying with mild urinary frequency. She has a prior history of stress urinary incontinence that spontaneously resolved 2 years ago. On pelvic examination, the patient has a grade 3 cystocele, a grade 2 rectocele, and a negative empty supine cough stress test with or without the cystocele reduced.

This patient reports complex symptoms. Given a prior history of SUI that has resolved, the clinician should suspect that the patient has underlying intrinsic sphincter deficiency or occult SUI that is no longer evident due to urethral kinking from the cystocele. During examination, the cystocele should be reduced (with a speculum, packing, or pessary) and the cough stress test repeated. If this is negative, the clinician may consider filling the bladder or performing urodynamics with prolapse reduction. Given that she reports mixed incontinence and obstructive symptoms, urodynamics would also be useful for assessing for detrusor overactivity and the ability of the bladder to empty. This comprehensive evaluation is useful for counseling patients on expected outcomes following intervention and management of expectations. Given her history of multiparity, it is also important to assess the perineal body during examination. If this is attenuated, the patient may benefit from a perineorrhaphy at the time of rectocele repair, if she indeed elects to undergo surgical intervention.

Commentary

Eric S. Rovner

This is an excellent chapter describing the initial evaluation of the patient with pelvic floor dysfunction. These authors provide a comprehensive description and rationale for the salient components of a good history, physical examination, and other preliminary lines of inquiry (e.g., questionnaires and diaries) which provide a basis for the initial diagnosis and interventional planning in most patients presenting with pelvic floor dysfunction. The importance of these components, especially taking a good history and doing a complete physical examination, when done well, cannot be overemphasized. It is easy to overlook the value and expertise required to do these most basic components of the patient intake process well. These skills were initially acquired as medical students and then developed as interns and residents in training and then continuously refined as active practitioners. To this end, the astute clinician practices, retains, and exploits these proficiencies on a daily basis and does not permit the "templating" and "box checking" of the modern electronic medical record to supplant this acquired expertise.

Patients with pelvic floor dysfunction represent a broad array of connected pathologies. As the authors point out, symptoms in one system or compartment (i.e., urinary) should lead to an exploration and solicitation of other potentially related symptoms and signs (defecatory, sexual, etc.). Although, as clinicians, we are acutely aware of the intimate relationship between the various domains of the pelvic floor, the patient may not realize that these disorders are very often connected and may not offer their full array of complaints unless directly queried. Such patients are often quite relieved when they are counseled that their seemingly disparate symptoms are related and can be addressed simultaneously in a well-constructed therapeutic plan.

The bladder has been historically and famously termed an "unreliable witness" for many reasons including the limitations of patient recall of symptoms, as well as a lack of exact correlation of individual symptoms to a definitive diagnosis [47]. This characterization has been historically utilized as justification to pursue invasive diagnostic testing such as urodynamics in many patients. However, the wise clinician can elicit relevant symptoms, signs, and physical examination findings, parse through these data, and often arrive at a provisional and even definitive diagnosis prior to pursuing additional testing in the majority of patients with pelvic floor dysfunction, thus avoiding the cost and inconvenience of such investigations. In fact, recent publications have questioned the widespread utility of urodynamics in particular even when contemplating surgery [48].

In an era of buzzwords including cost containment, and quality of care, a thorough "H and P" can preclude the need for invasive and expensive tests such urodynamics or imaging in many, if not most, uncomplicated cases. Recently published guidelines certainly support such an approach [49–51]. Though the pace of advanced technological innovation in the diagnosis of pelvic floor disorders and indeed in all of medicine is accelerating, and the momentum is sometimes difficult to resist, such investigations are only variably and infrequently indicated when a proper, well-done, and complete initial evaluation is performed. This is not to suggest that such testing is unnecessary, but rather it should be selectively utilized, always balancing the incremental information gleaned from these investigations with the cost, invasiveness, and discomfort resulting from their utilization. It is appropriately emphasized by these authors that additional invasive testing should be reserved for those patients who remain complex diagnostic dilemmas following a thorough initial evaluation and/or obtained in those patients in whom irreversible, invasive, and expensive interventions are being pursued (e.g., surgery) and further or definitive diagnostic clarity is necessary.

References

1. Wu JM, Vaughan CP, Goode PS, Redden DT, Burgio KL, Richter HE, Markland AD. Prevalence and trends of symptomatic pelvic floor disorders in U.S. women. Obstet Gynecol. 2014;123(1):141–8.
2. Herschorn S, Gajewski J, Schulz J, Corcos J. A population-based study of urinary symptoms and incontinence: the Canadian Urinary Bladder Survey. BJU Int. 2008;101(1):52–8.
3. Devore EE, Minassian VA, Grodstein F. Factors associated with persistent urinary incontinence. Am J Obstet Gynecol. 2013;209(2):145.e1–6.
4. Hu TW, Wagner TH, Bentkover JD, Leblanc K, Zhou SZ, Hunt T. Costs of urinary incontinence and overactive bladder in the United States: a comparative study. Urology. 2004;63(3):461–5.
5. Abrams P, Cardozo L, Fall M, Griffiths D, Rosier P, Ulmsten U, van Kerrebroeck P, Victor A, Wein A. The standardisation of terminology of lower urinary tract function: report from the Standardisation Subcommittee of the International Continence Society. Am J Obstet Gynecol. 2002;187(1):116–26.
6. Bo K, Frawley HC, Haylen BT, Abramov Y, Almeida FG, Berghmans B, et al. An International Urogynecological Association (IUGA)/International Continence Society (ICS) joint report on the terminology for the conservative and nonpharmacological management of female pelvic floor dysfunction. Int Urogynecol J. 2017;28(2):191–213.
7. Sakakibara R, Tateno F, Nagao T, Yamamoto T, Uchiyama T, Yamanishi T, Yano M, Kishi M, Tsuyusaki Y, Aiba Y. Bladder function of patients with Parkinson's disease. Int J Urol. 2014;21(7):638–46.
8. Itoh Y, Yamada S, Konoeda F, Koizumi K, Nagata H, Oya M, Suzuki N. Burden of overactive bladder symptom on quality of life in stroke patients. NeurourolUrodyn. 2013;32(5):428–34.
9. Lykke R, Blaakær J, Ottesen B, Gimbel H. Incidence of pelvic organ prolapse repair subsequent to hysterectomy: a comparison between radical hysterectomy and total abdominal hysterectomy. Int Urogynecol J. 2017;28(5):745–9.
10. Gill EJ, Hurt WG. Pathophysiology of pelvic organ prolapse. Obstet Gynecol Clin North Am. 1998;25(4):757–69.
11. Lethaby A, Ayeleke RO, Roberts H. Local oestrogen for vaginal atrophy in postmenopausal women. Cochrane Database Syst Rev. 2016;31(8):CD001500.
12. Loke YK, Singh S. Risk of acute urinary retention associated with inhaled anticholinergics in patients with chronic obstructive lung disease: systematic review. Ther Adv Drug Saf. 2013;4(1):19–26.
13. Elliott CS, Comiter CV. The effect of angiotensin inhibition on urinary incontinence: data from the National Health and Nutrition Examination Survey (2001–2008). NeurourolUrodyn. 2014;33(8):1178–81.
14. Twiss C, Triaca V, Rodríguez LV. Familial transmission of urogenital prolapse and incontinence. Curr Opin Obstet Gynecol. 2007;19(5):464–8.
15. Richter HE, Whitehead N, Arya L, Ridgeway B, Allen-Brady K, Norton P, Sung V, Shepherd JP, Komesu Y, Gaddis N, Fraser MO, Tan-Kim J, Meikle S, Page GP, Pelvic Floor Disorders Network. Genetic contributions to urgency urinary incontinence in women. J Urol. 2015;193(6):2020–7.
16. Cartwright R, Kirby AC, Tikkinen KA, Mangera A, Thiagamoorthy G, Rajan P, Pesonen J, Ambrose C, Gonzalez-Maffe J, Bennett P, Palmer T, Walley A, Järvelin MR, Chapple C, Khullar V. Systematic review and metaanalysis of genetic association studies of urinary symptoms and prolapse in women. Am J Obstet Gynecol. 2015;212(2):199.e1–24.
17. Lince SL, van Kempen LC, Vierhout ME, Kluivers KB. A systematic review of clinical studies on hereditary factors in pelvic organ prolapse. Int Urogynecol J. 2012;23(10):1327–36.
18. Rockwood TH, Church JM, Fleshman JW, et al. Fecal incontinence quality of life scale: quality of life instrument for patients with fecal incontinence. Dis Colon Rectum. 2000;43:9.
19. Rockwood TH, Church JM, Fleshman JW, et al. Patient and surgeon ranking of the severity of symptoms associated with fecal incontinence: the fecal incontinence severity index. Dis Colon Rectum. 1999;42(12):1525–32.
20. Jorge JMN, Wexner SD. Etiology and management of fecal incontinence. Dis Colon Rectum. 1993;36(1):77–97.
21. Barber MD, Kuchibhatla MN, Pieper CF, et al. Psychometric evaluation of 2 comprehensive condition-specific quality of life instruments for

women with pelvic floor disorders. Am J Obstet Gynecol. 2001;185:1388–95.
22. Jackson S, Donovan J, Brookers S, et al. The Bristol female lower urinary tract symptoms questionnaire: development and psychometric testing. Br J Urol. 1996;77:805–12.
23. Avery K, Donovan J, Peters TJ, et al. ICIQ: a brief and robust measure for evaluating the symptoms and impact of urinary incontinence. NeurourolUrodyn. 2004;23:322–30.
24. Uebersax JS, Wyman JF, Shumaker SA, et al. Short forms to assess life quality and symptom distress for urinary incontinence in women: the Incontinence Impact Questionnaire and the Urogenital Distress Inventory, Continence Program for Women Research Group. NeurourolUrodyn. 1995;14:131–9.
25. Wagner TH, Patrick DL, Bavendam TG, et al. Quality of life of persons with urinary incontinence: development of a new measure. Urology. 1996;47:67–71.
26. Coyne K, Revicki D, Hunt T, et al. Psychometric validation of an overactive bladder symptom and health-related quality of life questionnaire: the OAB-q. Qual Life Res. 2002;11:563–74.
27. Blaivas JG, Panagopoulos G, Weiss JP, et al. Validation of the overactive bladder symptom score. J Urol. 2007;178:543–7.
28. Bradley CS, Rovner ES, Morgan MA, et al. A new questionnaire for urinary incontinence diagnosis in women: development and testing. Am J Obstet Gynecol. 2005;192:66–73.
29. Stach-Lempinen B, Kujansuu E, Laippala P, et al. Visual analogue scale, urinary incontinence severity score and 15 D: psychometric testing of three different health-related quality-of-life instruments for urinary incontinent women. Scand J Urol Nephrol. 2001;35:476–83.
30. Krhut J, Zachoval R, Smith PP, Rosier PF, Valanský L, Martan A, Zvara P. Pad weight testing in the evaluation of urinary incontinence. NeurourolUrodyn. 2014;33(5):507–10.
31. Nitti VW, Mourtzinos A, Brucker BM, SUFU Pad Test Study Group. Correlation of patient perception of pad use with objective degree of incontinence measured by pad test in men with post-prostatectomy incontinence: the SUFU Pad Test Study. J Urol. 2014;192(3):836–42.
32. Groutz A, Blaivas J, Chaikin D, et al. Noninvasive outcome measures of urinary incontinence and lower urinary tract symptoms: a multicenter study of micturition diary and pad tests. J Urol. 2000;164:698–701.
33. Schick E, Jolivet-Tremblay M, Dupont C, Bertrand PE, Tessier J. Frequency-volume chart: the minimum number of days required to obtain reliable results. NeurourolUrodyn. 2003;22(2):92–6.
34. Tangalos EG, Smith GE, Ivnik RJ, et al. The Mini-Mental State Examination in general medical practice: clinical utility and acceptance. Mayo Clin Proc. 1996;71(9):829–37.
35. Dmochowski RR, Blaivas JM, Gormley EA, Juma S, Karram MM, Lightner DJ, Luber KM, Rovner ES, Staskin DR, Winters JC, Appell RA, Female Stress Urinary Incontinence Update Panel of the American Urological Association Education and Research, Inc., Whetter LE. Update of AUA guideline on the surgical management of female stress urinary incontinence. J Urol. 2010;183(5):1906–14.
36. Antovska V. Outcome assessment of the Marshall coughing test during cervix reposition maneuver in women with urinary stress incontinence with/without genital prolapse. ISRN Urol [Internet]. 2012 [cited 2018 Mar 26];2012:109858.
37. Li C, Gong Y, Wang B. The efficacy of pelvic floor muscle training for pelvic organ prolapse: a systematic review and meta-analysis. Int Urogynecol J. 2016;27(7):981–92.
38. Koh CE, Young CJ, Young JM, Solomon MJ. Systematic review of randomized controlled trials of the effectiveness of biofeedback for pelvic floor dysfunction. Br J Surg. 2008;95(9):1079–87.
39. Butrick CW. Pathophysiology of pelvic floor hypertonic disorders. Obstet Gynecol Clin North Am. 2009;36(3):699–705.
40. Gormley EA, Lightner DJ, Burgio KL, Chai TC, Clemens JQ, Culkin DJ, Das AK, Foster HE, Scarpero HM, Tessier CD, Vasavada SP, American Urological Association, Society of Urodynamics, Female Pelvic Medicine & Urogenital Reconstruction. Diagnosis and treatment of overactive bladder (non-neurogenic) in adults: AUA/SUFU guideline. J Urol. 2012;188(6 Suppl):2455–63.
41. Gormley EA, Lightner DJ, Faraday M, Vasavada SP, American Urological Association, Society of Urodynamics, Female Pelvic Medicine. Diagnosis and treatment of overactive bladder (non-neurogenic) in adults: AUA/SUFU guideline amendment. J Urol. 2015;193(5):1572–80.
42. Davis R, Jones JS, Barocas DA, Castle EP, Lang EK, Leveillee RJ, et al. Diagnosis, evaluation and follow-up of asymptomatic microhematuria (AMH) in adults: AUA guideline. J Urol. 2012;188(6 Suppl):2473–81.
43. Winters JC, Dmochowski RR, Goldman HB, Herndon CD, Kobashi KC, Kraus SR, Lemack GE, Nitti VW, Rovner ES, Wein AJ, American Urological Association, Society of Urodynamics, Female Pelvic Medicine & Urogenital Reconstruction. Urodynamic studies in adults: AUA/SUFU guideline. J Urol. 2012;188(6 Suppl):2464–72.
44. Staack A, Vitale J, Ragavendra N, Rodríguez LV. Translabial ultrasonography for evaluation of synthetic mesh in the vagina. Urology. 2014;83(1):68–74.
45. Gousse AE, Barbaric ZL, Safir MH, Madjar S, Marumoto AK, Raz S. Dynamic half Fourier acquisition, single shot turbo spin-echo magnetic resonance imaging for evaluating the female pelvis. J Urol. 2000;164(5):1606–13.
46. Cortes E, Reid WM, Singh K, Berger L. Clinical examination and dynamic magnetic resonance

imaging in vaginal vault prolapse. Obstet Gynecol. 2004;103(1):41–6.
47. Turner-Warwick R, Whiteside CG, Worth PH, Milroy EJ, Bates CP. A urodynamic view of the clinical problems associated with bladder neck dysfunction and its treatment by endoscopic incision and trans-trigonal posterior prostatectomy. Br J Urol. 1973;45:44–59.
48. Nager C, Brubaker L, Litman H, et al. A randomized trial of urodynamic testing before stress-incontinence surgery. NEJM. 2012;366:1987–97.
49. Dmochowski RR, Blaivas JM, Gormley EA, Juma S, Karram MM, Lightner DJ, Luber KM, Rovner ES, Staskin DR, Winters JC, Appell RA. Female stress urinary incontinence update panel of the American Urological Association Education and Research, Inc., Whetter LE. Update of AUA guideline on the surgical management of female stress urinary incontinence. J Urol. 2010;183(5):1906–14.
50. Kobashi KC, Albo ME, Dmochowski RR, et al. Surgical treatment of female stress urinary incontinence (SUI): AUA/SUFU guideline: published 2017. 2017. https://www.auanet.org/guidelines/incontinence-stress-urinary-incontinence.
51. Gormley EA, Lightner DJ, Burgio KL, Chai TC, Clemens JQ, Culkin DJ, Das AK, Foster HE, Scarpero HM, Tessier CD, Vasavada SP, American Urological Association, Society of Urodynamics, Female Pelvic Medicine & Urogenital Reconstruction. Diagnosis and treatment of overactive bladder (non-neurogenic) in adults: AUA/SUFU guideline. J Urol. 2012;188(6 Suppl):2455–63.

The Role of Urodynamics

2

J. Christian Winters and Madeline Rovira Koerner

Stress Urinary Incontinence with Pelvic Organ Prolapse

History

The patient is a 43-year-old female with a chief complaint of vaginal bulge. She has failed a pessary three times and is interested in discussing surgical management of her pelvic prolapse. The patient denies symptoms of stress urinary incontinence (SUI), urinary urgency (UU), or urgency urinary incontinence (UUI). The patient has had four pregnancies each resulting in a vaginal delivery. She is obese with a 23-pack/year smoking history. She had a hysterectomy 3 years ago.

Physical Exam

On physical exam, the patient is noted to have a BMI of 38. She has Stage III pelvic organ prolapse (POP) with the cuff at +1. She has urethral hypermobility and a positive stress test with her pessary in place. Her post-void residual (PVR) is 36.

Commentary by Kathleen C. Kobashi, Virginia Mason Medical Center, Department of Urology and Renal Transplantation, Seattle, WA, USA

J. C. Winters (✉) · M. R. Koerner
Louisiana State University Health Sciences Center, Department of Urology, New Orleans, LA, USA
e-mail: cwinte@lsuhsc.edu

Recommendation

For this patient with high-grade anterior compartment prolapse, the absence of mixed incontinence symptoms, no emptying LUTS, and no history of previous anti-incontinence intervention, a stress test with prolapse reduction is indicated prior to surgical counseling. In this clinical setting, a urodynamic study is optional to further characterize lower urinary tract function. This facilitates screening for occult SUI and the ability to selectively manage the urethra in the same operation.

In women with high-grade anterior or apical POP who present with associated symptoms of mixed urinary incontinence (MUI) or emptying disorders and/or complicated SUI, a multichannel pressure flow study with the prolapse reduced is indicated. This facilitates a more comprehensive understanding of complex symptomatology or history prior to surgical intervention. This approach in applying UDS testing on women with POP affords the clinician the ability to selectively perform UDS in more complex situations (Fig. 2.1).

Discussion

Stress urinary incontinence is the symptom of urinary leakage during events with increased abdominal pressure such as sneezing, coughing,

K. C. Kobashi, S. D. Wexner (eds.), *Female Pelvic Medicine*, https://doi.org/10.1007/978-3-030-54839-1_2

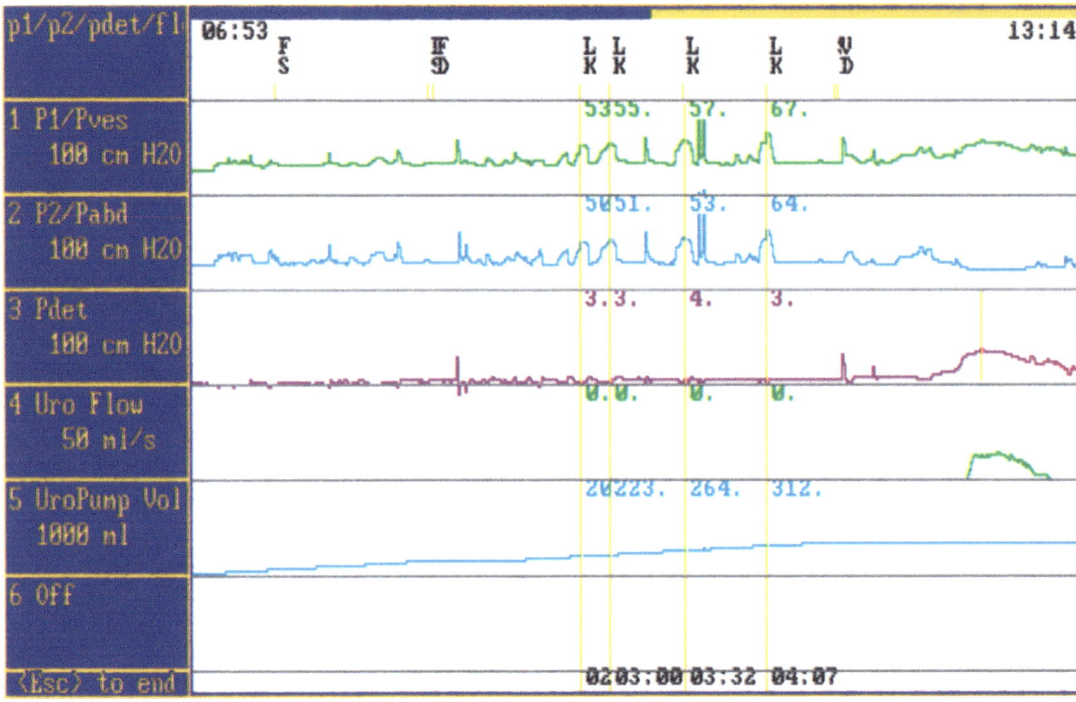

Fig. 2.1 Multichannel UDS done following prolapse reduction. During bladder filling, there are multiple leaks with Valsalva maneuvers (LK) and no evidence of detrusor overactivity. In addition, there are normal voiding pressures and a normal flow rate with complete bladder emptying. This study demonstrates SUI consistent with intrinsic sphincteric deficiency. In this patient, it is recommended to treat the demonstrable SUI with the prolapse reduced due to the high risk of SUI postoperatively if left untreated. In this scenario, the risks and benefits of a retropubic midurethral sling and autologous fascial sling were discussed

lifting, bending, exercise, laughing, or changing positions [1]. For patients who present for surgical management of SUI, the baseline evaluation includes focused history, pelvic exam (with assessment of urethra mobility), urinalysis, provocative stress test, and post-void residual measurement. Bladder diaries and questionnaires serve as useful adjuncts to the history [2–4].

A thorough history should characterize the incontinence including the frequency, severity, and bother of urinary symptoms as well as their impact on lifestyle and expectations for treatment [1]. PVR is a cost-effective screening tool with a high negative predictive value that provides information on the emptying status and allows for pre- to postoperative comparison. Further, it is a simple assessment that can suggest overflow incontinence, bladder outlet obstruction, and detrusor underactivity [3, 5]. Uroflow may be useful in the evaluation for possible voiding dysfunction. The negative predictive value of normal uroflow is more than 90%; a normal uroflow and normal PVR make voiding dysfunction unlikely [4].

For the uncomplicated patient with clinically demonstrable SUI, beyond this basic evaluation, urodynamic studies may change the clinical diagnosis but rarely alter the treatment plan and do not improve the treatment outcome [4–8]. When evaluating patients who had preoperative urodynamics (UDS) compared to a basic office evaluation, there are similar rates of treatment success, patient satisfaction at 12 months, and adverse events. Further there are similar changes in incontinence severity measures and quality-of-life metrics [2]. Compared with the basic office evaluation, this more extensive workup is not cost-effective [9, 10]. Urodynamic evaluation becomes more valuable with increasing patient complexity or when patients are considering invasive treatment, thus making the case for more selective application of studies.

Indications for urodynamic testing in patients presenting with SUI include prior urinary tract surgery or anti-incontinence procedure, mixed incontinence, known or suspected neurogenic bladder (NGB), negative stress test, elevated PVR, dysfunctional voiding, and Grade III or greater POP [1].

High-grade POP can mask SUI by kinking the urethra [11–14]. After POP repair, an estimated 25–40% of women will develop SUI [12]. For women considering a procedure to treat high-grade POP, physicians should evaluate for SUI by performing stress testing with the prolapse reduced such as with a pessary, ring forceps, or vaginal packing [5, 11, 13–17]. Even with this evaluation, it is important to consider masked SUI due to urethral compression from whatever method was used to reduce the prolapse. When SUI is demonstrated during the evaluation of POP, surgical intervention may be considered to perform concurrent anti-SUI surgery at the time of POP surgery [1, 3, 11–13, 16].

When using urodynamics to diagnose stress incontinence, the clinician should assess urethral function. This assessment most commonly consists of the Valsalva leak point pressure. Less commonly utilized, the maximal urethral closure pressure is an alternative method to measure urethral resistance and determine the degree of intrinsic sphincter deficiency. These tests may provide a measure of disease severity that can facilitate patient counseling and surgical decision-making [3, 5, 17, 18].

In the more complicated patient population, urodynamics may further aid in patient counseling by helping predict the postoperative disease course. Urodynamics may help identify patients at risk for persistent symptoms, postoperative dysfunctional voiding, urgency, or urinary urgency incontinence [9]. Reduced preoperative peak urine flow rates may be correlated with a higher risk for postoperative urinary retention. The urodynamic observation of detrusor overactivity can predict de novo urgency and urgency urinary incontinence following prolapse surgery [3, 9]. Poor preoperative detrusor contractility may also be associated with postoperative voiding dysfunction [9].

Overactive Bladder, Urgency Urinary Incontinence, and Urgency Urinary Incontinence Not Responsive to Medication

History

The patient is a 54-year-old woman presenting to clinic for evaluation of urinary urgency and frequency. The patient is consistent with timed voiding and avoids all caffeine. She has progressed through medical therapy with oxybutynin, trospium, and mirabegron and has been unhappy with her treatment results. At this time, she is interested in pursuing further therapy. Seven years ago, patient had a procedure performed to “stop me from peeing when I laugh” – she doesn’t remember what the procedure was called.

Physical Exam

Healthy appearing woman. No POP. PVR 27. Urinalysis without evidence of infection or bleeding.

Recommendation

Perform multichannel filling cystometry in this patient with urgency and frequency that is refractory to medical therapy who is considering surgical treatment. In addition, this patient has a history of anti-incontinence surgery, and UDS may be useful to rule out bladder outlet obstruction as a cause of storage symptomatology (Fig. 2.2).

Discussion

Overactive bladder (OAB) is a clinical syndrome defined by the presence of bothersome urinary symptoms that are not related to a neurologic con-

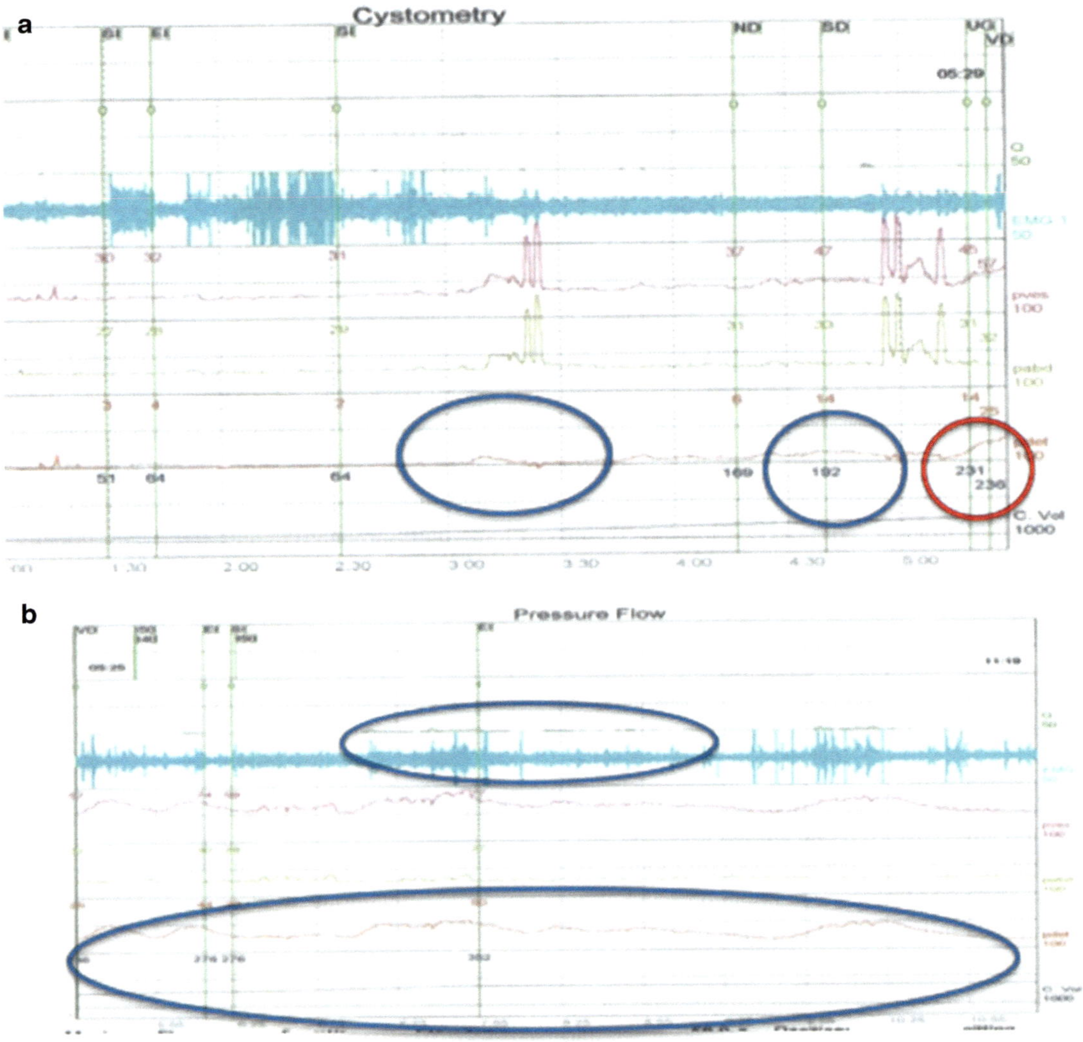

Fig. 2.2 A 54-year-old woman failed several courses of medical therapy for OAB symptoms and desires further treatment. She has a previous history of an unknown bladder suspension. A multichannel UDS was recommended due to her refractory OAB symptoms and previous history of anti-incontinence surgery. (**a**) This figure illustrates the multichannel filling cystometry of the UDS study. The findings confirm the presence of detrusor overactivity and terminal detrusor overactivity at capacity. Note the UDS observations of detrusor overactivity within the blue circles and terminal detrusor overactivity (in red) at bladder capacity. (**b**) This figure illustrates the voiding (pressure flow) portion of the UDS study. Note, in blue, there is very low urinary flow accompanied by high detrusor pressures during voiding. The high detrusor pressure with low urinary flow is indicative of bladder outlet obstruction. In addition, there is intermittent low flow with incomplete emptying as a result of the obstruction. The recommended treatment is surgical intervention to relieve bladder outlet obstruction, most commonly a sling incision. Following this, a reassessment of bladder symptoms should follow

dition. Symptoms include urgency, frequency, and nocturia with or without urinary incontinence. Initial evaluation involves a focused history with a physical examination and urinalysis to rule out infectious cause of symptoms. Urgency is essential to the diagnosis [19, 20]. In most patients with overactive bladder, history and physical exam is sufficient to start treatment with lifestyle change and oral medications; urodynamics, cystoscopy, and ultrasound are not necessary in evaluation of an uncomplicated patient [3, 20].

For patients with worsening overactive bladder symptoms, equivocal emptying measures following bladder outlet surgery, concern for upper tract damage, or failure to respond to first-line behavioral and medical therapies, there may be a role for further evaluation with urodynamics, cystoscopy, and a pressure flow study. UDS allows clinicians to evaluate for functional bladder outlet obstruction and for concomitant SUI [3, 5, 19]. This additional information may allow for improved physician counseling and appropriate setting of patient expectations heading into treatment [5].

When considering invasive treatment with considerable potential morbidity for urgency incontinence, clinicians may utilize multichannel filling cystometry to assess bladder storage and filling pressures. This allows the clinician to identify urodynamic abnormalities including altered compliance or detrusor overactivity (DO) – the presence of involuntary contractions during filling cystometry [3, 19]. Of significance, lack of DO on a single urodynamic study does not exclude DO as a cause of urgency incontinence or mixed incontinence [3].

Assessment of detrusor function allows for some prediction of surgical outcome. In women with POP, the presence or absence of DO predicted persistence of symptoms of UU and UUI following surgery. UU and UUI often resolved in patients without DO and persisted in patients with DO [16]. In contrast, preoperative detrusor underactivity was correlated with large PVR postoperatively [16]. For patients with overactive bladder, response to treatment with Botox or sacral neuromodulation was not dependent on the preoperative finding of DO [19].

Assessment of urethral function may clarify the diagnosis for patients with MUI or UUI not responsive to medical therapy [18]. Pressure flow studies may be used for patients with UUI to evaluate for bladder outlet obstruction following bladder outlet procedures; these studies are most useful when compared preoperatively with postoperatively [5].

When treating patients with OAB, it is important to remember that an OAB diagnosis does not require UDS. Further, the lack of symptoms on a urodynamic study does not eliminate the possibility that those symptoms are present in a normal, daily environment. The value of UDS in this setting may be to best rule out what patients do not have and to use this information in the design of an individualized treatment plan.

Neurogenic Bladder

History

The patient is a 24-year-old woman with a history of motor vehicle accident leading to a thoracic spinal cord injury 8 weeks ago. Since the time of the accident, the patient has learned self-catheterization which she performs four to six times daily. She has had no recent febrile infections.

Physical Exam

Thin female sitting in wheelchair. Patient has normal upper extremity function. Her PVR is 96.

Recommendation

Initial evaluation of this patient with a spinal cord injury should be deferred for several more weeks. After 12 weeks post injury, videourodynamic evaluation would be recommended to assess urinary storage (compliance, capacity, +/− detrusor overactivity) and emptying status. For patients on clean intermittent catheterization (CIC), a 3-day volume diary is quite useful in determining the urodynamic fill volume. Assessment of detrusor leak point pressure (DLPP) is useful in incontinent patients with NGB. Before urodynamics on patients with spinal cord injury, the clinician should assess for the occurrence of autonomic dysreflexia and be prepared to intervene appropriately should this occur.

The Role of Videourodynamics

Complex multichannel UDS is not a "static" study. It is a combination of urodynamic tests designed to answer the urodynamic question composed by the clinician after a basic office assessment and/or empiric therapy. One of the urodynamic tests include adding fluoroscopy to the multichannel UDS. The major advantage of fluoroscopy is to provide anatomic detail to the functional assessment of the lower urinary tract. Initial evaluation of neurogenic bladder and symptoms of impaired bladder emptying in young men and women are the most common reasons to perform fluoroscopy at the time of multichannel UDS. In patients with neurogenic bladder, the presence of a trabeculation, cellules, or a small contracted bladder often correlates with disorders of bladder compliance. In addition, the presence of vesicoureteral reflux fluoroscopy can be highly effective at confirming the diagnosis of detrusor sphincter dyssynergia and/or bladder neck dyssynergia (Fig. 2.3a). Oftentimes, the electromyography (EMG) findings are non-specific. However, the presence of a "spinning top" urethra in patients with neurogenic voiding disorders facilitates the diagnosis. In younger men and women without neurogenic LUTS, fluoroscopy can greatly aid in the detection of dysfunctional voiding or primary bladder neck obstruction (Fig. 2.3b). Oftentimes the UDS study may demonstrate obstruction, and fluoroscopy can greatly facilitate in determining the cause of obstruction.

Neurogenic bladder patients present with numerous underlying pathologies and varied patterns of symptoms. Neurogenic bladder patients may lack normal awareness or sensation of bladder dysfunction and therefore may not report classic lower urinary tract symptoms. In this population, dysfunctional storage or voiding may present with incontinence, infection, stones, or renal insufficiency [18].

The goal of treating this patient population is not only to maintain continence and ensure adequate bladder emptying but to protect the upper urinary tracts. A PVR may be considered at the time of diagnosis in all patients with NGB disorders and can be a useful, noninvasive means of monitoring disease progression and treatment efficacy [20].

The AUA/SUFU Adult Urodynamics Guidelines recommend evaluation of patients with neurogenic bladder based on disease risk. These guidelines define "relevant neurologic conditions" as those disease processes posing risk to the upper urinary tracts or risk for renal impairment [3]. See Table 2.1, reproduced from the guideline statements, for more information. In general, patients with higher risk for upper tract complication "relevant neurogenic bladder" should receive multichannel urodynamic evaluation. Patients with lower risk for upper tract complication may receive PVR followed by empiric therapy with urodynamics reserved for circumstances of failed empiric therapy.

PVR may be assessed in isolation or as part of a complete urodynamic study and may be repeated, as indicated, throughout ongoing follow-up for close monitoring of bladder function in those patients whose disease course varies across time [3, 5, 15, 18]. When elevated PVR is symptomatic, disease treatment may aim at PVR reduction [18]. A PVR greater than 300 mL may be associated with an increased risk for urinary tract infection, upper tract dilation, and renal insufficiency [5].

Regardless of symptoms, clinicians should perform complex cystometrogram (CMG) on all patients during the initial evaluation of patients with neurologic conditions that pose a potential risk to the upper urinary tracts. It is necessary to define the lower urinary tract dysfunction in order to protect the upper tracts, prevent stone formation, and minimize risk of infection or stone formation [18]. When patients are found to have poor compliance or elevated leak point pressures, treatment of neurogenic lower urinary tract dysfunction should be directed toward lowering storage pressures, and depending on severity, urodynamics should be repeated to confirm a favorable treatment effect [3]. In neurogenic bladder patients with conditions not predisposing to upper tract dysfunction, CMG is an optional adjunct to urologic evaluation [3, 15].

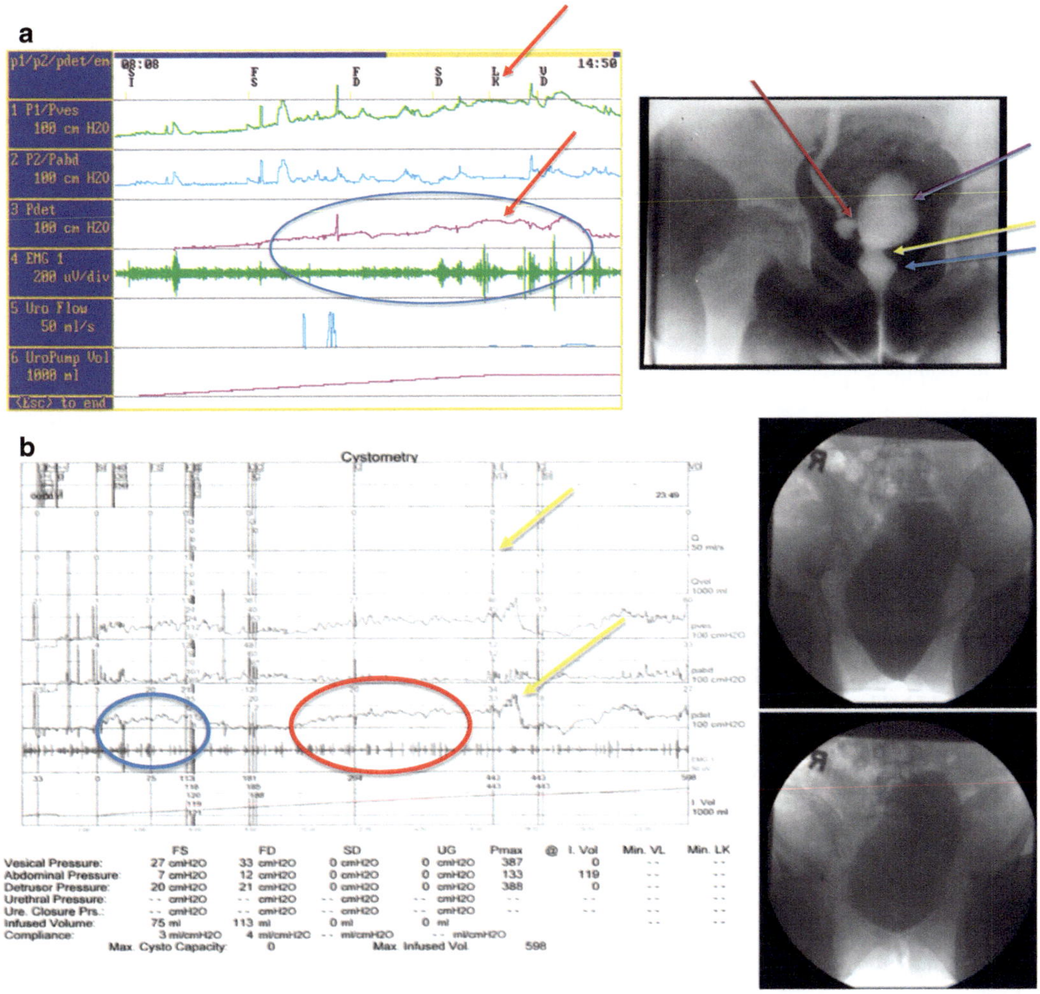

Fig. 2.3 (**a**) Left: Complex multichannel UDS on a 27-year-old quadriplegic male 6 years s/p fall injury at work with multiple vertebral thoracic and lumbar levels of injury. He is currently leaking between catheterizations and complaining of recurrent admissions for pyelonephritis. Note the UDS illustrates abnormally poor bladder compliance and a detrusor leak point pressure of greater than 60 cm water. These findings both implicate propensity to upper tract complications (such as recurrent sepsis). Right: Fluoroscopic images obtained during UDS study. This illustration demonstrates the tremendous anatomic detail provided by using fluoroscopy during the UDS study. Adding the anatomic images to the functional assessment above provides the clinician with more complete information about LUT abnormalities, which substantially aids in guiding further therapies. In the patient above, the blue arrow illustrates a "spinning top" urethra which is highly suggestive of external sphincter dyssynergia, and the yellow arrow illustrates narrowing of the bladder neck which indicates an element of bladder neck dyssynergia. One also notes the small contracted bladder (purple arrow) and the right vesicoureteral reflux (red arrow) which is most likely due to chronically elevated bladder storage pressures. A clinician cannot obtain this information without fluoroscopic assessment of the LUT. (**b**) Left: A 42-year-old female complaining of incomplete emptying, straining to void, and urgency incontinence and was recently evaluated for declining renal function with an US revealing mild bilateral hydronephrosis. A neurologic workup including MRI was normal. There was no associated prolapse or significant pelvic floor dysfunction, and the PVR was greater than 300 cc. The above multichannel UDS was performed revealing detrusor overactivity (blue), abnormality in bladder compliance (red), and significantly elevated voiding pressures with essentially no urinary flow (yellow). Right: These illustrations highlight the value in fluoroscopy in facilitating the diagnosis of the cause of voiding dysfunction in men and women. In this female, during the voiding phase despite significant elevations in voiding pressure, there is no urinary flow. The images demonstrate clearly that the bladder neck is not opening, and the etiology of the obstruction is likely primary bladder neck obstruction, which can only be diagnosed with fluoroscopy. This detail greatly improves diagnostic accuracy, and this patient did improve greatly after a bladder neck incision

Table 2.1 Risk of upper urinary tract damage in common neurogenic lower urinary tract conditions [3]

Classification of common neurogenic lower urinary tract (NLUT) conditions by upper tract risk	
Relevant NLUT disorders with risk of upper tract complication	Other NLUT disorders with little risk of upper tract complication
Spinal cord injury	Parkinson's disease
Transverse myelitis	Brain tumor
Myelomeningocele	Cerebrovascular accident
Radical pelvic surgery	Lumbar disc disease
Men with multiple sclerosis	Women with multiple sclerosis
Any neurogenic bladder disorder with upper tract complications	

Clinicians should also consider pressure flow analysis in patients with elevated PVR, empiric treatment failure, hydronephrosis, pyelonephrosis, complicated UTI, or frequent autonomic dysreflexia [5, 15]. These conditions may result from elevated storage pressures, and multichannel UDS is the optimal way to detect these. Multichannel pressure-flow studies allow for differentiation between bladder outlet obstruction and detrusor hypocontractility or acontractility.

To delineate the specific site of obstruction, clinicians may perform urodynamics with fluoroscopy videourodynamic studies (VUDS) in patients with neurologic diseases predisposing to upper tract dysfunction. This may also be considered in patients at risk for neurogenic bladder or in those who have an elevated PVR or symptoms [3, 15]. Using fluoroscopy at the time of urodynamics allows for grading vesicoureteral reflux, identifying anatomic abnormalities during reflux, and defining the urodynamic parameters present during reflux [3, 15]. VUDS can clarify the site of urinary tract obstruction at the bladder neck versus external sphincter and can identify diverticula or stones [15]. Defining these voiding characteristics allows clinicians to determine the target site for treatment [15]. When considering VUDS, clinicians must weigh the benefits of diagnostic accuracy against the cost and feasibility at smaller neurogenic bladder care centers [5].

EMG is indicated at the time of CMG, with or without pressure flow studies, in patients predisposed to upper tract damage or those with neurologic disease and elevated PVR or bothersome voiding symptoms [3, 15]. EMG allows evaluation of the coordination between perineal contractions and detrusor contractions [3]. This is useful for diagnosing detrusor external sphincter dyssynergia – involuntary contractions of the external urethral sphincter during detrusor contractions [2, 3, 15, 18]. Caution is necessary when interpreting EMG as this is a non-specific measure of pelvic floor muscle activity and can be distorted by artifact [5]. The addition of fluoroscopy demonstrating the presence of a spinning top urethra greatly aids in detection.

Commonly Encountered Neurogenic Bladder Conditions

Spinal Cord Injury

Patients with spinal cord injury are considered to be at high risk for urinary tract dysfunction and damage to the upper urinary tracts. As such, guidelines recommend baseline urodynamic evaluation using multichannel UDS and PVR with ongoing follow-up and further urodynamic evaluation as clinically indicated [3, 21].

Urinary symptom presentation is somewhat predictable based on lesion location. Suprasacral lesions typically present with up to three months of spinal shock during which the bladder is areflexic, lacking sensation, and with a closed bladder neck – patients often present with urinary retention and overflow incontinence. Following spinal shock, as spinal reflexes return with reflex bladder contractions, patients often develop detrusor overactivity with or without detrusor external sphincter dyssynergia [22, 23]. These patients may be predisposed to elevated storage pressures and reflex voiding with increased detrusor leak point pressures [21, 24]. Sacral lesions present with highly compliant, acontractile bladders [21]. Although lesions are characteristic of the lesion location, it is of paramount importance that spinal cord injuries are often incomplete and UDS is essential in determining the dysfunction present.

In the workup of a spinal cord injury patient, initial UDS should be deferred during the first six to twelve weeks following injury while the patient is in spinal shock. Although it is interesting that Cameron et al. reported a significant percentage of patients had adverse UDS findings at three months – suggesting benefit to earlier assessment. Following this period, baseline urodynamic studies characterize voiding dysfunction and identify patients with risk for upper tract complications [21, 22]. Follow-up urological evaluation is recommended for patients with spinal cord injuries though there is no consensus as to the frequency or the essential components of this workup [21, 25, 26]. Annual UDS have been recommended for patients with ongoing detrusor hyperactivity or those who empty their bladder by reflex voiding or straining to void [24]. However, to date, most clinicians selectively perform repeat studies in the setting of adverse findings on initial urodynamics (such as poor compliance or elevated detrusor leak point pressure), change in upper tract imaging surveillance, hydronephrosis, recurrent pyelonephritis, and/or refractory incontinence [22].

Cerebrovascular Accident

Following cerebrovascular accident (CVA), patients are considered to be at low risk for upper tract dysfunction and deterioration [3]. The most common urodynamic finding is detrusor overactivity with sphincteric synergistic emptying. Thus, this rarely leads to bladder pressures high enough or sustained long enough to lead to risk of upper tract damage [20]. The primary treatment for OAB is as reflected in guidelines. Behavioral modification and antimuscarinic medications are often introduced early [27]. If these measures fail, patients are usually offered botulinum toxin as neuromodulation is not indicated for neurogenic bladder conditions [28]. Of note, a number of studies are demonstrating efficacy of neurolodulation for neurogenic bladder patients [23, 28–31]. Treatment of LUTS after CVA can be more complicated by a high association of detrusor underactivity which necessitates attention to detrusor contractility (emptying status) while treating OAB symptoms [27].

Spinal Dysraphism

Spinal dysraphism refers to a collection of neural tube defects. These are categorized as open defects when the cord is visible and without skin covering at the time of birth and closed when the skin remains intact [32]. There is no association between open or closed spinal dysraphism with particular urodynamic findings [33].

Urodynamic evaluation is necessary in all patients with spinal dysraphism; the European Association of Urology Guidelines on Neurogenic Lower Urinary Tract Dysfunction recommends urodynamics every one to two years in patients with spinal dysraphism [33]. UDS are more likely to identify significant results in spinal dysraphism patients who are wheelchair bound or presenting with urinary symptoms than in ambulatory patients. Wheelchair-bound and symptomatic patients require active surveillance and therapeutic intervention when their upper tracts are at risk. If a patient is ambulatory and without urinary symptoms, it is safe to lengthen the interval between urodynamic evaluations [33].

Spina bifida patients often present with increased detrusor leak point pressure, vesicoureteral reflux, and detrusor sphincter dyssynergia [34]. In children, UDS has been recommended as often as every six months due to rapidly changing bladder pathology [34]. Videourodynamics is recommended with the initial adult evaluation. After this, urodynamic evaluation is recommended annually for adults with elevated storage pressure or for those with a history of hydronephrosis or decreased GFR. UDS is recommended for evaluation of new urinary symptoms including persistent urinary tract infection, leaking between catheterization, or unexpected changes in continence. Patients without urinary tract symptoms may undergo urodynamic evaluation at a longer interval, every two to three years [34].

Multiple Sclerosis

Bladder dysfunction, both storage and voiding, is reported in up to 97% of patients with multiple sclerosis (MS), a disease characterized by demyelinating plaques in white matter of the central nervous system [35, 36]. Among patients with urinary symptoms, 99% of these patients will have a urodynamic abnormality – most commonly, neurogenic detrusor overactivity followed by detrusor sphincter dyssynergia and detrusor hypocontractility [37]. Despite the frequency of bladder dysfunction, upper tract changes and sequelae are quite rare [36].

overactivity and low PVR. In contrast, PVR greater than 100 mL, presence of detrusor sphincter dyssynergia, an open bladder neck at the start of bladder filling, internal sphincter denervation, and neurogenic motor potentials are all suggestive of multiple system atrophy [41].

As with all patients, elderly patient with urinary complaints may require UDS for diagnostic clarity beyond a basic office evaluation. In this population, attention must be paid to mental status and patient ability to clearly describe symptoms, mobility and associated limitations, and medications and their potential contributions to symptoms.

Commentary

Kathleen C. Kobashi

Urodynamics (UDS) is an important tool in the evaluation of non-index patients with urinary incontinence and voiding dysfunction. Though UDS is not advocated in the evaluation of the straightforward patient with clear-cut symptoms by any of the applicable AUA/SUFU guidelines (UDS, overactive bladder, or stress urinary incontinence), it is a useful adjunct to the evaluation of patients with less evident clinical pictures. Patients who have a mixed picture, high-grade prolapse, incomplete emptying, and prior pelvic reconstruction or whose diagnoses are not confirmed on initial assessment are examples of those in whom UDS may be helpful.

This chapter nicely presents several commonly encountered but potentially complicated scenarios and discusses the indications for UDS and how the study can be helpful. When presented with a patient in whom several diagnoses are possible, confirmation of the diagnosis is crucial in order to facilitate appropriate treatment planning and assist in thorough counseling about potential outcomes. While diagnoses such as high-grade pelvic prolapse can contribute to symptoms such as voiding dysfunction and incomplete emptying, they can concomitantly mask others, like stress incontinence. In patients with mixed incontinence and voiding dysfunction following an anti-incontinence surgery, elucidation of the components that make up the overall picture can facilitate decisions regarding the order in which the issues should be addressed. UDS in the assessment of patients with neurogenic bladder are key in prognostication for both the upper and lower urinary tracts and in clarifying the situation in patients in whom sensation may not correlate with function. Similarly, in the geriatric population, cognition and processing of sensation may also play a role in continence, and UDS can be a helpful adjunct in the diagnostic assessment.

While it is important to be good stewards of healthcare dollars and avoid overutilization of costly resources, UDS can be invaluable in the evaluation of the non-index patient with urinary incontinence or voiding dysfunction. A good rule of thumb before embarking on a UDS study is for the clinician to consider the unanswered questions for which UDS may be helpful. If UDS would not change the course, it may not be necessary to perform the study. However, in cases in which it could facilitate decision-making, prognostication, or patient counseling, it is a valuable tool to have in the armamentarium.

References

1. Dmochowski RR, Blaivas JM, Gormley EA, Juma S, Karram MM, Lightner DJ, et al. Update of AUA guideline on the surgical management of female stress urinary incontinence. JURO. Elsevier Inc. 2010;183(5):1906–14.
2. Nager CW, Brubaker L, Daneshgari F, Litman HJ, Dandreo KJ, Sirls L, et al. Design of the Value of Urodynamic Evaluation (ValUE) trial: a non-inferiority randomized trial of preoperative urodynamic investigations. Contemp Clin Trials. 2009;30(6):531–9.
3. Collins CW, Winters JC, American Urological Association, Society of Urodynamics Female Pelvic Medicine and Urogenital Reconstruction. AUA/SUFU adult urodynamics guideline. Urol Clin North Am. 2014;41(3):353–62.
4. Rachaneni S, Latthe P. Does preoperative urodynamics improve outcomes for women undergoing surgery for stress urinary incontinence? A systematic review and meta-analysis. BJOG. 4th ed. 2014;122(1):8–16.
5. Gomelsky A, Khaled D, Krlin R. A Critical Appraisal of the AUA Urodynamics Guidelines. AUA Update Series. 2017;36(12).

6. Nager CW, Brubaker L, Litman HJ, Zyczynski H, Varner RE, Amundsen CL, et al. A randomized trial of urodynamic testing before stress-incontinence surgery. N Engl J Med. 2012;366:1987–97.
7. Sirls LT, Richter HE, Litman HJ, Kenton K, Lemack GE, Lukacz ES, et al. The effect of urodynamic testing on clinical diagnosis, treatment plan and outcomes in women undergoing stress urinary incontinence surgery. JURO. Elsevier Inc. 2013;189(1):204–9.
8. Nambiar A, Bosch R, Cruz F, Lemack G, Thiruchelvam N, et al: EAU Guidelines on assessment and nonsurgical management of urinary incontinence. Eur Urol, https://doi.org/10.1016/j.eururo.2017.12.031.
9. Serati M, Giarenis I, Meschia M, Cardozo L. Role of urodynamics before prolapse surgery. Int Urogynecol J Pelvic Floor Dysfunct. 2014;26(2):165–8.
10. Weber AM, Walters MD. Cost-effectiveness of urodynamic testing before surgery for women with pelvic organ prolapse and stress urinary incontinence. Am J Obstet Gynecol. 2000;183(6):1338–47.
11. Ballert KN, Biggs GY, Isenalumhe A, Rosenblum N, Nitti VW. Trauma/reconstruction/diversion managing the urethra at transvaginal pelvic organ prolapse repair: a urodynamic approach. JURO Am Urol Assoc. 2009;181(2):679–84.
12. Drain A, Khan A, Ohmann EL, Brucker BM, Smilen S, Rosenblum N, et al. Voiding dysfunction use of concomitant stress incontinence surgery at time of pelvic organ prolapse surgery since release of the 2011 notification on serious complications associated with transvaginal mesh. JURO. Elsevier Ltd. 2017;197(4):1092–8.
13. Barnes NM, Dmochowski RR, Park R, Nitti VW. Pubovaginal sling and pelvic prolapse repair in women with occult stress urinary incontinence: effect on postoperative emptying and voiding symptoms. Urology. 2002;59(6):856–60.
14. Brown ET, Krlin RM, Winters JC. Urodynamics: examining the current role of UDS testing. What is the role of urodynamic testing in light of recent AUA urodynamics and overactive bladder guidelines and the VALUE study? Curr Urol Rep. 2013;14(5):403–8.
15. Winters JC, Dmochowski RR, Goldman HB, Herndon CDA, Kobashi KC, Kraus SR, et al. Urodynamic studies in adults: AUA/SUFU guideline. JURO. Elsevier Inc. 2012;188(S):2464–72.
16. Araki I, Haneda Y, Mikami Y, Takeda M. Incontinence and detrusor dysfunction associated with pelvic organ prolapse: clinical value of preoperative urodynamic evaluation. Int Urogynecol J Pelvic Floor Dysfunct. 2009;20(11):1301–6.
17. Visco AG, Brubaker L, Nygaard I, Richter HE, Cundiff G, Fine P, et al. The role of preoperative urodynamic testing in stress-continent women undergoing sacrocolpopexy: the Colpopexy and Urinary Reduction Efforts (CARE) randomized surgical trial. Int Urogynecol J Pelvic Floor Dysfunct. 2008;19(5):607–14.
18. Patel BN, Kobashi KC. Practical use of the new American Urological Association adult urodynamics guidelines. Curr Urol Rep. 2013;14(3):240–6.
19. Rovner ES, Goudelocke CM. Urodynamics in the evaluation of overactive bladder. Curr Urol Rep. 2010;11(5):343–7.
20. Yared J, Gormley EA. The role of urodynamics in elderly patients. Clin Geriatr Med. 2015;31(4):567–79.
21. Goldmark E, Niver B, Ginsberg DA. Neurogenic bladder: from diagnosis to management. Curr Urol Rep. 2014;15(10):739–8.
22. Dray EV, Cameron AP. Identifying patients with high-risk neurogenic bladder. Urol Clin North Am. 2017;44(3):441–52.
23. Li L-F, Leung GK-K, Lui W-M. Sacral nerve stimulation for neurogenic bladder. World Neurosurg. 2016;90(C):236–43.
24. Nosseir M, Hinkel A, Pannek J. Clinical usefulness of urodynamic assessment for maintenance of bladder function in patients with spinal cord injury. NeurourolUrodyn. 2007;26(2):228–33.
25. Shin JC, Lee Y, Yang H, Kim DH. Clinical significance of urodynamic study parameters in maintenance of renal function in spinal cord injury patients. Ann Rehabil Med. 2014;38(3):353–7.
26. Cameron AP, Rodriguez GM, Schomer KG. Review article systematic review of urological followup after spinal cord injury. JURO. Elsevier Inc. 2012;187(2):391–7.
27. Natsume O. Detrusor contractility and overactive bladder in patients with cerebrovascular accident. Int J Urol. 2008;15(6):505–10.
28. Sanford MT, Suskind AM. Neuromodulation in neurogenic bladder. Transl Androl Urol. 2016;5(1):117–26.
29. Monteiro ÉS, de Carvalho LBC, Fukujima MM, Lora MI, do Prado GF. Electrical stimulation of the posterior tibialis nerve improves symptoms of poststroke neurogenic overactive bladder in men: a randomized controlled trial. Urology. 2014;84(3):509–14.
30. Schneider MP, Gross T, Bachmann LM, Blok BFM, Castro-Diaz D, Del Popolo G, et al. Tibial nerve stimulation for treating neurogenic lower urinary tract dysfunction: a systematic review. Eur Urol. 2015;68(5):859–67.
31. Joussain C, Denys P. Electrical management of neurogenic lower urinary tract disorders. Ann Phys Rehabil Med. 2015;58(4):245–50.
32. Veenboer PW, de Kort LMO, Chrzan RJ, de Jong TPVM. Urinary considerations for adult patients with spinal dysraphism. Nat Rev Urol. Nature Publishing Group. 2015;12(6):331–9.
33. Veenboer PW, Bosch JLHR, Rosier PFWM, Dik P, van Asbeck FWA, de Jong TPVM, et al. Cross-sectional study of determinants of upper and lower urinary tract outcomes in adults with spinal dysraphism-new recommendations for urodynamic followup guidelines? JURO. Elsevier Ltd. 2014;192(2):477–82.
34. Mourtzinos A, Stoffel JT. Management goals for the spina bifida neurogenic bladder: a review

Principles in Using Anorectal Manometry

Normal defecatory process relies on several intricate mechanisms such as the rectal wall, anal sphincter complex, and pudendal nerves. Endoanal ultrasound can be used to evaluate the integrity of anal sphincters and determine the length of anal canal. ARM complements endoanal ultrasound as it provides objective assessment of anorectal functional physiology by measuring the pressure generated in the low rectum and anal canal (Fig. 3.1).

Although interobserver reliability and reproducibility in ARM have been demonstrated in several small series [7, 8], variation in techniques in using ARM exists in different institutions [9]. In recent years, guidelines and expert consensus statements have been published to try to minimize variability in clinical practice and to standardize reporting [10–12].

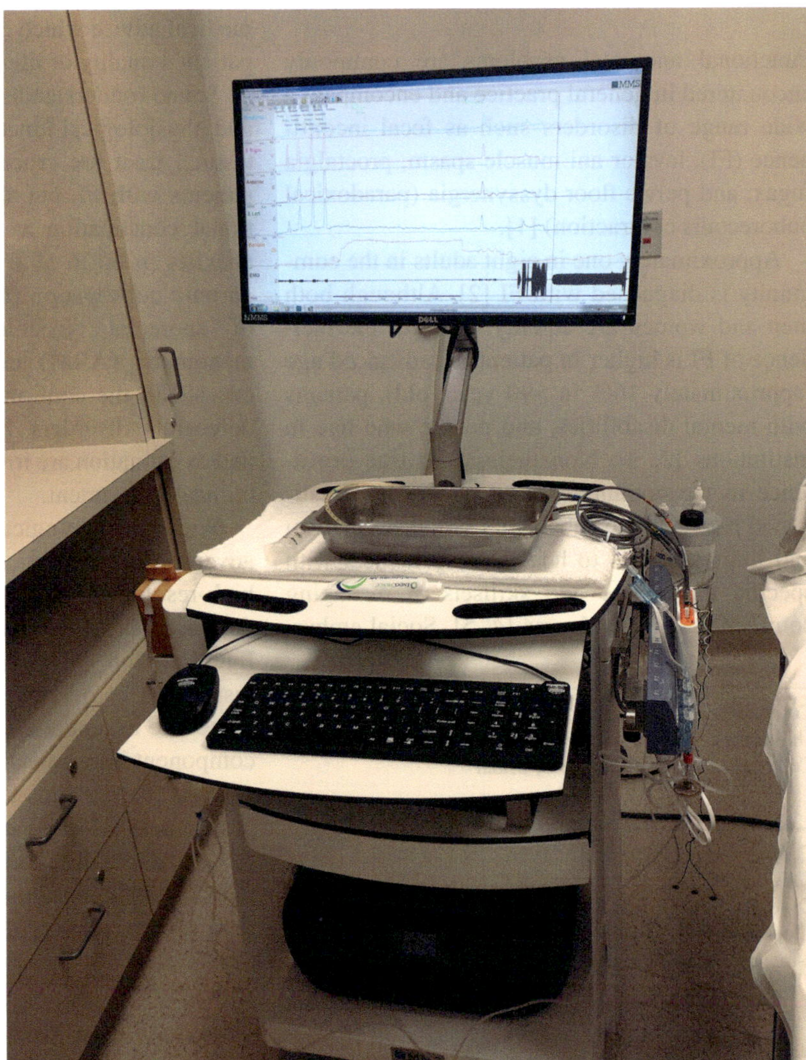

Fig. 3.1 Basic setup of anorectal manometry

Indications

ARM can be a useful diagnostic tool in patients with FI, chronic constipation, or pelvic floor dyssynergia. In patients with persistent anal fissure after unilateral internal sphincterotomy, it can help to identify individuals who may be suitable for contralateral internal sphincterotomy if the resting anal sphincter pressure remains high. It can also be used in screening for Hirschsprung's disease which is characterized by absence of rectoanal inhibitory reflex (RAIR). It can also be used to evaluate patients with ileal J-pouch dysfunction [13, 14].

Techniques

Anorectal manometry measures rectal and anal sphincter luminal pressure via an air-charged or water-perfused catheter with a variably located pressure sensor (Fig. 3.2). Air-charged catheters have the advantage of being single-use and negate the need to use water irrigation during the procedure as compared to water-perfused catheter. Nonetheless, they have been shown to provide similar measurements [15]. The more advanced solid-state catheter is equipped with more sensors at shorter intervals, hence providing better resolution and spatiotemporal measurement. Computerized software can depict colored pressure gradient and plot for easier interpretation. In addition, three-dimensional (3D) topographic pressure map can be generated using HDARM which can demonstrate the location of sphincter defect [16]. In addition to the initial cost, the ongoing costs of cleaning and maintenance are the major shortcomings of solid-state catheter.

Oral mechanical cathartic bowel preparation is unnecessary, although a disposable enema can be given if the patient has significant amount of stool in the rectum; a left lateral position is preferable. Examination begins with general inspection of the perianal region and perineum, particularly paying attention to previous surgical scar at the perineum and shape of the anus. A patulous anal opening is indicative of significant injuries to the anal sphincters and/or nerves. Several reflexes can be elicited such as the anocutaneous and bulbocavernosus reflex, to exclude spinal cord injury. Digital rectal examination is performed to exclude a rectal mass and assess anal sphincter tone.

A lubricated catheter is inserted a few centimeters above anal sphincter complex; either a pull-through or stationary technique can be used [12]. After a period of relaxation and anal pressure stabilization, the resting anal pressure is measured during approximately 20 seconds. The patient is asked to contract the anal sphincters for up to 30 seconds, followed by 1 minute of rest. Meanwhile, the catheter is manually withdrawn at 1 cm intervals. Next, squeeze pressure measurements are performed after pressure normalization (Table 3.1).

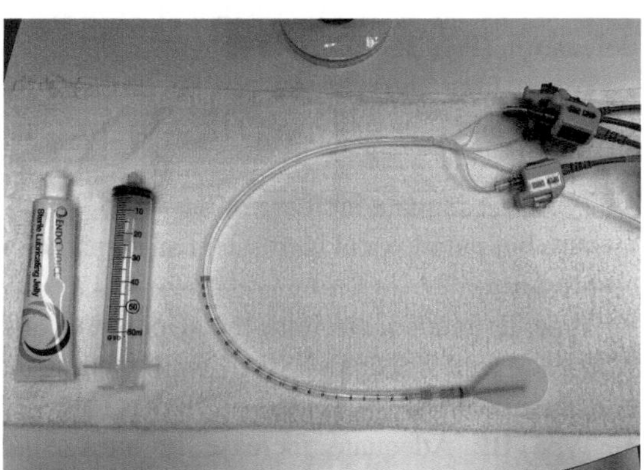

Fig. 3.2 Air-charged catheter with latex balloon

Table 3.1 Reference range of anorectal manometry (ARM) results at the Cleveland Clinic

	Measurement
Anal canal length	Male 4–5 cm Female 3–4 cm
Normal resting pressure	>40 mmHg
Normal squeeze pressure	>100 mmHg
Volume studies	
Rectoanal inhibitory reflex	10–60 ml
Average volume of first sensation	10–60 ml
Average volume of first urge	10–100 ml
Maximum tolerated volume	200–300 ml
Rectal compliance	5–15 ml/mmHg

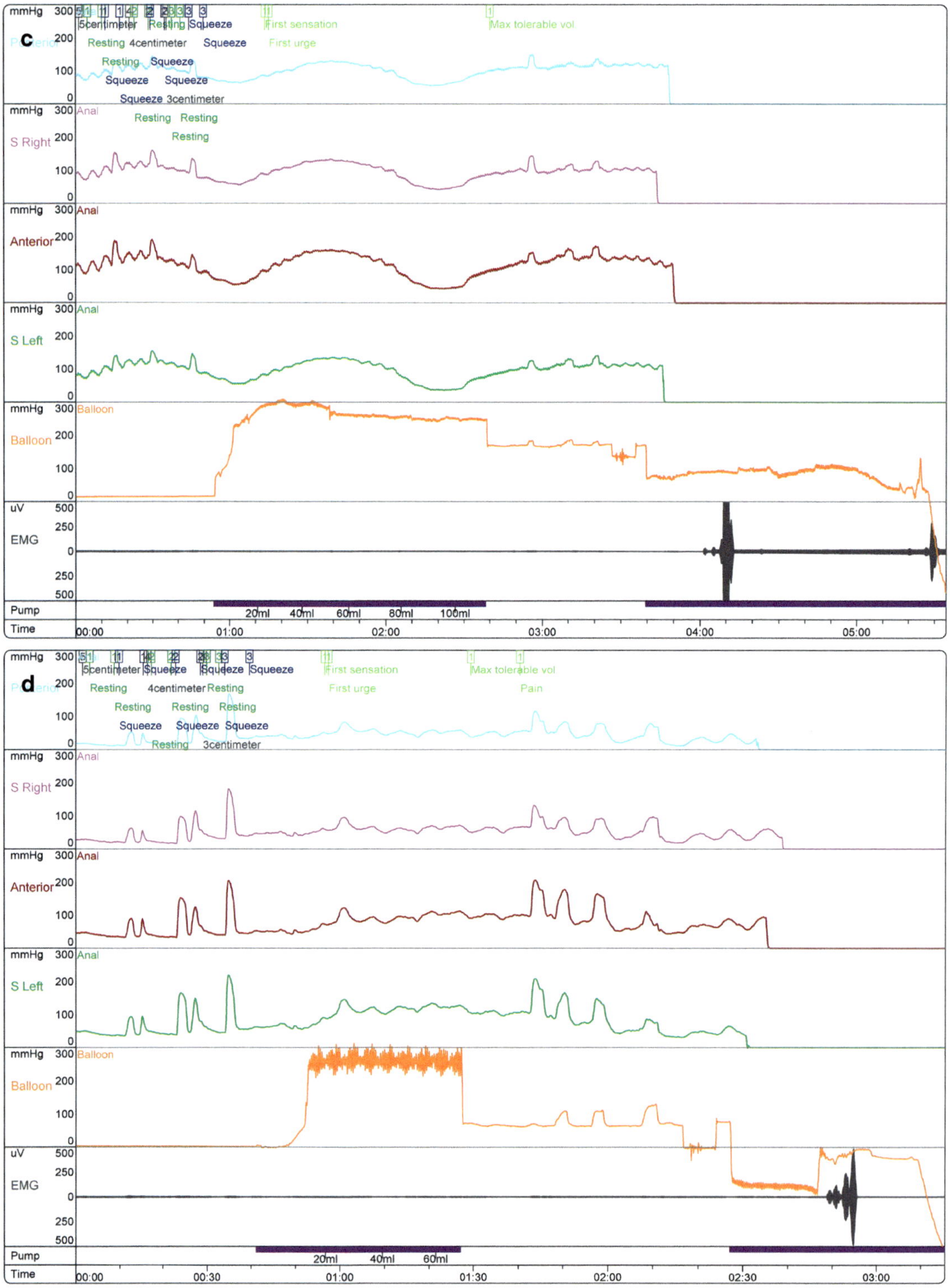

Fig. 3.3 (continued)

- Type IV: Inadequate intra-rectal pressure and absent or inadequate relaxation of the anal sphincter

Electromyography using surface electrodes can be used to quantify striated pelvic floor muscle activity, and pudendal terminal nerve latency testing can also be employed [35, 36] (Fig. 3.3d).

Interpretation of Defecography

Defecography provides a dynamic anatomical and functional evaluation of pelvic organs during defecation. It is primarily used to investigate patients suffering from rectal and/or vaginal prolapse and chronic constipation. Compared to conventional fluoroscopic defecography, dynamic magnetic resonance (MR) defecography can demonstrate superb resolution of pelvic floor muscle anatomy and surrounding soft tissue, especially in assessing other pelvic organ prolapse [37, 38]. MR defecography can be performed in an open-configuration magnetic unit which allows more physiological image acquisition as patient is in an erect sitting position. Similar to ARM, it should be performed in a relatively relaxed and comfortable environment. It is essential to explain to the patients each step of the procedure to try to help optimize compliance with testing and thus the accuracy of the results.

In preparation for fluoroscopic defecography, barium contrast paste is administered into the rectum in addition to oral and vaginal barium contrast. When using conventional fluoroscopic defecography, the patient is instructed to sit on a radiolucent commode which allows lateral projection of X-ray to center at the pelvis. A series of radiological images are captured during the following maneuvers: rest, squeeze, strain, defecating, and following evacuation.

It is essential to recognize several key anatomical landmarks and measurements such as anorectal angle and pubococcygeal and ischiococcygeal lines [18]. The anorectal angle is measured between a line drawn at the central axis of anal canal and a line drawn parallel to posterior rectal wall (at rest; normal range, 90°–110°) or at the center of distal rectum (during evacuation). This angle is largely maintained by the puborectalis muscle at rest. During evacuation, the anorectal angle becomes more obtuse as the puborectalis muscle relaxes. In the case of obstructive defecation due to paradoxical movement of pelvic floor musculatures, the anorectal angle is less exaggerated during evacuation.

The pubococcygeal line is measured from the inferior border of the symphysis pubis to the last coccygeal joint, whereas the ischiococcygeal line is measured from the inferior border of ischium to the last coccygeal joint. These two lines can be used to classify the severity of small bowel (enterocele) and large bowel (sigmoidocele) herniation into three grades: grade I, above pubococcygeal line; grade II, between pubococcygeal and ischiococcygeal lines; and grade III, below ischiococcygeal line [39]. Perineal descent is represented by the difference in position of anorectal junction at rest and during maximal straining in relation to the pubococcygeal line (Fig. 3.4). Exaggerated perineal descent (>3.5 cm) is associated with weakening of pelvic floor musculature secondary to repetitive straining. Although it can be observed in patients with chronic constipation, however, it does not correlate with severity of symptoms or quality of life [40].

Summary

Objective functional assessment given by ARM and defecography provides additional values in tailored management in various defecatory disorders and FI which are often overlooked in our society. Nonetheless, a thorough history and physical examination remain essential in the initial assessment. Multidisciplinary collaboration and holistic approaches are required to manage patients who have multiple pelvic compartment issues.

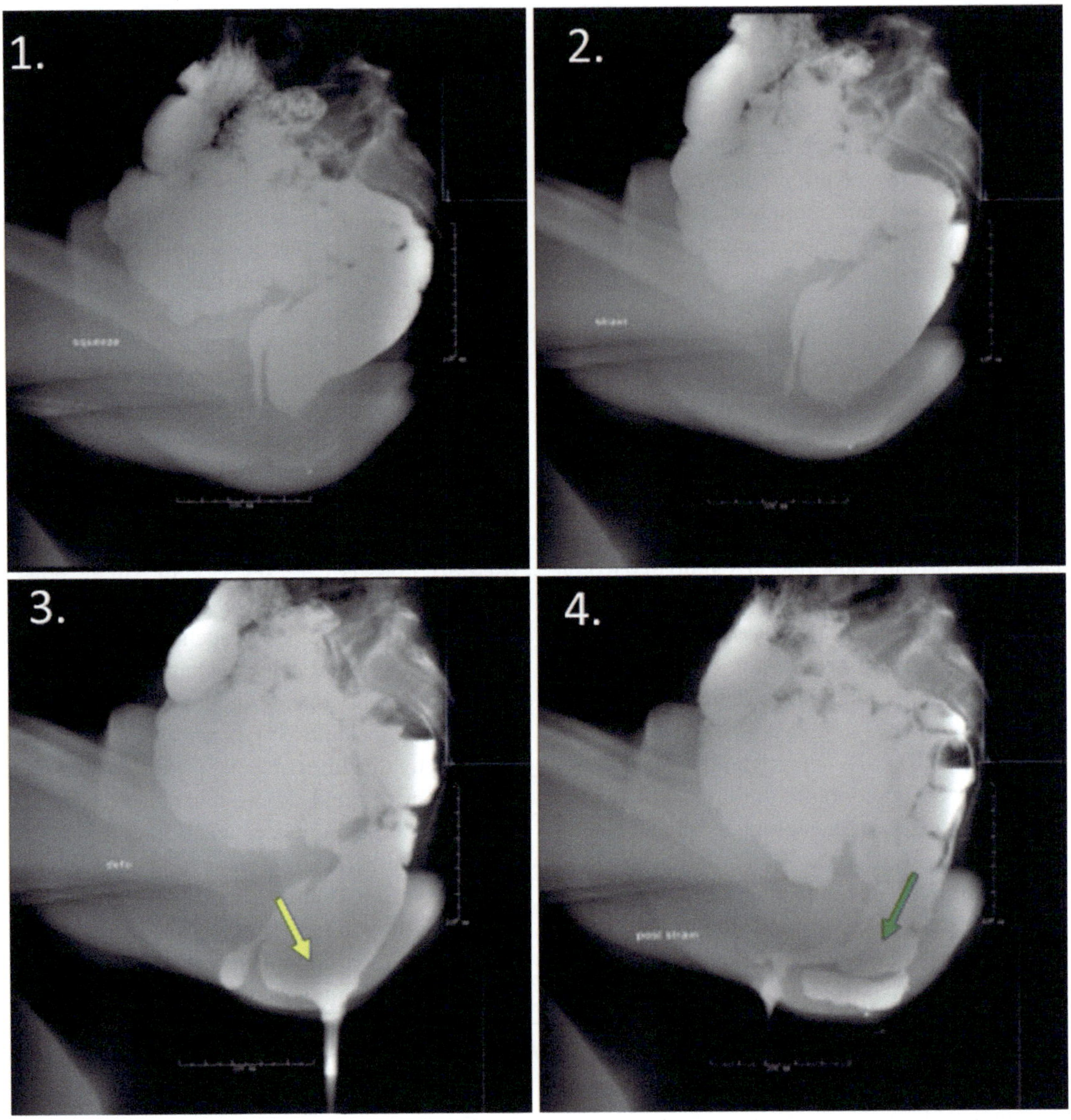

Fig. 3.4 Fluoroscopic defecography (series 1–4) demonstrating exaggerated perineal descent, large rectocele (yellow arrow), and sigmoidocele (green arrow)

Commentary

J. Marcio N. Jorge

This chapter addresses the main aspects of physiologic testing in complex functional colorectal disorders. Despite affecting both men and women, constipation and incontinence are more prevalent in the latter group. This is probably due to the effects of pregnancy and childbirth on the pelvic floor and the higher prevalence of constipation in this gender group.

Patients with fecal incontinence and rectal prolapse are among those with the worst quality of life seen in our specialty. Embarrassment poses a major difficulty in addressing evaluation and proper treatment. As emphasized by the authors, although history and physical examination are irreplaceable, anorectal physiology testing can be crucial to better understand the mechanisms involved and to uncover the etiology.

The initial therapeutic schema includes dietary assessment, a diary of defecation and symptoms, and, when indicated, psychological evaluation. Patients referred for colorectal physiologic testing often present with refractory and severe idiopathic symptoms, and a combination of anorectal physiology studies is usually indicated due to the complex etiology of these functional disorders.

In practice, anorectal manometry, videodefecography, colonic transit time, and endoanal ultrasound are considered the most useful tests. Through this physiologic investigation, treatable conditions of the colon, rectum, and anus can be diagnosed in 67% and 55% of patients with constipation and fecal incontinence, respectively [41]. In patients with rectal pain, however, these tests permit definite diagnosis in only 18%, and this condition remains poorly understood and refractory to therapy. In addition, these tests can be helpful preoperatively, when anal continence status may be endangered due to the nature of the procedure or a pre-existing disorder that affects the mechanism of continence.

A history and physical examination often dictate additional tests. Electroneuromyography including conventional anal electromyography (EMG) and pudendal nerve terminal motor latency (PNTML) testing can be helpful to uncover neuromuscular disease. However, pudendal neuropathy is a common finding with increasing age and parity and in many comorbidities including chronic constipation and diabetes. Thus, the therapeutic decision is not usually affected by this finding. As discussed by the authors, these tests should be reserved for patients with complex diagnostic dilemmas [42].

Most tests are performed with minimal preparation. A disposable enema is administered 4 hours prior to the test to remove any significant amount of stool and to allow for a more comfortable exam for both the patient and physician.

Anorectal manometry is often indicated to evaluate functional disorders but is also useful in the preoperative assessment of other disorders when there is a risk of postoperative incontinence either due to the preoperative continence status or the procedure itself. More recently, parameters such as the fatigue index to detect earlier external sphincter dysfunction have been incorporated [43]. Accordingly, 3D high-definition anorectal manometry, a more refined technique, has shown significant correlation between the fecal incontinence score and voluntary contraction variables including the mean anal pressure during sustained squeeze – the most discriminant parameter [44]. The sphincter asymmetry index can help to identify sphincter defects; however, anal ultrasound is preferred if available [45].

Videodefecography provides a wide range of information to assist the surgeon in the evaluation and management of patients with evacuatory and other associated pelvic floor disorders [46]. As pointed out in this chapter, wide ranges of normal values for each of these parameters are observed, and the exact value of any of these isolated parameters is of relatively little consequence. Instead, the role of static proctography is to provide a basis for relative comparison among resting, squeezing, and pushing values in a single patient. Causative or associated abnormalities, such as nonrelaxing puborectalis (puborectalis indentation), rectocele, internal rectal prolapse, sigmoidocele, and enterocele can all be diagnosed by defecography. These findings, particularly a small rectocele and an intussusception, may be found in up to 70% of asymptomatic individuals [46]. Failure to recognize these variants of normal can easily lead to overdiagnosis and overtreatment. Therefore, a treatment decision should be made based upon both clinical history and evaluation of rectal emptying during videodefecography. Most individuals evacuate their rectum within 15–20 seconds; factors affecting rectal emptying rate include consistency of contents and patients' embarrassment. Patients must be reassured and fully informed regarding the importance of the defecographic findings in their therapeutic approach. Dynamic evaluations of defecation using computerized tomography, resonance, and ultrasound are compatible, with the advantage of evaluating extra-rectal structures. However, in order to better evaluate rectal emptying and the clinical relevance of a diagnostic finding, conventional defecography remains the preferred method in many centers [46, 47].

Defecographic criteria of nonrelaxing puborectalis syndrome include failure to open the anorectal angle, persistence of the puborectalis impression during attempted defecation, an overly capacious rectum, a long and persistently closed anal canal, ballooning of the rectum, and the presence of compensatory anterior and posterior rectoceles. These findings can be associated with non-emptying, incomplete emptying, or even total evacuation after prolonged and difficult attempts. However, although useful, both defecography and electromyography have their limitations. Voluntary contraction of the pelvic floor due to embarrassment may simulate a functional disorder on defecography. Likewise, the inability to relax the sphincter may occur during pushing as a response to fear or pain during electromyographic assessment. These factors may cause false-positive findings of nonrelaxing puborectalis syndrome in patients without symptoms of obstructed evacuation. Sensitivity, specificity, and predictive values of both electromyography and defecography are suboptimal, and the combination of these tests may be necessary to permit optimal data accrual [48]. Nevertheless, defecography is likely superior as it can detect associated abnormalities and demonstrate both the dynamics of evacuation and rectal emptying. Although false-positive results may ensue due to the patient's fear of evacuating in front of others, they can be asked to evacuate in the privacy of a bathroom followed by fluoroscopic reassessment of the evacuated rectum. Finally, the diagnosis of nonrelaxing puborectalis syndrome should be reserved for patients whose clinical symptoms of pelvic outlet obstruction are supported by physiologic confirmation. In order to differentiate an incidental finding from a clinically significant sigmoidocele, a classification system has been proposed [49]. This classification system is based on the degree of descent of the lowest portion of the sigmoid loop during maximum straining in relation to the following pelvic anatomic landmarks: pubis, coccyx, and ischium. First-degree sigmoidocele corresponds to an intrapelvic loop of sigmoid which does not surpass the pubococcygeal line; second-degree sigmoidocele is noted when the sigmoid loop is situated below the pubococcygeal line but remains above the ischiococcygeal line; and third-degree sigmoidocele is considered if the sigmoid loop transcends the ischiococcygeal line. This classification system yielded excellent correlation between the mean level of sigmoidocele, degree of sigmoid redundancy, and clinical symptoms.

Physiologic testing permits objective assessment of subjective and highly prevalent functional colorectal symptoms. A judicious indication and association and interpretation of the tests discussed in this chapter will ensure a better perspective of treating the refractory, at times, incapacitating symptoms. Finally, because the pelvic floor is an integrated functional structure, these disorders should be addressed using a multidisciplinary and integrated approach.

References

1. Bharucha AE, Wald A, Enck P, Rao S. Functional anorectal disorders. Gastroenterology. 2006;130:1510–8.
2. Ng KS, Sivakumaran Y, Nassar N, Gladman MA. Fecal incontinence: community prevalence and associated factors--a systematic review. Dis Colon Rectum. 2015;58:1194–209.
3. Madoff RD, Parker SC, Varma MG, Lowry AC. Faecal incontinence in adults. Lancet. 2004;364:621–32.
4. O'Connell PR. Needs assessment for treatment of fecal incontinence. Dis Colon Rectum. 2017;60:358–9.
5. Garcia JA, Crocker J, Wyman JF, Krissovich M. Breaking the cycle of stigmatization: managing the stigma of incontinence in social interactions. J Wound Ostomy Continence Nurs. 2005;32:38–52.
6. Noelting J, Eaton JE, Choung RS, et al. The incidence rate and characteristics of clinically diagnosed defecatory disorders in the community. Neurogastroenterol Motil. 2016;28:1690–7.
7. Freys SM, Fuchs KH, Fein M, et al. Inter- and intraindividual reproducibility of anorectal manometry. Langenbecks Arch Surg. 1998;383:325–9.
8. Gosling J, Plumb A, Taylor SA, Cohen R, Emmanuel AV. High-resolution anal manometry: repeatability, validation, and comparison with conventional manometry. Neurogastroenterol Motil. 2019;31:e13591.
9. Carrington EV, Heinrich H, Knowles CH, et al. Methods of anorectal manometry vary widely in clinical practice: results from an international survey. Neurogastroenterol Motil. 2017;29:e13016.

10. Rao SS, Azpiroz F, Diamant N, et al. Minimum standards of anorectal manometry. Neurogastroenterol Motil. 2002;14:553–9.
11. Carrington EV, Scott SM, Bharucha A, et al. Expert consensus document: advances in the evaluation of anorectal function. Nat Rev Gastroenterol Hepatol. 2018;15:309–23.
12. Azpiroz F, Enck P, Whitehead WE. Anorectal functional testing: review of collective experience. Am J Gastroenterol. 2002;97:232–40.
13. Quinn KP, Tse CS, Lightner AL, et al. Nonrelaxing pelvic floor dysfunction is an underestimated complication of ileal pouch-anal anastomosis. Clin Gastroenterol Hepatol. 2017;15:1242–7.
14. Hull TL, Fazio VW, Schroeder T. Paradoxical puborectalis contraction in patients after pelvic pouch construction. Dis Colon Rectum. 1995;38:1144–6.
15. Fang JC, Hilden K, Tuteja AK, Peterson KA. Comparison of air-coupled balloon esophageal and anorectal manometry catheters with solid-state esophageal manometry and water-perfused anorectal manometry catheters. Dig Dis Sci. 2004;49:1657–63.
16. Vitton V, Ben Hadj Amor W, Baumstarck K, et al. Comparison of three-dimensional high-resolution manometry and endoanal ultrasound in the diagnosis of anal sphincter defects. Colorectal Dis. 2013;15:e607–11.
17. Bordeianou LG, Carmichael JC, Paquette IM, et al. Consensus statement of definitions for anorectal physiology testing and pelvic floor terminology (revised). Dis Colon Rectum. 2018;61:421–7.
18. Penninckx F, Lestar B, Kerremans R. The internal anal sphincter: mechanisms of control and its role in maintaining anal continence. Baillieres Clin Gastroenterol. 1992;6:193–214.
19. Li Y, Yang X, Xu C, Zhang Y, Zhang X. Normal values and pressure morphology for three-dimensional high-resolution anorectal manometry of asymptomatic adults: a study in 110 subjects. Int J Colorectal Dis. 2013;28:1161–8.
20. Noelting J, Ratuapli SK, Bharucha AE, et al. Normal values for high-resolution anorectal manometry in healthy women: effects of age and significance of rectoanal gradient. Am J Gastroenterol. 2012;107:1530–6.
21. Felt-Bersma RJ, Gort G, Meuwissen SG. Normal values in anal manometry and rectal sensation: a problem of range. Hepatogastroenterology. 1991;38:444–9.
22. Prichard D, Harvey DM, Fletcher JG, Zinsmeister AR, Bharucha AE. Relationship among anal sphincter injury, patulous anal canal, and anal pressures in patients with anorectal disorders. Clin Gastroenterol Hepatol. 2015;13:1793–800.e1.
23. Felt-Bersma RJ, Klinkenberg-Knol EC, Meuwissen SG. Anorectal function investigations in incontinent and continent patients. Differences and discriminatory value. Dis Colon Rectum. 1990;33:479–85; discussion 85–6.
24. Bordeianou L, Lee KY, Rockwood T, et al. Anal resting pressures at manometry correlate with the fecal incontinence severity index and with presence of sphincter defects on ultrasound. Dis Colon Rectum. 2008;51:1010–4.
25. Gibbons CP, Read NW. Anal hypertonia in fissures: cause or effect? Br J Surg. 1986;73:443–5.
26. Prohm P, Bonner C. Is manometry essential for surgery of chronic fissure-in-ano? Dis Colon Rectum. 1995;38:735–8.
27. Ram E, Alper D, Stein GY, Bramnik Z, Dreznik Z. Internal anal sphincter function following lateral internal sphincterotomy for anal fissure: a long-term manometric study. Ann Surg. 2005;242:208–11.
28. Carapeti EA, Kamm MA, McDonald PJ, et al. Randomised controlled trial shows that glyceryl trinitrate heals anal fissures, higher doses are not more effective, and there is a high recurrence rate. Gut. 1999;44:727–30.
29. Thornton MJ, Kennedy ML, King DW. Prospective manometric assessment of botulinum toxin and its correlation with healing of chronic anal fissure. Dis Colon Rectum. 2005;48:1424–31.
30. Meinds RJ, Trzpis M, Broens PMA. Anorectal manometry may reduce the number of rectal suction biopsy procedures needed to diagnose Hirschsprung disease. J Pediatr Gastroenterol Nutr. 2018;67:322–7.
31. Kakodkar R, Gupta S, Nundy S. Low anterior resection with total mesorectal excision for rectal cancer: functional assessment and factors affecting outcome. Colorectal Dis. 2006;8:650–6.
32. Felt-Bersma RJ, Sloots CE, Poen AC, Cuesta MA, Meuwissen SG. Rectal compliance as a routine measurement: extreme volumes have direct clinical impact and normal volumes exclude rectum as a problem. Dis Colon Rectum. 2000;43:1732–8.
33. Kamm MA, Lennard-Jones JE. Rectal mucosal electrosensory testing--evidence for a rectal sensory neuropathy in idiopathic constipation. Dis Colon Rectum. 1990;33:419–23.
34. Rao SS, Patcharatrakul T. Diagnosis and treatment of dyssynergic defecation. J Neurogastroenterol Motil. 2016;22:423–35.
35. Diamant NE, Kamm MA, Wald A, Whitehead WE. Aga technical review on anorectal testing techniques. Gastroenterology. 1999;116:735–60.
36. Cheong DM, Vaccaro CA, Salanga VD, Wexner SD, Phillips RC, Hanson MR, Waxner SD. Electrodiagnostic evaluation of fecal incontinence. Muscle Nerve. 1995;18(6):612–9.
37. Mortele KJ, Fairhurst J. Dynamic MR defecography of the posterior compartment: indications, techniques and MRI features. Eur J Radiol. 2007;61:462–72.
38. Roos JE, Weishaupt D, Wildermuth S, et al. Experience of 4 years with open MR defecography: pictorial review of anorectal anatomy and disease. Radiographics. 2002;22:817–32.
39. Jorge JM, Yang YK, Wexner SD. Incidence and clinical significance of sigmoidoceles as determined

by a new classification system. Dis Colon Rectum. 1994;37(11):1112–7.

40. Alves-Ferreira PC, Gurland B, Zutshi M, Hull T. Perineal descent does not imply a more severe clinical disorder. Colorectal Dis. 2012;14:1372–9.
41. Wexner SD, Jorge JMN. Colorectal physiological tests: use or abuse of technology? Eur J Surg. 1994;160:167–74.
42. Jorge JMN, Wexner SD. Physiologic evaluation. In: Wexner SD, Vernava AM, editors. Clinical decision making in colorectal surgery. New York: Igaku-Shoin; 1995. p. 11–22.
43. Marcello PW, Barrett RC, Coller JA, Schoetz DJ Jr, Roberts PL, Murray JJ, Rusin LC. Fatigue rate index as a new measurement of external sphincter function. Dis Colon Rectum. 1998;41:336–43.
44. Mion F, Garros A, Subtil F, Damon H, Roman S. Anal sphincter function as assessed by 3D high definition anorectal manometry. Clin Res Hepatol Gastroenterol. 2018;42:378–81.
45. Jorge JMN, Habr-Gama A. The value of sphincteric asymmetry index analysis in anal incontinence. Int J Colorectal Dis. 2000;15:303–10.
46. Jorge JM, Habr-Gama A. Clinical applications and techniques of cinedefecography. Am J Surg. 2001;182:93–101.
47. Matsuoka H, Wexner SD, Desai MB, Nakamura T, Nogueras JJ, Weiss EG, Adami C, Billotti VL. A comparison between dynamic pelvic resonance imaging and videoproctography in patients with constipation. Dis Colon Rectum. 2001;44:571–6.
48. Jorge JMN, Wexner SD, Ger GC, Jagelman DG. Cinedefecography and EMG in the diagnosis of nonrelaxing puborectalis syndrome. Dis Colon Rectum. 1993;36:668–76.
49. Jorge JMN, Yang Y-K, Wexner SD. Incidence and clinical significance of sigmoidoceles as determined by a new classification system. Dis Colon Rectum. 1994;37:1112–7.

4 Quantitative and Qualitative Analysis of Fecal Incontinence

Allison Pang, Julie Ann Van Koughnett, and Marylise Boutros

Introduction

Fecal incontinence (FI) is an anorectal disorder characterized by the impaired ability to control the release of gas and stool. This decreased control can range in severity and can often greatly impact quality of life (QoL). The incidence of FI ranges from 2% to 15% among non-institutionalized adults in the United States. However, it is often underreported due to the complexity of symptoms, the difficulty patients face to quantify their symptoms, and their hesitancy to seek care due to embarrassment [1, 2]. Although there are several physiologic tests that measure FI, none of them have been shown to accurately reflect disease severity or to quantify the exact response to therapy. This finding is likely due to the important, and often underestimated, contribution of the patients' own perception of their symptoms. Acknowledging this subjectivity is essential in the assessment of FI. The evaluation of a patient's FI is dependent on two important components: symptom severity and impact on QoL. In order to assess the effect that a treatment has on FI, it is important to document these two components pre- and post-treatment. To accomplish this, both questionnaires and scoring systems must be used. This chapter is an updated review from a previous publication written by the authors on the quantitative and qualitative analysis of FI [3].

Case Scenario: Part A

A 73-year-old woman presents with a 5-year history of progressive FI. She has type 1 diabetes with good glycemic control. She describes her current symptoms as having four to six episodes of accidental liquid stool leakage per week, which forces her to wear sanitary pads almost every day. She has two formed bowel movements every day; however, prior to a bowel movement, she experiences urgency that sometimes leads to fecal soiling. She has no nocturnal incontinence. There is no blood or mucus associated with bowel movements. She is continent to gas. She does not experience urinary incontinence. These symptoms have caused her to alter her daily activities, most pronounced during the weekdays. A recent

Commentary by Ann C. Lowry, University of Minnesota, Department of Colon and Rectal Surgery, Minneapolis, MN, USA

A. Pang · M. Boutros (✉)
Jewish General Hospital, Division of Colon and Rectal Surgery, Montreal, QC, Canada
e-mail: marylise.boutros@mcgill.ca

J. A. Van Koughnett
London Health Sciences Centre – University Hospital, Departments of Surgery and Oncology, London, ON, Canada

K. C. Kobashi, S. D. Wexner (eds.), *Female Pelvic Medicine*,
https://doi.org/10.1007/978-3-030-54839-1_4

colonoscopy was reportedly normal. Her obstetrical history includes four vaginal deliveries, one of which resulted in a second-degree perineal tear that was repaired with sutures. She has had previous anorectal surgery including a fistulotomy in her late 20s for an uncomplicated fistula-in-ano. She has no other relevant history, including no history of back injury and no neurologic problems. On physical exam, her abdominal exam is normal. Perineal inspection revealed a thin perineal body. Digital rectal exam revealed a moderately patulous anus with weak resting and squeeze sphincter tone.

Study Questions

- *What are the common symptom severity scores that are used to assess the severity of FI?*
- *How would the use of a symptom severity score be utilized to guide the care of this patient?*
- *In this scenario, what would be the benefits of using a FI severity score with a summary score?*

Quantifying and Qualifying Fecal Incontinence: The Use of Weighted and Non-weighted Symptom Severity Scores and Quality-of-Life Measures

Symptom severity scores can be useful for the evaluation of subjective and complex symptoms. When used in the context of FI, these instruments are often used to assess the frequency and type(s) of stool leakage and, in turn, are helpful in assessing treatment outcomes. There are two types of severity scores for FI – grading scales and summary scores (see below). Many of these scoring systems have been validated through research studies; however, an important aspect to consider in assessing self-reported FI severity is whether the questionnaire has been weighted or not.

A weighted questionnaire assigns a certain value to each question. These "weights" can either be self-determined by the patient or externally assigned. An example of a self-determined weighted score is the Anal Sphincter Replacement Scoring System [4], which asks the patient to follow fairly complicated directions to assign a weight to each incontinence item description. This questionnaire can be quite time-consuming with a high cognitive burden for the patient. An example of an externally developed weighted score is the Vaizey/St. Mark's FI score [5]. This questionnaire was designed to assign a lesser weight for the use of pads and constipating medications when compared to incontinent episodes. However, the final score may not necessarily reflect the patients' perceived impact of FI on their daily activities. As a result, this externally developed weight has the potential to add physician subjectivity to the tool. Another example of a weighted scale is the Fecal Incontinence Severity Index (FISI), which asks patients to rank order the type/frequency combinations from the most severe to the least severe [6]. It is important to understand, however, that when the FISI was initially being evaluated, the weight assigned by patients and physicians did not always correlate. For these reasons, a weighted scoring tool can be problematic when quantifying/qualifying FI.

In contrast, non-weighted questionnaires use simple numerics to describe the severity of FI such that there is no judgment as to which type of incontinence is worse. Although only vague quantifiers are used, non-weighted tools are often the simplest and the most frequently cited and utilized. For example, the Cleveland Clinic Florida-Fecal Incontinence Score (CCF-FIS) asks the patient to score each equally weighted item on a scale of 0 (never) to 4 (more than once per day) [7]. Thus, there is no judgment by the physician as to which type of incontinence is worse, and in this way, the severity of the symptoms is based on the patient's personal experience. The drawback of such a scale is the difficulty in comparing severity between individuals. However, it does allow patients to summarize their symptoms, which can be rather challenging without the aid of a scoring tool. The problem with weighting is that the weight assigned by patients may differ from weights assigned by physicians.

QoL measures help understand and measure the subjective perception of a patients' health state on their emotional and social life. Furthermore, they allow physicians to better evaluate patient functioning and thus complement severity scores when assessing a patient. There are three main types of QoL measures: generic scales, specialized scales, and condition-specific scales. Generic scales are often based on health-related questions which span a wide range of QoL issues and can therefore be applied to a broad population. They can compare a target population to other populations. A common example of a generic QoL scale is the 36-Item Short-Form Health Survey (SF-36) [8]. The responsiveness of a generic scale is fair, meaning that responses to the questionnaire can identify gross changes, but the questions may not be specific enough to detect subtle changes in QoL. Specialized scales are developed around a specific condition instead of a specific population. As such, they are generally more detailed and more responsive to change. An example of a commonly used specific scale is the Gastrointestinal Quality of Life Index (GIQLI) [9]. It includes 36 items divided between 5 domains: symptoms, physical dysfunction, emotional dysfunction, social dysfunction, and a single-item question on the effect of medical treatment. Lastly, condition-specific scales describe a specific element of a condition, such as FI. Condition-specific scales, like the FISI, are the most sensitive to changes.

Grading Scales for Fecal Incontinence

Grading scales are simple tools that assign a value to each specific type of FI in an ordinal fashion. They do not qualify the patients' experience, nor the subjective severity of their FI. The original scoring of FI was described by Sir Alan Parks, when he created a simple four-category grading scale to assess pre- and postoperative outcomes after anal surgery (see Table 4.1) [10]. A few years later, Broden et al. described a second grading scale that was based on degrees of FI – none, medium, or severe – rather than on the type of incontinence [11]. The grading scales that followed were all similar in their composition of three to five broad grades, ranging from "excellent" to "poor" continence. They are summarized in Table 4.2. These scales did not include either the grading of the frequency of FI or the impact of incontinence on the patient. Due to their simplicity and their broad categorization of FI, grading scales do not have the ability to differentiate between the nuances and variability of FI. As a consequence, their ability to detect minor clinical changes is less exact.

Table 4.1 Park's scoring of fecal incontinence [10]

Category A	Category B	Category C	Category D
Continent to solid and liquid stool and flatus	Continent to solid and liquid stool but not to flatus	Continent to solid but not to liquid stool or flatus	Incontinent to solid and liquid stool and flatus

Table 4.2 Examples of severity grading scores of fecal incontinence

Author	Year	Spectrum
Browning and Parks [10]	1975	Normal to no control of solid stool
Rudd [11]	1979	Perfect continence to unsatisfactory requiring colostomy
Keighley and Fielding [23]	1983	Minor leakage to severe incontinence
Corman [24]	1985	Excellent to poor continence
Hiltunen et al. [25]	1986	Gross fecal incontinence to full continence
Broden et al. [26]	1988	No fecal incontinence to incontinence to stool at all times
Rainey et al. [27]	1990	Continent of solid +/− flatus to incontinent to all stool
Womack et al. [28]	1988	Continent to incontinent
Williams et al. [29]	1991	Continent to frequent incontinence

Summary Scores for Fecal Incontinence

Summary scores for FI, unlike grading scales, assign specific values to different aspects of FI, thus attempting to reflect the severity of symptoms. This strategy includes questions on the frequency of incontinence. At the end of the questionnaire, a summary score is calculated based on the addition of values in each category. In doing this, there is a greater ability to discriminate differences between patients, to detect clinically important changes, and to assess treatment outcomes. For this reason, summary scoring systems have become the more preferred way of measuring FI. Table 4.3 presents a summary of the most common FI summary scoring systems currently found in the literature; three of the scores are weighted (see Table 4.3). The CCF-FIS, Vaizey/St. Mark's FIS, and the FISI are the most published and widely used of all FI scores.

The difficulty with severity measures of FI is that we do not always know if they accurately and reliably capture severity or how well they correlate with each other. Hussain et al. found that both the CCF-FIS and Vaizey/St. Mark's scores demonstrated excellent intra- and interobserver reliability [12]. More recently, a comparative analysis of summary scoring systems found that the CCF-FIS correlated the most closely between the subjective perception of symptom severity reported by patients and the clinical assessment by investigators [13]. Importantly, the CCF-FIS includes two categories that address impact on QoL – "changes in lifestyle" and "wearing a pad." Without resorting to physician-designed weighted scores, these two categories give the investigator a starting point in the measurement of a patients' subjective experience and

Table 4.3 Examples of severity summary scores of fecal incontinence

Name	Author	Year	Spectrum of episodes	Validity tested	Reliability tested
Incontinence score system	Miller et al. [30]	1988	<1/month to >1/week	Yes	No
Anal incontinence score (also known as modified Miller scale)	Rothenberger [31]	1989	<1/month to >1/week	Yes	No
Pescatori grading and scoring of fecal incontinence	Pescatori et al. [32]	1992	<1/week to daily	Yes	No
Cleveland Clinic Florida-fecal incontinence score (CCF-FIS)	Jorge and Wexner [7]	1993	<1/month to >2/day	Yes	Yes
Continence scoring system	Lunnis et al. [33]	1994	<1/month to most days	Yes	No
Vaizey/St. Mark's score	Vaizey et al. [5]	1999	<1/month to >1/day	Yes	Yes
Fecal incontinence severity index (FISI)[a]	Rockwood et al. [6]	1999	1–3/month to >2/day	Yes	Yes
Mayo fecal incontinence questionnaire	Reilly et al. [34]	2000	n/a	Yes	No
Fecal incontinence questionnaire intended for phone/mail	Malouf et al. [35]	2000	<1/month to daily	Yes	No
American Medical Systems scale	O'Brien et al. [36]	2000	Never to >1/day	Yes	Yes
Outcome tool for surgical management of fecal Incontinence	Hull et al. [37]	2001	<1/month to >1/week	Yes	No
Clinical bowel function scoring system	Bai et al. [38]	2002	Variable	Yes	No
Anal sphincter replacement scoring system[a]	Violi et al. [4]	2002	Never to always	No	No
Fecal incontinence and constipation assessment (FICA) scale	Bharucha et al. [2]	2004	<1/month to ≥2–3/week	Yes	Yes
Revised fecal incontinence scale (RFIS)[a]	Sansoni et al. [39]	2013	Never to always	Yes	Yes
Visual analogue scale for fecal incontinence (VASFI)	Devesa et al. [16]	2013	Perfect continence to total incontinence	Not tested	Not tested
Rapid assessment fecal incontinence score (RAFIS)	De la Portilla et al. [17]	2015	No leaks to several leaks daily + visual analogue scale	Yes	Yes

[a]Weighted scores

how their FI impacts their QoL. Similarly, the Vaizey/St. Mark's score uses the same two categories of questions but also includes the use of constipating medications. The addition of these impact measurements adds an important dimension to the summary scoring system. The exclusive assessment of the impact of FI on the patient's QoL will be discussed in more detail later in the chapter.

All summary scores share similar limitations, the most important one being the difficulty in correlating between investigator and patient perception. For example, scoring systems generally regard type and frequency as major categories in the measurement of FI, whereas, patients' perceptions may in fact view the urgency of bowel movements and the amount of incontinence as equally relevant issues, categories which are not yet routinely reflected in the commonly used scoring systems [14, 15]. The CCF-FIS, which has garnered the widest acceptance, is commended for evaluating both lifestyle alteration and the qualitative aspects of FI. However, the final score is a single number, and a single number does not always describe the true degree of dysfunction that a patient might be experiencing. Ideally, a score that represents both the severity of the condition and its impact on QoL can give the care provider better insight into the patient's experience with FI. Of equal importance, the questionnaire should be quick and simple for patients to complete. Visual analogue scales (VAS) are reproducible and easy to use. For this reason, Devesa et al. studied whether VAS could substitute validated summary scores [16]. Their study concluded that visual analogue scales alone cannot replace summary scores, such as the CCF-FIS, nor can they replace QoL scores such as the Fecal Incontinence Quality of Life (FIQL) scale. However, they did show that VAS have a strong correlation with "embarrassment" and "coping/behavior" categories.

The most recently validated summary score in the literature is quite different than previously published scores. It is known as the Rapid Assessment Fecal Incontinence Score (RAFIS) and was developed by a group in Spain [17]. It was first presented as a case–control study. RAFIS jointly measures severity and impact of FI in a simple way – the questionnaire includes a VAS as well as an ordinary scale. However, as with other existing scores, FI severity was only based on the frequency of leaks rather than on the amount. Nevertheless, the use of the RAFIS in a clinical study was found to have excellent intraobserver agreement and internal consistency with a Pearson's correlation of 0.92 and a Cronbach's α of 0.93. In their study, the RAFIS was also found to be a valid and reliable tool to assess FI; however, a test-retest was not able to be performed due to logistical reasons. Lastly, the study showed significant correlation between the RAFIS and every subscale of the FIQL score, except for the category of "depression." Therefore, the RAFIS shows great potential for describing several dimensions of FI; furthermore, the questionnaire is especially attractive due to its simplicity of use.

Thresholds

It can be difficult to know which score to use when assessing patients with FI. It can also be challenging to fully comprehend the effect of FI on QoL. Therefore, when using a validated scoring tool, the treating physician must know at what point FI affects QoL based on a threshold score. Knowing this threshold is important. In 2001, Rothbarth et al. performed a study to calculate the threshold for the CCF-FIS in women who had undergone an anterior sphincter repair for FI from obstetrical trauma [18]. Functional outcome was measured by the CCF-FIS, which was compared to both the GIQLI and the Medical Outcomes Study Short-Form General Health Survey. They found that a CCF-FIS of ≥ 9 was associated with a GIQLI score less than the mean and, therefore, associated with significantly worse QoL. This finding also meant that this threshold could be used for decision-making purposes. Other groups have done similar studies, for example, Brown et al. provided evidence that a CCF-FIS of ≥ 10 was associated with women seeking care due to worse QoL [19]. To summarize, the threshold of a FI scoring tool reflects the discriminatory ability of the scoring tool and, therefore, allows physicians to use the threshold score to predict changes in QoL and to determine which patients will benefit the most from treatment.

Question Recall: Answers

There are two main types of symptom severity scores that can be used for FI – grading scales and summary scores. One important aspect to also consider is whether or not the questionnaire in use has been weighted, and how closely the score reflects a patient's own personal experience. The CCF-FIS, the Vaizey/St. Mark's score, and the FISI are the most published and widely used of all FI severity questionnaires.

A symptom severity score helps medical professionals better quantify a patient's FI symptoms and, overall, allows them to better understand how these symptoms affect QoL. This is where the symptom severity threshold plays an important role. These thresholds give medical professionals an idea of how much a patient is suffering and how aggressively patients should be treated. For example, in the above presented clinical scenario, the CCF-FIS is 10. This score equates to having "moderate FI." However, we also know that with a score of 10, patients likely have an associated decreased QoL and seek care due to this fact.

Summary scores, unlike grading scales, assign specific values to a variety of FI symptoms, as well as to certain lifestyle alterations that patients make to compensate for these symptoms. The goal of summary scores is to capture the global severity of FI, hopefully being able to better discriminate differences between patients and to reliably assess treatment outcomes.

Case Scenario: Part B

This same 73-year-old patient went on to further explain that she is normally quite active and enjoys walking with her husband and playing tennis with her friends. She is also an active member of her church and takes part in many of their social activities. Over the past year, as her symptoms of fecal incontinence have worsened, she stopped playing tennis and only goes out on short walks. Taking part in any of her usual social activities causes her great anxiety due to the unpredictability of her bowel movements. She is unable to travel long distances, as she feels more comfortable being in close proximity to a bathroom. Furthermore, she reveals that she is occasionally incontinent to flatus, and this bothers her most while out in social settings. Overall, her mood is lower than usual, and she finds herself becoming more withdrawn from her friends and family because of her worsening symptoms.

Study Questions

- *How can the impact of FI on QoL be assessed?*
- *What are the different types of QoL scales currently in use to qualify the impact of FI on a patient's overall well-being?*
- *How would you use the FIQL scale in the care of this patient?*

Assessment of the Impact of Fecal Incontinence on Quality of Life

QoL instruments are designed to measure the subjective perception of a patients' health on their emotional state and social life. Measuring QoL can be difficult by using questionnaires alone. The physician must be mindful of who is determining the quality of life of the patient – is it the clinician, the patient, or the target population? A summary of various FI-specific QoL scores is found in Table 4.4.

The most widely cited and validated QoL score used for fecal incontinence is the FIQL scale. This is an example of a condition-specific scale that was developed by the American Society of Colon and Rectal Surgeons (ASCRS) in 2000 [20]. It has been thoroughly studied and found to be a reliable and valid questionnaire. The scale consists of 4 domains, lifestyle, coping/behavior,

Table 4.4 Quality-of-life scores (generic and disease-specific)

Score	Author	Year	Summary score	Validity tested	Reliability tested	Generic, specialized, or condition-specific
Short Form-36 (SF-36)	Ware and Sherbourne [8]	1992	Yes	/	/	Generic
European Organization for Research and Treatment of Cancer (EORTC) and EORTC QLQ-CR38	Aaronson et al. [40]	1993 1999	Yes	Yes	Yes	Generic (EORTC) Condition EORTC QLQ-CR38
Gastrointestinal quality of life (GIQL)	Eypasch et al. [9]	1995	Yes	Yes	Yes	Specialized
Functional assessment of Cancer therapy-colorectal (FACT-C)	Ward et al. [41]	1999	Yes	Yes	Yes	Condition
Fecal incontinence quality of life (FIQL)	Rockwood et al. [20]	2000	Yes	Yes	Yes	Condition
Quality of life scale for fecal incontinence in pediatrics	Bai et al. [38]	2000	Yes	Yes	No	Condition
Manchester Health questionnaire	Bugg et al. [42]	2001	Yes	Yes	Yes	Condition
Pelvic floor impact questionnaire and disease inventory	Barber et al. [43]	2001	Yes	Yes	No	Specialized
Hirschsprung's disease and anorectal malformations quality of life (HAQL)	Hanneman et al. [22]	2001	Yes	Yes	Yes	Condition
Direct questioning of objectives (DQO) scale	Byrne et al. [21]	2002	Yes	No	No	Condition
TyPE specification	Wexner et al. [44]	2002	No	Yes	No	Condition
Modified Manchester health questionnaire for phone interview	Kwon et al. [45]	2005	No	Yes	No	Condition
Simple QoL fecal incontinence questionnaire	Kyrsa et al. [46]	2009	No	Yes	No	Condition
Low anterior resection syndrome (LARS) score	Emmertsen and Laurberg [47]	2012	Yes	Yes	Yes	Condition-specific

depression/self-perception, and embarrassment and a total of 29 items. Incontinent patients have significantly worse FIQL scores than continent patients. The FIQL correlates well with both the SF-36 QoL score and the Wexner/CCF score [20]. Condition-specific scores, like the FIQL, are important because they are developed around a specific condition rather than a specific population. Other gastrointestinal-specific scales include the International Consultation on Incontinence Modular Questionnaire-Bowels (ICIQ-B), the MSKCC Bowel Function Instrument, the Modified Manchester Health Questionnaire (MMHQ), Gastrointestinal Quality of Life (GIQL) [9], the LARS score, and the Direct Questioning of Objectives (DQO) scale [21].

Generic QoL scores are designed for use in broad populations but have been used to also measure the impact of FI. As mentioned previously, one of the most common generic scores utilized as part of the assessment of patients with FI is the SF-36. Other examples can be found in Table 4.4. The advantage of these generic scores is that they allow for the comparison of FI between different populations. However, similar to assessing severity with grading scores, generic QoL scores often lack the ability to detect subtle changes within a specific population.

There is a limitation with using QoL questionnaires among populations with different and complex colorectal and pelvic dysfunction, especially when comparing populations of different economic backgrounds and cultures. One must be thoughtful when choosing a questionnaire to ensure it is appropriate for the patient or population being assessed. There are indeed specialized subgroups that have their own FI questionnaires, for example, the Hirschsprung's Disease and Anorectal Malformations QoL scale [22]. It is also important to note that FI can develop as a result of colorectal and pelvic surgery. It is a significant characteristic of low anterior resection syndrome (LARS) after rectal surgery and of bowel dysfunction after proctectomy and pouch formation. Therefore, not all condition-specific QoL questionnaires are equal in the qualitative assessment of FI.

Question Recall: Answers

The impact of FI on QoL can be assessed by a variety of well-validated questionnaires and scoring tools. However, again, the scores can be weighted or non-weighted, meaning that one must be mindful of who is actually determining the QoL of the patient.

There are different types of scoring systems used for assessing QoL in the context of FI. They are generic, specific, or condition-specific QoL questionnaires, and the most cited and validated score for FI is the FIQL scale. The FIQL scale is condition-specific, meaning that it has been specifically developed for FI. It assesses the patients' lifestyle changes, coping behaviors, extent of depression/self-perception, and level of embarrassment, thereby summarizing the total effect of their FI on QoL. The FIQL would be an ideal questionnaire for the patient in the presented clinical scenario.

Summary

The quantitative and qualitative assessment of FI can be very useful for evaluating treatment outcomes, but, as explained in this chapter, this can also be quite challenging. FI severity can be measured with a variety of grading and summary scores. These scores are often in the form of questionnaires and are usually easy for patients to use. Most importantly, these scores allow physicians, healthcare professionals, and patients to communicate the symptoms of FI in a simple and standardized fashion. This is extremely beneficial as FI is often underreported, and due to the sensitive nature of having incontinence, it can also be difficult for patients to quantify and qualify their symptoms without specific prompting. Patient FI diaries, however, are still useful in the office setting and allow the physician to obtain a "gestalt" of the severity of the patient's symptoms. Most of the severity scores presented in this chapter are well cited in the literature, and their validity and reliability as questionnaires have been well documented. The impact of FI on QoL is also a subject of much interest and importance. FI can truly be a life-altering disease, and its impact on a patient's life should always be assessed. A list of generic and condition-specific QoL scores is also summarized in this chapter.

The most widely cited and utilized symptom scoring tools for FI share important similarities. First, the symptoms are patient-reported and are clinically relevant. Second, the tool is physician validated, ideally using multiple methods of validation. Third, the results of these symptom scoring tools are reliable at capturing the severity of patient symptoms, ideally being able to detect small but clinically relevant differences. Fourth, a clinically validated and robust threshold can be calculated for each of these summary scores, helping guide care and treatment options. Lastly, these symptom scoring tools are practical and easy to use for both patients and physicians, and the results are relatively easy to interpret. The establishment of an ideal measurement tool for FI, that can calculate both symptom severity and QoL, would allow healthcare providers to easily communicate and better direct the treatment of FI.

Commentary

Ann C. Lowry

A scoring system for fecal incontinence (FI) that incorporates all the relevant factors is simple to complete and interpret which would benefit both clinicians and researchers. An instrument resulting in a single score reflecting both severity and quality of life would be ideal. Unfortunately, the perfect system does not exist. In their excellent chapter, Pang and colleagues provide a thorough summary of available instruments and address the important issue of measurement of severity and quality of life related to the disease. They point out that simplification to a visual analogue scale (VAS) scoring system was not adequate. Further complicating the effort, the surgical, gastroenterology, and gynecology literature all vary in their focus.

Like many functional disorders, it is well established that no objective measure accurately reflects the severity of fecal incontinence. Therefore, severity must be measured through recording of relevant symptoms. As the authors point out, most severity scoring systems include frequency and type of incontinence. It is unclear whether frequency alone is sufficient or if it needs to be addressed in the context of the patient's bowel habits. Are two episodes of incontinence per week equivalent in patients who have three bowel movements a week and ones who have ten bowel movements a week? Rarely are the amount of incontinence, urgency, awareness, unpredictability, discomfort, and wiping issues included; all of these symptoms have been cited as important issues for patients [48]. Two scoring systems (FISI. and St. Mark) include urgency, and FISI. includes volume of stool loss. Studies show that unpredictability is very distressing to patients but is not included in any of the instruments. While amount seems intuitively to be important, one study showed that it was not a significant factor in distress related to FI in multivariate analysis [49]. Further post hoc analysis revealed that the lack of significance was related to very high correlation with other significant items. Thus, whether quantity of leakage is an important factor is unclear.

Some commonly included items may not reflect severity. An example is the use of pads. Patients may wear pads for the urinary incontinence, and successfully treated patients may wear pads from lack of confidence in their symptom resolution.

Another unresolved issue is whether to use weighting of items to establish a final score. As discussed in the chapter, patients and physicians weigh frequency and type differently. For example, patients rate leakage of liquid stool as more severe, while physicians label leakage of solid stool as more severe [50]. Patients tend to rate items on the impact on the quality of their life, while physicians are more likely to consider the relationship of a symptom to either the degree of anal sphincter weakness or to the difficulty of correcting it.

The collection of data for severity scoring may be through daily diaries, weekly questionnaires, or longer interval recall questionnaires. Many investigators believe that daily diaries are necessary to obtain accurate data, but Noelting and colleagues [51] found a strong correlation between daily diaries and weekly questionnaires. The concern about longer intervals such as the 1-year recall for FISS is that it may not reflect current status or be as responsive to changes related to treatment.

The work on thresholds and minimal important differences (MIDs) is critical to research and approval of new therapies particularly high cost ones. It is possible to have statistically significant outcomes that have little meaning in terms of the patient's quality of life. In addition, it is important to the design of research studies on FI. These thresholds or MIDs are available for only a few scales.

The wish for the simplicity of a single score drives the combination of severity and quality-of-life items. While correlated, those concepts are independent. Clinicians are aware that incontinence of flatus may be very distressing to one patient but barely noticeable to another. Therefore, the severity items and quality-of-life items need to be scored separately. An option is an instrument such as the Modified Manchester Health Questionnaire which includes both types of items but only scores the quality-of-life items. Presumably the severity items could also be scored if they were validated. At present, it is uncertain if the length of the instrument reduces willingness to complete. The literature supports that condition-specific quality-of-life surveys are more responsive than general or specialized scale. Several studies correlated various severity scales with condition-specific quality-of-life scales. As noted in the chapter, the Cleveland Clinic Florida-Fecal Incontinence Score (CCF-FIS) has had the highest correlation. However, the significance of that is uncertain since the CCF-FIS includes a quality-of-life question.

Data collection is also an issue with quality-of-life instruments. Mail surveys are troubled by lack of response. Kwon and colleagues [52] studied telephone administration and found good correlation although the severity items were scored lower on the written form. Rockwood's commentary on the article highlights some remaining challenges, however, in survey development and choice of mode of administration.

Clearly, there is still more work to be done to develop the ideal method of evaluating FI severity and the impact on quality of life. Collaboration of the various medical and surgical specialties with interest in pelvic floor disorders, patients, and psychometricians is the most likely to succeed in the development of "ideal" tools for the quantitative and qualitative analysis of FI. The authors' effort to elucidate the issues is a helpful start to that effort.

References

1. Bedard K, Heymen S, Palsson OS, Bharucha AE, Whitehead WE. Relationship between symptoms and quality of life in fecal incontinence. Neurogastroenterol Motil. 2018;30(3):e13241.
2. Bharucha AE, Locke GR 3rd, Seide BM, Zinsmeister AR. A new questionnaire for constipation and faecal incontinence. Aliment Pharmacol Ther. 2004;20(3):355–64.
3. Van Koughnett JA, Boutros M, Wexner SD. Signs and symptoms in coloproctology: data collection and scores. In: Colon, rectum and anus: anatomic, physiologic and diagnostic bases for disease management, coloproctology 1. Cham: Springer International Publishing; 2017.
4. Violi V, Boselli AS, De Bernardinis M, et al. A patient-rated, surgeon-corrected scale for functional assessment after total anorectal reconstruction. An adaptation of the Working Party on Anal Sphincter Replacement scoring system. Int J Colorectal Dis. 2002;17(5):327–37.
5. Vaizey CJ, Carapeti E, Cahill JA, Kamm MA. Prospective comparison of faecal incontinence grading systems. Gut. 1999;44(1):77–80.
6. Rockwood TH, Church JM, Fleshman JW, et al. Patient and surgeon ranking of the severity of symptoms associated with fecal incontinence: the fecal incontinence severity index. Dis Colon Rectum. 1999;42(12):1525–32.
7. Jorge JM, Wexner SD. Etiology and management of fecal incontinence. Dis Colon Rectum. 1993;36(1):77–97.
8. Ware JE Jr, Sherbourne CD. The MOS 36-item short-form health survey (SF-36). I. Conceptual framework and item selection. Med Care. 1992;30(6):473–83.
9. Eypasch E, Williams JI, Wood-Dauphinee S, et al. Gastrointestinal Quality of Life Index: development, validation and application of a new instrument. Br J Surg. 1995;82(2):216–22.
10. Browning GG, Parks AG. Postanal repair for neuropathic faecal incontinence: correlation of clinical result and anal canal pressures. Br J Surg. 1983;70(2):101–4.

11. Rudd WW. The transanal anastomosis: a sphincter-saving operation with improved continence. Dis Colon Rectum. 1979;22(2):102–5.
12. Hussain ZI, Lim M, Stojkovic S. The test-retest reliability of fecal incontinence severity and quality-of-life assessment tools. Dis Colon Rectum. 2014;57(5):638–44.
13. Seong MK, Jung SI, Kim TW, Joh HK. Comparative analysis of summary scoring systems in measuring fecal incontinence. J Korean Surg Soc. 2011;81(5):326–31.
14. Bharucha AE, Dunivan G, Goode PS, et al. Epidemiology, pathophysiology, and classification of fecal incontinence: state of the science summary for the National Institute of Diabetes and Digestive and Kidney Diseases (NIDDK) workshop. Am J Gastroenterol. 2015;110(1):127–36.
15. Cotterill N, Norton C, Avery KN, Abrams P, Donovan JL. A patient-centered approach to developing a comprehensive symptom and quality of life assessment of anal incontinence. Dis Colon Rectum. 2008;51(1):82–7.
16. Devesa JM, Vicente R, Abraira V. Visual analogue scales for grading faecal incontinence and quality of life: their relationship with the Jorge-Wexner score and Rockwood scale. Tech Coloproctol. 2013;17(1):67–71.
17. de la Portilla F, Calero-Lillo A, Jimenez-Rodriguez RM, et al. Validation of a new scoring system: rapid assessment faecal incontinence score. World J Gastrointest Surg. 2015;7(9):203–7.
18. Rothbarth J, Bemelman WA, Meijerink WJ, et al. What is the impact of fecal incontinence on quality of life? Dis Colon Rectum. 2001;44(1):67–71.
19. Brown HW, Wexner SD, Lukacz ES. Factors associated with care seeking among women with accidental bowel leakage. Female Pelvic Med Reconstr Surg. 2013;19(2):66–70.
20. Rockwood TH, Church JM, Fleshman JW, et al. Fecal Incontinence Quality of Life Scale: quality of life instrument for patients with fecal incontinence. Dis Colon Rectum. 2000;43(1):9–16; discussion 16–17.
21. Byrne CM, Pager CK, Rex J, Roberts R, Solomon MJ. Assessment of quality of life in the treatment of patients with neuropathic fecal incontinence. Dis Colon Rectum. 2002;45(11):1431–6.
22. Hanneman MJ, Sprangers MA, De Mik EL, et al. Quality of life in patients with anorectal malformation or Hirschsprung's disease: development of a disease-specific questionnaire. Dis Colon Rectum. 2001;44(11):1650–60.
23. Keighley MR, Fielding JW. Management of faecal incontinence and results of surgical treatment. Br J Surg. 1983;70(8):463–8.
24. Corman ML. Gracilis muscle transposition for anal incontinence: late results. Br J Surg. 1985;72 Suppl:S21–2.
25. Hiltunen KM, Matikainen M, Auvinen O, Hietanen P. Clinical and manometric evaluation of anal sphincter function in patients with rectal prolapse. Am J Surg. 1986;151(4):489–92.
26. Broden G, Dolk A, Holmstrom B. Recovery of the internal anal sphincter following rectopexy: a possible explanation for continence improvement. Int J Colorectal Dis. 1988;3(1):23–8.
27. Rainey JB, Donaldson DR, Thomson JP. Postanal repair: which patients derive most benefit? J R Coll Surg Edinb. 1990;35(2):101–5.
28. Womack NR, Morrison JF, Williams NS. Prospective study of the effects of postanal repair in neurogenic faecal incontinence. Br J Surg. 1988;75(1):48–52.
29. Williams NS, Patel J, George BD, Hallan RI, Watkins ES. Development of an electrically stimulated neoanal sphincter. Lancet. 1991;338(8776):1166–9.
30. Miller R, Bartolo DC, Locke-Edmunds JC, Mortensen NJ. Prospective study of conservative and operative treatment for faecal incontinence. Br J Surg. 1988;75(2):101–5.
31. Rothenberger DA. Anal incontinence. In: Current surgical therapy. 3rd ed. Philadephia: BC Decker; 1989.
32. Pescatori M, Anastasio G, Bottini C, Mentasti A. New grading and scoring for anal incontinence. Evaluation of 335 patients. Dis Colon Rectum. 1992;35(5):482–7.
33. Lunniss PJ, Kamm MA, Phillips RK. Factors affecting continence after surgery for anal fistula. Br J Surg. 1994;81(9):1382–5.
34. Reilly WT, Talley NJ, Pemberton JH, Zinsmeister AR. Validation of a questionnaire to assess fecal incontinence and associated risk factors: Fecal Incontinence Questionnaire. Dis Colon Rectum. 2000;43(2):146–53; discussion 153–144.
35. Malouf AJ, Norton CS, Engel AF, Nicholls RJ, Kamm MA. Long-term results of overlapping anterior anal-sphincter repair for obstetric trauma. Lancet. 2000;355(9200):260–5.
36. O'Brien PE, Dixon JB, Skinner S, Laurie C, Khera A, Fonda D. A prospective, randomized, controlled clinical trial of placement of the artificial bowel sphincter (Acticon Neosphincter) for the control of fecal incontinence. Dis Colon Rectum. 2004;47(11):1852–60.
37. Hull TL, Floruta C, Piedmonte M. Preliminary results of an outcome tool used for evaluation of surgical treatment for fecal incontinence. Dis Colon Rectum. 2001;44(6):799–805.
38. Bai Y, Chen H, Hao J, Huang Y, Wang W. Long-term outcome and quality of life after the Swenson procedure for Hirschsprung's disease. J Pediatr Surg. 2002;37(4):639–42.
39. Sansoni J, Hawthorne G, Fleming G, Marosszeky N. The revised faecal incontinence scale: a clinical validation of a new, short measure for assessment and outcomes evaluation. Dis Colon Rectum. 2013;56(5):652–9.
40. Aaronson NK, Ahmedzai S, Bergamn B, et al. The European Organization for Research and Treatment of Cancer QLQ-C30: a quality-of-life instrument for use in international clinical trials in oncology. J Natl Cancer Inst. 1993;85(5):365–76.

41. Ward WL, Hahn EA, Mo F, Hernandez L, Tulsky DS, Cella D. Reliability and validity of the Functional Assessment of Cancer Therapy-Colorectal (FACT-C) quality of life instrument. Qual Life Res. 1999;8(3):181–95.
42. Bug GJ, Kiff ES, Hosker G. A new condition-specific health-related quality of life questionnaire for the assessment of women with anal incontinence. BJOG. 2001;108(10):1057–67.
43. Barber MD, Kuchibhatla MN, Pieper CF, Bump RC. Psychometric evaluation of 2 comprehensive condition-specific quality of life instruments for women with pelvic floor disorders. Am J Obstet Gynecol. 2001;185(6):1388–95.
44. Wexner SD, Baeten C, Bailey R, et al. Long-term efficacy of dynamic graciloplasty for fecal incontinence. Dis Colon Rectum. 2002;45(6):809–18.
45. Kwon S, Visco AG, Fitzgerald MP, Ye W, Whitehead WE, Pelvic Floor Disorders Network. Validity and reliability of the Modified Manchester Health Questionnaire in assessing patients with fecal incontinence. Dis Colon Rectum. 2005;48(2):323–31; discussion 331–324.
46. Krysa J, Lyons M, Williams AB. A simple quality of life questionnaire for patients with faecal incontinence. Int J Colorectal Dis. 2009;24(10):1213–7.
47. Emmertsen KJ, Laurberg S. Low anterior resection syndrome score: development and validation of a symptom-based scoring system for bowel dysfunction after low anterior resection for rectal cancer. Ann Surg. 2012;255(5):922–8.
48. Sung VW, Rogers RG, Bann CM, et al. Symptom outcomes important to women with anal incontinence: a conceptual framework. Obstet Gynecol. 2014;123(5):1023–30.
49. Bedard K, Heymen S, Palsson OS, Bharucha AE, Whitehead WE. Relationship between symptoms and quality of life in fecal incontinence. Neurogastroenterol Motil. 2018;30(3).
50. Rockwood TH, Church JM, Fleshman JW, et al. Patient and surgeon ranking of the severity of symptoms associated with fecal incontinence: the fecal incontinence severity index. Dis Colon Rectum. 1999;42(12):1525–32.
51. Noelting J, Zinsmeister AR, Bharucha AE. Validating endpoints for therapeutic trials in fecal incontinence. Neurogastroenterol Motil. 2016;28(8):1148–56. https://doi.org/10.1111/nmo.12809.
52. Kwon S, Visco AG, Fitzgerald MP, Ye W, Whitehead WE, Pelvic floor disorders N. Validity and reliability of the Modified Manchester Health Questionnaire in assessing patients with fecal incontinence. Dis Colon Rectum. 2005;48(2):323–31; discussion 331–324.

5 Imaging in Pelvic Floor Medicine: Roles of Fluoroscopy, Ultrasound, CT, and MRI

Sophia D. Delpe, Casey G. Kowalik, and Roger R. Dmochowski

Background

Many patients presenting with periurethral lesions are asymptomatic and therefore do not seek treatment for these lesions. Rarity, lack of symptoms, and nonspecific clinical presentation often lead to delayed diagnosis. Delay in treatment in symptomatic patients can be upward of 6 years [1].

Urethral diverticula (UD) are rare and reported worldwide at an incidence of 0.02–6% [2, 3]. UD are congenital or acquired protrusion of the urethra through the periurethral fascia, accounting for up to 84% of periurethral masses [4–7]. Acquired cases may be secondary to periurethral infection or trauma [8–10]. It has been documented that up to 40% of women reporting lower urinary tract symptoms with unexplained etiologies have urethral diverticular disease.

Though most urethral diverticula are benign lesions, there is a long-term risk of malignant transformation in up to 9% of cases [11], although experientially, the actual rates are much lower. Given these findings, it is prudent that urethral diverticular disease remains high on the differential diagnosis for timely and successful diagnosis. Surgeons must identify paravaginal lesions on physical exam and confirm their diagnosis with imaging to avoid a missed diagnosis or inappropriate disease management.

While treatment options for urethral diverticula include fulguration of urethral os, endoscopic de-roofing, marsupialization, and transvaginal excision [12], management of urethral carcinoma requires staging and more extensive surgical excision with the potential need for partial urethrectomy or cystourethrectomy with pelvic lymph node dissection.

Case Scenario

Patient KJ is a 56-year-old female who was evaluated for dysuria, recurrent urinary tract infections, and urinary retention. She also endorsed straining, hesitancy, double voiding, nocturia, and intermittent hematuria. She denied urinary incontinence or any other systemic symptoms.

On physical examination, she had normal external genitals with an orthotopic meatus. There was some fullness noted on palpation of ventral urethra with tenderness to palpation. No fluid was expressed from urethral meatus during palpation.

Commentary by Polina Reyblat, Kaiser Permanente, Los Angeles Medical Center, Department of Urology, Los Angeles, CA, USA

S. D. Delpe (✉) · R. R. Dmochowski
Vanderbilt University Medical Center, Department of Urology, Nashville, TN, USA
e-mail: Sophia.d.delpe@vanderbilt.edu

C. G. Kowalik
University of Kansas Health System, Department of Urology, Kansas City, KS, USA

K. C. Kobashi, S. D. Wexner (eds.), *Female Pelvic Medicine*,
https://doi.org/10.1007/978-3-030-54839-1_5

Office cystoscopy was done which demonstrated papillary fronds in the right mid-urethra. No diverticular os was noted.

At this point in the evaluation, imaging should be considered to further evaluate her report of hematuria as well as the office cystoscopy findings. This chapter will explore different imaging modalities available for the evaluation and diagnosis of paravaginal masses.

Imaging Techniques

Voiding Cystourethrogram (VCUG)

Urethral diverticula are not always seen on voiding cystourethrograms (VCUG). If the os of the diverticulum is large enough and adequate pressure is applied to the urethra, the diverticulum can often be opacified with contrast (Fig. 5.1). It is diagnostic in 55–87% of cases. While it reliably provides information on the size of the diverticulum in 72% of cases, often times details about configuration and location of communication with urethra are not provided [13, 14].

Positive pressure urethrography (PPU) can augment VCUG and is done by simultaneous obstruction of the bladder neck and external urethral meatus using a double-balloon catheter [15]. This technique has been shown to have an accuracy of 90% for detection of urethral diverticula [15].

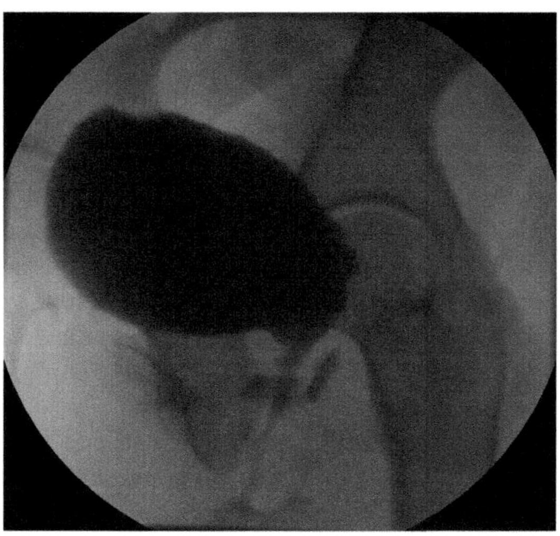

Fig. 5.1 Oblique view of a VCUG demonstrating a "saddlebag" urethral diverticulum. (Courtesy of Matthew Morgan, MD)

VCUG done in conjunction with PPU may provide more information but is often poorly tolerated by patients due to pain and discomfort, and general anesthesia should be considered. Additionally, applying pressure to the urethra in such a fashion can lead to extravasation and fibrosis [16, 17].

Computed Tomography

Traditional computed tomography (CT) is limited in the evaluation of female urethral disease. CT scans can characterize cystic paraurethral lesions and identify tissue thickening and enhancement. Additionally, diverticular calculi are able to be visualized in the dependent portion of the diverticulum. Enhancing solid components may be suggestive of neoplasm (Fig. 5.2). In these instances, CT can be used for preoperative staging [18].

Combining voiding cystourethroscopy with CT scan can provide two-dimensional and three-dimensional reformatting to your evaluation allowing for detailed description of periurethral lesions. Prior to CT exam, the bladder is filled with diluted contrast (50 mL of iodinated contrast diluted with 500 mL of normal saline) via a bladder catheter. The lower urinary tract is scanned during voiding with the patient in prone or supine position. A multidetector CT scanner is used with thin-section spiral scanning to generate 2D and 3D images. This does, however, expose patients to additional ionizing radiation and takes significant post-processing time [19–21].

Magnetic Resonance Imaging (MRI)

Magnetic resonance imaging (MRI) is the most accepted imaging modality for the diagnosis of lower pelvic anatomy such as periurethral masses. It enables more detailed anatomic evaluation compared to CT scan allowing for more

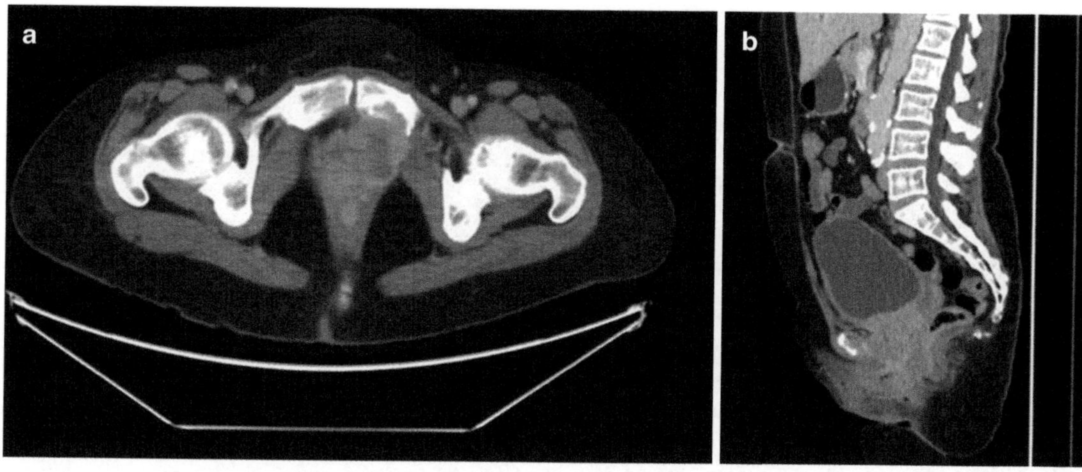

Fig. 5.2 Contrast CT images of urethral carcinoma. (**a**) Axial view of infiltrative enhancing mass measuring 5.8 × 5.7 × 6.6 cm with invasion into the left pubic bone. (**b**) Mass invades the base and posterior wall of the bladder and abutment of the anal canal

detailed classification of urethral lesions including location, number, size, configuration, and communication while sparing the patient ionizing radiation [22, 23]. The specificity, sensitivity, NPV, and PPV have been reported as 83%, 100%, 100%, and 92%, respectively [22, 23].

MRI can be performed with an endoluminal or torso phased array coil. Endoluminal coils include endovaginal, endourethral, or endorectal [24]. This allows for improvement in resolution by decreasing noise-to-signal ratio [25]. The evaluation of urethral or periurethral lesions is performed on a 1.5-T MR imager with a pelvic phased array coil. The protocol recommended for evaluation consists of coronal, axial, and sagittal fat-saturated fast spin-echo T2 sequences. The use of endoluminal MR has the advantage of estimating the complexity of urethral involvement and identifying the diverticular os [26, 27]. T2, fine-section, post-micturition MRI has also led the way with great detail regarding extent and configuration of diverticula. The timing of this imaging maximizes the chance of urine in the diverticulum. Sensitivity and specificity of this technique approaches 100%, with intraobserver concordance of 93% [23, 27, 28].

There is a wide differential diagnosis for cystic periurethral masses diagnosed on MRI including ectopic ureter, urethral carcinoma (Fig. 5.3), urethral diverticulum (Fig. 5.4), Skene's gland cyst (Fig. 5.5), vaginal cyst, leiomyoma, fibroepithelial polyp, endometriosis, urethral caruncle, and urethral mucosal prolapse. While MRI has been proven to be the best imaging modality, interpretation of obtained images requires expertise. Diagnostic errors were published in a 2010 series which included Bartholin cyst, periurethral sterile abscess, and post-collagen injection being

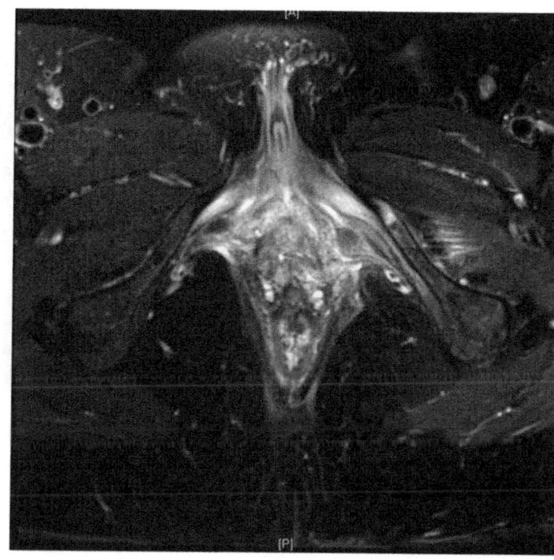

Fig. 5.3 Axial T2-weighted MR image of enhancing periurethral mass with extensive encasement of the urethra suspicious for urethral carcinoma

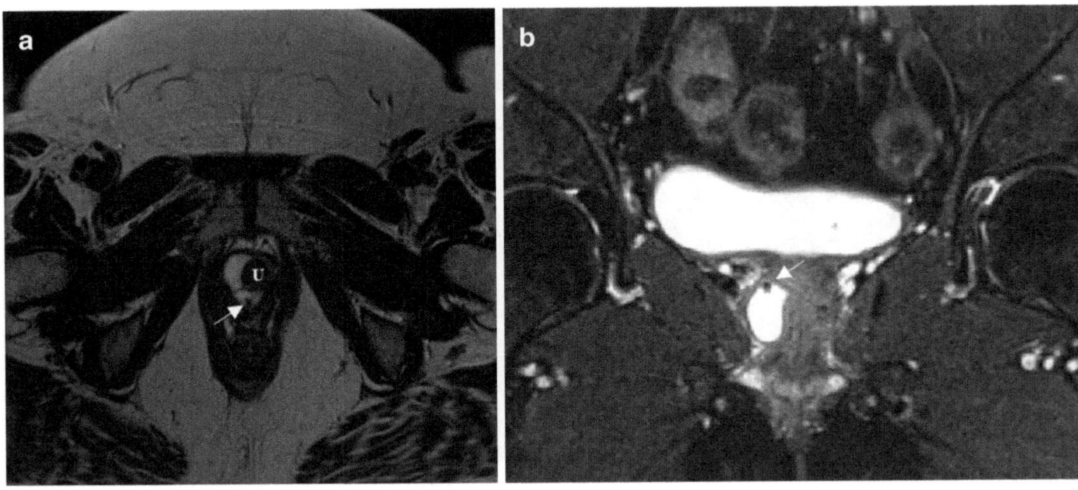

Fig. 5.4 MR images of urethral diverticulum. (**a**) Axial T2-weighted MRI shows homogenously enhancing elongated structure with thin septation along the right aspect of the mid-urethra consistent with urethral diverticulum. (**b**) Sagittal T2-weight MR image. No definitive connection between the diverticulum and urethra was seen on imaging, but was confirmed surgically. Arrow indicates small stone within the diverticulum. U urethra

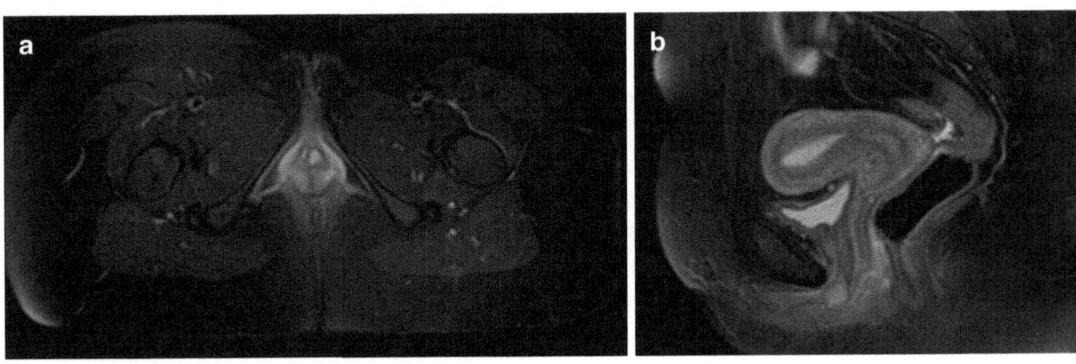

Fig. 5.5 MR images of Skene's gland cyst. (**a**) Axial T2-weighted image with fat saturation showing 1 cm homogenous cystic structure along the left aspect of the urethra with slight deviation of the urethra to the right. (**b**) Axial T2-weighted image with fat saturation showing the same highlighting the location at the urethra meatus consistent with a Skene's gland cyst

misdiagnosed as urethral diverticula on MRI report. Additionally, there was a failure to diagnose an existing diverticulum in 7% of cases and failure to diagnose cancer in 5% of cases [29]. Careful review of all imaging by operating surgeon is imperative for proper surgical planning.

Ultrasound

Various ultrasound techniques have been described for use in Female Pelvic Medicine and Reconstructive Surgery including transperineal, endovaginal, and endoanal in addition to transabdominal and transvaginal. Use of three-dimensional ultrasound allows for reproducible multiplanar reconstruction and visualization of spatial distribution of pelvic floor structures (Fig. 5.6) [30]. In the evaluation of urethral diverticulum, transvaginal US can be done with or without contrast enhancement. The degree of success with this imaging modality approaches 66% [31, 32]. On ultrasonography, diverticula can be imaged as hypoechoic or anechoic lesions

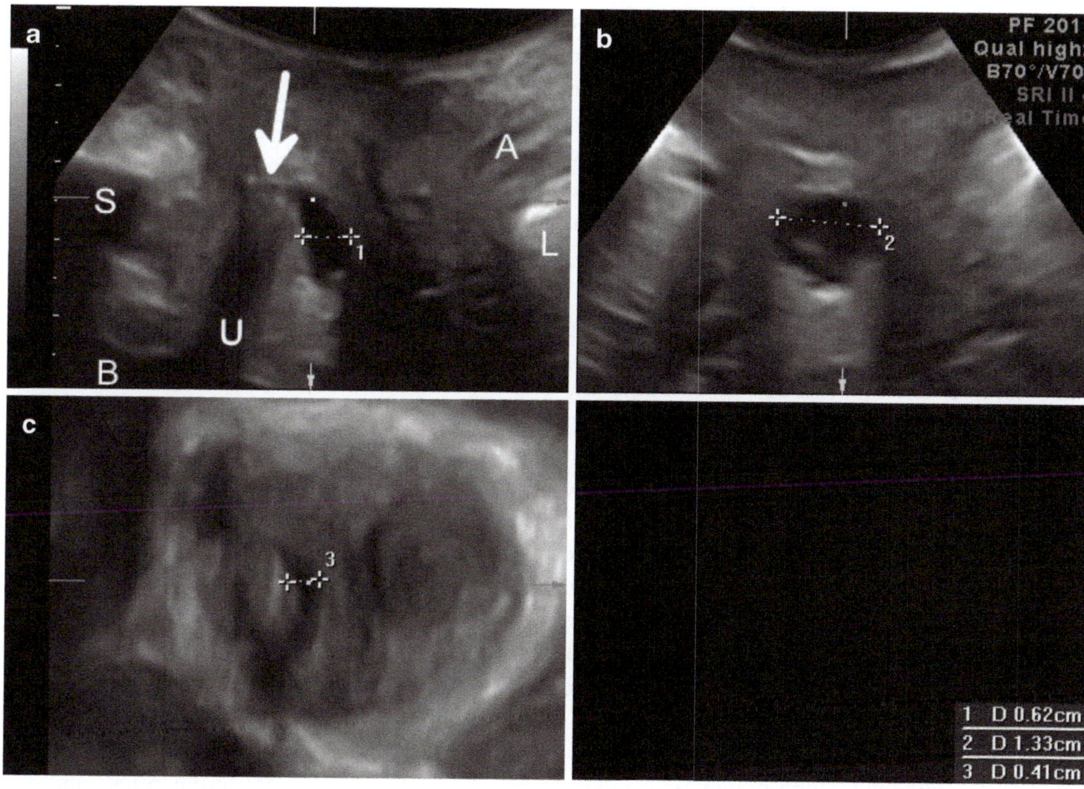

Fig. 5.6 Sectional plane views of a typical posterior urethral diverticulum. (**a**) The midsagittal plane, (**b**) the coronal plane, and (**c**) the axial plane. The diverticulum is the anechoic structure measured with calipers. The arrow indicates the tract which was confirmed by cystoscopy at 6 o'clock, about 1 cm from the external urethral meatus. S symphysis pubis, U urethra, B bladder, A anal canal, L levator ani. (Courtesy of Hans Peter Dietz, MD)

with transmission of signal throughout the diverticulum. Limiting factors to US are that it is heavily operator dependent and it does not give adequate information about soft tissue masses. This imaging modality is not the standard of care; however, it has been reported to have superior efficacy to VCUG in regard to extent and location of periurethral lesions [22].

Videocystometrography or Videourodynamics (VUDS)

This technique combines VCUG with cystometrogram allowing the clinician to have visual diagnostic evidence in addition to information about potential voiding dysfunction. It is diagnostic in 62–95% of patients [13, 31]. Stress urinary incontinence is present in up to 49% of these cases and can be demonstrated on VUDS [13, 33]. Though stress incontinence may not be present on initial presentation, Malde and associates demonstrated that with increasing complexity of lesions (ventral diverticulum vs. saddle diverticulum vs. circumferential diverticulum) increases the incidence of de novo SUI. Rates of de novo SUI ranged from 0% in simple diverticular excisions vs. 20% in complex diverticular excisions [34].

Case Scenario Cont.

As a part of KJ's hematuria workup, an IV contrast CT scan was obtained which demonstrated a periurethral mass demonstrating a possible urethral diverticulum versus a urethral cyst. No lymphadenopathy is noted. A small hepatic lesion was noted and thought to be a hemangioma.

Although formal guidelines do not exist for the evaluation of gross hematuria, microscopic hematuria guidelines can be extrapolated from the American Urological Association (AUA) [35]. Prior to imaging, BUN, creatinine, and eGFR should be obtained. In patients who have normal renal function and no contrast allergies, "Multi-phasic computed tomography (CT) urography (without and with intravenous (IV) contrast), including sufficient phases to evaluate the renal parenchyma to rule out a renal mass and an excretory phase to evaluate the urothelium of the upper tracts, is the imaging procedure of choice because it has the highest sensitivity and specificity for imaging the upper tracts." Magnetic resonance urography is an acceptable alternative in patients who have contraindications for CT. In patients with renal insufficiency who cannot undergo IV contrast or gadolinium administration, non-contrast CT or ultrasound can be paired with fluoroscopic retrograde urography.

To better delineate the periurethral anatomy, an MRI was obtained. Upon review with radiology, it was determined that the MRI demonstrated a 5 × 3.3 3.2 cm thick-walled enhancing mass encasing the entire urethra protruding into the base of the bladder abutting the anterior vaginal wall suspicious for malignancy (Fig. 5.7).

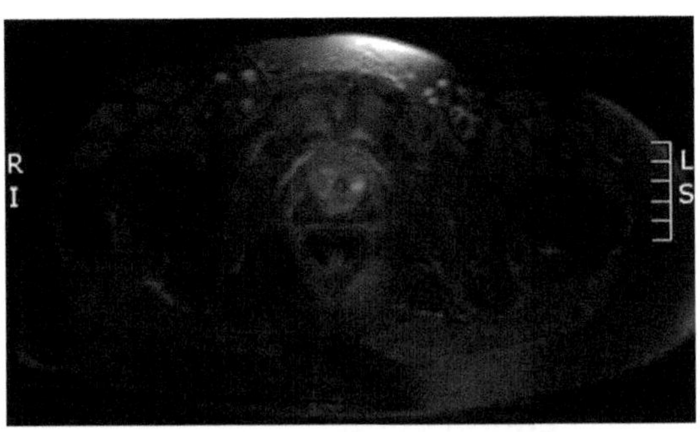

Fig. 5.7 T1 axial MR image of enhancing circumferential periurethral mass suggestive of malignancy

With these findings, she was taken to the operating room where transurethral resection of the frondular mid-urethral lesion was done. Under anesthesia, the lesion was noted to be more proximal.

Pathology returned as high-grade, papillary urothelial carcinoma with glandular differentiation suspicious for lamina propria invasion. She subsequently underwent anterior exenteration, radical cystectomy, urethrectomy, and bilateral pelvic lymph node dissection.

Summary

Female urethral disease and paravaginal masses are rare clinical entities which require a high index of suspicion for diagnosis and prevention of delay in treatment. Diagnosis and treatment are facilitated by imaging to help properly classify lesions and determine operative management. While MRI is the standard imaging modality, other imaging options that include VCUG, CT scan, videourodynamics, and US have been used. Each of these imaging modalities offers unique perspectives on periurethral/paravaginal lesions. A skilled clinician is needed in order to accurately interpret the images. Review of imaging by the surgeon is also imperative to ensure concordance with the radiologist's findings prior to surgical intervention. Though not a radiographic measure, cystourethroscopy should be considered in all patients with periurethral or paravaginal lesions for a complete evaluation. 15–70% of diverticular os can be visualized with cystoscopy [27, 32]. Associated inflammation and small size of the os may make it difficult to visualize. Endoscopic examination may be enhanced by manual compression of the anterior vagina to express fluid or pus, making identification of the os easier (Table 5.1).

Table 5.1 Summary of imaging options

Imaging modality	Pros	Cons	Findings
Micturition cystourethrography Double-balloon urethrography	In-office procedure Relative ease	Decreased sensitivity Ionizing radiation One-dimensional difficult visualization of complex diverticula Double-balloon urethrography painful and technically difficult	Visualization of contrast-filled lumen
Computed tomography +/− cystourethrography	Identification of diverticular stones Staging imaging for urethral/diverticular cancer + cystourethrography 2D and 3D reformatting	Low of sensitivity for small lesions Ionizing radiation + cystourethrography additional time needed for post-processing	Fluid-filled lesion Enhancement of lesion Urethral stones
MRI Endoluminal coil Torso phased array coil	Great visualization of soft tissue lesions and small periurethral diverticula Good visualization of non-communicating diverticula	Costly Requires skilled clinicians for interpretation Endoluminal coil not readily available	Visualization of cystic fluid-filled lesions Enhancement Visualization of anatomy of complex periurethral lesions
US	Noninvasive Inexpensive Access and availability No ionizing radiation	Nonspecific findings, low sensitivity	Visualization of fluid-filled lesion
Videourodynamics +/− cystourethrography	Office procedure Identification of pre-existing voiding dysfunction	No prediction of postoperative voiding function	No potential for diagnosis or evaluation of urethral diverticulum without cystourethrography

Commentary

Polina Reyblat

This is a detailed review of the imaging modalities available for evaluation of the periurethral lesions. The authors highlight a wide differential diagnosis for periurethral masses and dissect the details of the available imaging modalities. A predominant majority of the entities on the differential are of the benign nature, yet the rare cases of malignancy are not to be underestimated. Due to rarity of these conditions, little is known about the natural course of the periurethral lesions in general and urethral diverticula in particular. Most frequently, the workup is initiated upon a physical exam finding or triggered by vague lower urinary tract symptoms refractory to symptom-specific treatment. Given the rarity of these lesions and variable presentation of each entity on the differential, it is critical that we highlight these in clinical training and expose our trainees to a multitude of clinical exams to build their competence and confidence in ability to differentiate between a normal and abnormal on a given physical exam.

As we review and compare specific imaging options available, it becomes clear that only three-dimensional studies allow evaluation not only of the lesion in question but the organs and tissues around it and therefore aid in identification of a lesion suspicious for malignancy. Evaluations based on plain radiography, while less costly and easier to obtain, are limited by biplanar representation of the lesion and depend on the contrast reaching into the lesion. These studies often can be inconclusive and lead to additional studies (CT or MRI). Double-balloon urethrography, while showing good correlation to MRI [36], will miss lesions other than a diverticulum, i.e., cysts, bulking agent, and possible malignancy. The study is painful for the patient to undergo and challenging and time-consuming for the practitioner to perform and exposes patients and providers to additional ionizing radiation. While, academically, it is an interesting study, it should probably be reserved for rare instances where other modalities are not available or not feasible to obtain.

Given the rarity of these conditions, most published series are small and single institutional. Dr. Anne Cameron analyzed data from 25 studies and performed meta-analysis of over 800 patients [37]. The outcomes of this and most other papers focus on the surgical outcomes. Success is defined predominantly by the resolution of the lesions on the imaging [38]. Resolution of symptoms following surgical intervention is less clear. The information on malignancy within the diverticula is even more limited and seen predominantly as case reports. We also lack data on the natural history of the urethral diverticula that are not being surgically removed. This could only be accomplished by a multi-institutional registry within a research network. Lack of information on the natural course of these lesions limits our ability to effectively counsel patients and provide recommendations for the incidentally found asymptomatic urethral diverticula. In our era of the shared decision-making, how do we guide our patients through the available treatment options? Are the perioperative risks worth it? Is the risk of harboring malignancy high enough to strongly recommend surgery? If the surveillance is selected, what would be our recommendations for the follow-up and imaging and at what the long-term cost to the patient and our healthcare system?

In summary, periurethral lesions are rare and frequently challenging to diagnose. We need to have a heightened awareness of "wolf in sheep clothes" of a small proportion of these. A variety of imaging modalities are available to characterize these lesions. The imaging, frequently more than one modality, needs to be tailored to the individual history and careful physical exam findings. Careful interpretation of the available data and high index of suspicion will lead the clinician to a correct diagnosis and will help guide patients through available treatment options.

References

1. Greenwell TJ, Spilotros M. Urethral diverticula in women. Nat Rev Urol. 2015;12:671–80.
2. Anderson MJ. The incidence of diverticula in female urethra. J Urol. 1967;98:96–8.
3. El-Nasher SA, et al. Incidence of female urethral diverticulum: a population-based analysis and literature review. Int Urogynecol J. 2014;25:73–9.
4. Lee JW, Fynes MM. Female urethral diverticula. Best Pract Res Clin Obstet Gynaecol. 2005;19(6):875–93.
5. Quiroz L, Gutman R. Diagnosis and management of urethral diverticulum in women. UpToDate. 2008;16(3).
6. Antosh DD, Gutman RE. Diagnosis and management of female urethral diverticulum. Female Pelvic Med Reconstr Surg. 2011;17(6):264–71.
7. Leach GE, Bavendam TG. Female urethral diverticula. Urology. 1987;30(5):407–15.
8. Silk MR, Lebowitz JM. Anterior urethral diverticulum. J Urol. 1969;101(1):66–7.
9. Aldridge CW Jr, Beaton JH, Nanzig RP. A review of office urethroscopy and cystometry. Am J Obstet Gynecol. 1978;131(4):432–7.
10. Lapides J. Transurethral treatment of urethral diverticula in women. J Urol. 1979;121(6):736–8.
11. Sachin M, et al. Urethral diverticulectomy with Martius labial fat pad interposition improves symptom resolution and reduces recurrence. BJU Int. 2017;199:158–63.
12. Woodhosue CR. Urethral diverticulum in females. Br J Urol. 1980;52:305–10.
13. Dai Y, et al. Diagnosis of female urethral diverticulum using transvaginal contrast enhanced sonourethrography. Int Urogynecol J. 2013;24:1467–72.
14. Chang YL. Presentation of urethral diverticulum is usually not typical. Urol Int. 2008;80:41–5.
15. Drutz HP. Urethral diverticula. Obstet Gynecol Clin North Am. 1989;16:923–9.
16. Dwarkasing RS, et al. MRI evaluation of urethral diverticula and differential diagnosis in symptomatic women. Am J Roentgenol. 2011;197:676–82.
17. Chancellor MB, et al. Intraoperative endoluminal ultrasound evaluation of urethral diverticula. J Urol. 1995;153:72–5.
18. Prasad SR, Menias CO, Narra VR, et al. Cross- sectional imaging of the female urethra: technique and results. Radiographics. 2005;25:749–61.
19. Chou CP, Huang JS, Wu MT, et al. CT voiding urethrography and virtual urethroscopy: preliminary study with 16-MDCT. AJR Am J Roentgenol. 2005;184:1882–8.
20. Kim SH, Kim SH, Park BK, et al. CT voiding cystourethrography using 16-MDCT for the evaluation of female urethral diverticula: initial experience. AJR Am J Roentgenol. 2005;184:1594–6.
21. Chou CP, Huang JS, Yu CC, Pan HB, Huang FD. Urethral diverticulum: diagnosis with virtual CT urethroscopy. AJR Am J Roentgenol. 2005;184:1889–90.

22. Woodhouse CR, et al. Urethral diverticulum in females. Br J Urol. 1980;52:305–10.
23. Foster RT. The utility of magnetic resonance imaging for diagnosis and surgical planning before transvaginal periurethral diverticulectomy in women. Int Urogynecol J Pelvic Floor Dysfunct. 2007;18:315–9.
24. Macura KJ, Genadry R, Borman TL, Mostwin JL, Lardo AC, Bluemke DA. Evaluation of the female urethra with intraurethral magnetic resonance imaging. J Magn Reson Imaging. 2004;20:153–9.
25. Elsayes KM, Mukundan G, Narra VR, Abou El Abbass HA, Prasad SR, Brown JJ. Endovaginal magnetic resonance imaging of the female urethra. J Comput Assist Tomogr. 2006;30:1–6.
26. Blander DS, Rovner ES, Schnall MD, et al. Endoluminal magnetic resonance imaging in the evaluation of urethral diverticula in women. Urology. 2001;57:660–5.
27. Kim B, Hricak H, Tanagho EA. Diagnosis of urethral diverticula in women: value of MR imaging. AJR Am J Roentgenol. 1993;161:809–15.
28. Chung DE. Urethral diverticula in women: discrepancies between magnetic resonance imaging and surgical findings. J Urol. 2010;183:2265–9.
29. Portnoy O, et al. Correlation between MRI and double-lumen urethrography findings in the diagnosis of female periurethral lesions. Eur J Radiol. 2013;82:2183–8.
30. Santoro GA. Perineal body anatomy seen by three-dimensional endovaginal ultrasound of asymptomatic nulliparae. Colorectal Dis. 2016;18:400–9.
31. Tancer MI, et al. Suburethral diverticulae. Clin Obstet Gynaecol. 1982;25:831–7.
32. Romanzi JL, et al. Urethral diverticula in women: diverse presentations resulting in diagnostic delay and management. J Urol. 2000;164:428–33.
33. Malde S. Preliminary report on the effect of urethral diverticulum magnetic resonance imaging configuration on the incidence of new onset urodynamic stress urinary incontinence following excision. Urol Ann. 2017;9(4):321–3.
34. Ockrim JL, et al. A tertiary experience of urethral diverticulectomy: diagnosis, imaging and surgical outcomes. BJU Int. 2009;103:1550–4.
35. Davis R, Jones SJ, Barocas DA, et al. Diagnosis, evaluation, and follow-up of asymptomatic microhematuria (AMH) in adults: AUA guideline. American Urological Association Education and Research, Inc. 2012:1–30.
36. Portnoy O, Kitrey N, Eshed I, et al. Correlation between MRI and double-balloon urethrography findings in the diagnosis of female periurethral lesions. Eur J Radiol. 2013;82(12):2183–8.
37. Cameron AP. Urethral diverticulum in the female: a meta-analysis of modern series. Minerva Ginecol. 2016;68(2):186–210.
38. Ko KJ, Suh YS, Kim TH, et al. Surgical outcomes of primary and recurrent female urethral diverticula. Urology. 2017;105.

The Importance of a Multidisciplinary Approach to Pelvic Floor Disorders

6

Lauren E. Stewart and Charles R. Rardin

Case Scenario

A 57-year-old P3 female presents with constant pelvic and rectal pain, which becomes excruciating during attempts at bowel movement, regardless of stool consistency. Bowel movements occur two to three times per week and are often hard. She denies anal incontinence.

She also describes overactive bladder (OAB) with urgency and frequency, mild nocturia, and a sense of incomplete bladder emptying. She denies urinary incontinence. She is not currently in a sexual relationship but recalls that dyspareunia has been a limiting factor in the past.

Her medical history is notable for mild relapsing-remitting multiple sclerosis, stable on medical therapy. Her surgical history is notable for an abdominal hysterectomy (for abnormal uterine bleeding) 20 years prior and synthetic pubovaginal sling placed 11 years earlier, which was uneventful and resolved her stress incontinence. She underwent an anterior and posterior vaginal colporrhaphy 4 years ago and notes this event as the onset of her current pelvic pain and dyschezia.

Her physical and neurologic exam is noncontributory; her abdominal exam is benign. Her pelvic organ prolapse quantification (POP-Q) exam is as follows:

$$Aa = -3 \quad Ba = -1 \quad C = -7$$
$$GH = 3 \quad PB = 4 \quad TVL = 9$$
$$Ap = -3 \quad Bp = -3$$

Her postvoid residual by catheterization is 145 cc; no significant resistance to passage of catheter is noted. The anterior and apical compartments of the vagina are nontender; no mesh is visible or palpable, and the periurethral sulci are nontender. As demonstrated in the POP-Q exam, the bladder neck is well supported, but proximal to that, anterior vaginal compartment laxity is seen. She has no tenderness of the posterior vagina, but her levator tone is globally increased, and palpation of the levator complex recreates some aspects of her pain. Her rectal exam demonstrates normal sphincter tone, without evidence of sphincter defects and without tenderness. Recto-vaginal examination suggests peritoneal contents sliding between the vaginal vault and the upper rectum with strain.

Commentary by Jason Kim, Women's Pelvic Health and Continence Center, Stony Brook University Hospital, Department of Urology, Stony Brook, NY, USA

L. E. Stewart
Female Pelvic Medicine and Reconstructive Surgery, Departments of Urology and Obstetrics and Gynecology, NYU Grossman School of Medicine/NYU Langone Health, New York, NY, USA

C. R. Rardin (✉)
Woman and Infants Hospital, Department of Obstetrics and Gynecology, Providence, RI, USA
e-mail: crardin@wihri.org

K. C. Kobashi, S. D. Wexner (eds.), *Female Pelvic Medicine*,
https://doi.org/10.1007/978-3-030-54839-1_6

This case serves to demonstrate the complex interplay of multiple organ systems in patients with pelvic floor disorders. She describes complaints that relate to urology, gynecology, colorectal surgery, and gastroenterology; diagnostic evaluation may well include all these areas, as well as radiology, neurology, and physical therapy, and therapeutic options may extend to include sex therapy and pharmacology. It is exceedingly unlikely that an individual provider can bring to bear expertise in all these domains. As this is the case, many centers have striven to develop coordinate multispecialty pelvic floor disorder centers.

Background

Disorders of the female pelvic floor are extremely common and represent a diverse group of diagnoses known to contribute to impaired quality of life. Epidemiologic studies suggest that roughly 25% of American women suffer from one or more pelvic floor disorders, and population-based estimates predict that the number of women seeking care for these conditions will double by 2050 [1–3]. It is therefore becoming increasingly important that we consider how best to provide effective and value-driven care to these patients.

Traditionally, the female pelvic floor has been described as consisting of three distinct compartments: the anterior compartment containing the bladder and urethra, the vaginal or apical compartment containing the vagina and uterus, and the posterior compartment containing the rectum and anus [4]. Because modern medical specialties are similarly compartmentalized, the workup and management of pelvic floor disorders fall under the purview of several distinct medical specialties including urology, gastroenterology, colorectal surgery, pelvic floor physical therapy, and female pelvic medicine and reconstructive surgery. In fact, there remains no one medical specialty with expertise in the workup and management of all pelvic floor disorders. As such, care for women with pelvic floor disorders has been historically fragmented. Similarly, research into the development, diagnosis, and treatments for pelvic floor disorders has tended to demonstrate a "separate silo" result.

Importantly, most pelvic floor disorders are thought to share common underlying etiologies. While no direct causal relationships have been established, evidence of denervation of the pelvic floor musculature can be found in nearly all patients with pelvic floor dysfunction [5]. Because of this common pathophysiology, it is not surprising that patients frequently have more than one coexisting pelvic floor disorder, and these often involve more than one pelvic compartment [6–10]. For example, one survey of community-dwelling women found that 60% of those with prolapse, overactive bladder, or urinary or fecal incontinence had coexisting defecatory dysfunction [11]. This high frequency of concurrent diagnoses combined with the historically compartmentalized approach to care puts patients at risk of receiving incomplete evaluations and potentially ineffective or inappropriate interventions [8]. These data highlight the importance of restructuring care for patients with pelvic floor disorders.

Over the past two decades, the concept of multidisciplinary care or the collaboration of medical specialists from different fields has been introduced as a way to improve the care provided to women with pelvic floor disorders. While systematic, comparative data from our field is scarce, evidence drawn from other fields suggests that a multidisciplinary care model can improve the accuracy of diagnosis, efficiency of workup, and appropriateness of interventions, as well as several patient-centered outcomes such as quality of life [12]. In fact, the multidisciplinary care model has been so successful in improving oncologic outcomes that regular multidisciplinary "tumor board" meetings are now a national requirement for cancer center accreditation [13]. Accordingly, there has been a strong push to consider implementation of multidisciplinary care models in numerous areas of medicine including in the care of pelvic floor disorders. The case presented at the outset describes a patient with a complex history of multi-compartment pelvic floor dysfunction, and we review the available evidence in support of a multidisciplinary approach to her care.

For women with complex, multifactorial, or otherwise unclear diagnoses such as the above patient, one can easily imagine that a multidisciplinary approach could be beneficial. This patient has multi-compartment pelvic floor dysfunction with chronic constipation, defecatory dysfunction and dyschezia, detrusor overactivity, incomplete bladder emptying possibly related to a prior anti-incontinence procedure, and levator myalgia, among other potential diagnoses. A review of the literature describing the propensity for these disorders to coexist as well as the outcomes of multidisciplinary management further supports the utilization of a multidisciplinary approach.

Association Between Pelvic Organ Prolapse and Defecatory Disorders

While this patient's exam does not suggest a diagnosis of pelvic organ prolapse, she does have a history of surgically corrected posterior vaginal prolapse which is temporally related to the onset of her pelvic/anorectal pain. The available data, which is largely observational, suggests that there is a high degree of overlap between pelvic organ prolapse and defecatory dysfunction with as many as 67% of prolapse patients experiencing defecatory symptoms [6, 9, 14–16]. Jelovsek et al. reported that among women with pelvic organ prolapse, 36% had one or more subtypes of constipation, 19% had fecal incontinence, and 25% had anorectal pain disorders [15]. Similarly, Jackson et al. found that 21% of women with urinary incontinence and/or pelvic organ prolapse also had fecal incontinence [17].

Despite the frequency with which defecatory disorders and pelvic organ prolapse coexist, the data is extremely heterogeneous with respect to the degree to which prolapse and prolapse repair impact defecatory symptoms [18, 19]. For instance, in a retrospective cohort of patients undergoing anterior/apical prolapse repair, all women experienced improvement of bowel symptoms postoperatively, but those who received concomitant posterior repair had a significantly greater improvement [20]. However, a subsequent retrospective cohort of women undergoing sacrocolpopexy with or without posterior repair showed no difference in postoperative defecatory symptoms [21]. Several prospective trials have had similarly conflicting results, and an ancillary analysis of a randomized controlled trial comparing different methods of posterior colporrhaphy suggested that nearly 50% of patients experience persistent defecatory symptoms at 1 year postoperatively [22–24].

Concerns that posterior colporrhaphy can cause de novo defecatory complaints, such as the painful defecation experienced by the case patient, are frequently raised, but a review of the literature shows similarly conflicting results [25]. In one randomized controlled trial comparing three surgical techniques for posterior colporrhaphy, de novo defecatory dysfunction and de novo pain with defecation were uncommon, occurring in 11% and 4% of patients, respectively [26, 27]. In those instances when painful defecation does ensue after posterior colporrhaphy, it is not clear exactly what pathophysiologic mechanism accounts for this change, although, as discussed below, there is mounting evidence that chronic spasm of the levator ani muscles may be the underlying cause [28]. In line with this theory is the fact that historically, the surgical strategy for posterior colporrhaphy involved plication of the levator ani muscles in the midline in order to reduce the posterior vaginal prolapse. Nonetheless, the differential diagnosis for painful defecation includes such diagnoses as anal fissure, hemorrhoids, solitary rectal ulcer, rectal prolapse or intussusception, and inflammatory bowel disease, further necessitating the involvement of a multidisciplinary team in the care of this patient [29].

Overall, it is clear that there is a high degree of overlap between pelvic organ prolapse and functional disorders of defecation; however, the data are not clear on how best to work up and manage patients with these coexisting conditions [19]. The available literature suggests that de novo pelvic pain and painful defecation following posterior colporrhaphy are uncommon but do occur, raising the possibility that this patient's pain is either directly related to her pelvic floor surgery or is the result of a pre-existing structural or functional defecatory disorder which was unmasked or exacerbated by her posterior colporrhaphy. These gaps in our knowledge and understanding of the complexity of pelvic floor function highlight an opportunity for a collaborative, multidisciplinary approach to future research.

Impact of the Levator Ani Complex on Global Pelvic Floor Function

While the differential diagnosis for this patient's complaints is quite broad and certainly warrants a workup to rule out organic etiologies, levator ani dysfunction should be considered as a possible contributor to each of her relatively diverse group of symptoms. Pelvic floor hypertonicity, also frequently referred to as levator spasm, levator myalgia, puborectalis syndrome, or levator ani syndrome, has been implicated in symptoms involving all three compartments of the pelvic floor. In fact, women with levator ani hypertonicity/dysfunction can present with a broad range of symptoms including voiding dysfunction, defecatory dysfunction, sexual dysfunction, and pain [30]. Disorders related to pelvic floor hypertonicity are broadly classified as functional pelvic floor disorders rather than structural disorders as they typically cannot be explained by any identifiable pathology [28, 31]. In line with this classification is data suggesting that workup for pelvic pain reveals no organic etiology in about 85% of cases [28]. The pathophysiology of this disorder is not well understood, but it is thought to involve chronic tension or spasm of the muscles of the pelvic floor [29].

When discussing levator ani dysfunction, it is important to note that nomenclature is not uniform across medical specialties, although all describe the same pathophysiology. For instance, in the gastroenterological and colorectal surgery literature, the disorder is frequently referred to as levator ani syndrome, and the recommended diagnostic criteria include localization of pain to the rectum and tenderness during posterior traction of the puborectalis muscle without reference to tenderness of other muscles in the levator ani complex [32]. In the women's health literature, levator hypertonicity is widely recognized as a common cause of chronic pelvic pain, but there is less consensus regarding a name or diagnostic criteria, although tenderness upon palpation of the levator ani muscles is generally considered the hallmark exam finding. It has been suggested that this disorder be referred to as nonrelaxing pelvic floor dysfunction since this name also describes the pathophysiology of the disorder [30]. In addition to the lack of consensus regarding nomenclature and diagnostic criteria, there is also significant symptom overlap with other functional pelvic floor disorders. These characteristics make systematic research of this disorder difficult.

Regardless of the name chosen to describe this syndrome, it is well known to contribute to chronic pelvic and anorectal pain. The pain typically begins insidiously without a clear inciting event [30, 33]. However, as was seen in the above case, some patients can clearly relate the onset of their pain with a particular provocation; trauma, surgery, and childbirth are the most common inciting events [33]. Chronic pelvic pain is a notoriously difficult condition to treat; however, once organic etiologies have been ruled out and the pain can be related to spasm of the levator ani muscles, several treatment options become available. Close collaboration with behavioral therapists and pelvic floor physical therapists can be extremely useful for these patients as there is a high prevalence of depression and anxiety in patients with chronic pain syndromes, and pelvic floor physical therapy with specialized techniques such as biofeedback has been shown to improve pain [30, 34, 35]. Additionally, for patients who experience inadequate relief with the more conservative measures, levator trigger point injections with local anesthetic, steroids, and/or onabotulinumtoxinA have been shown to reduce muscle tension and decrease pain [36–38].

Although the possibility of voiding dysfunction secondary to the case patient's prior midurethral sling placement should be considered and ruled out, increased levator ani tone has been associated with incomplete bladder emptying, urinary frequency, and urgency [30]. This is thought to be because chronic muscle tension leads to the inability of the levator ani to relax during normal voiding. This tension is transferred to the urethra, as demonstrated on urodynamics where chronic pelvic pain patients are seen to have elevated urethral pressures, making it more difficult for the bladder to overcome urethral resistance in order to empty completely [39, 40]. This pathophysiology has been acknowledged by the International Continence Society who defines dysfunctional voiding as intermittent and/or fluctuating flow due to involuntary, intermittent contractions of the periurethral striated or levator muscles during voiding [41]. Involvement of a trained pelvic floor physical therapist in the care of women with voiding dysfunction due to levator hypertonicity should be considered first line as physical therapists are trained in a number of modalities shown to improve pelvic floor relaxation [42]. In particular, learned pelvic floor relaxation techniques, myofascial release, massage, electrogalvanic therapy, and biofeedback have been shown to be beneficial [34, 43–46].

Defecatory dysfunction is another commonly reported symptom among women with levator ani hypertonicity. Patients typically give a history of chronic constipation or straining with stool. This history typically prompts a gastroenterological workup for organic etiologies of constipation including various metabolic, neurologic, and iatrogenic causes [47]. On the differential for constipation is puborectalis dyssynergia, also called dyssynergic defecation, a condition commonly seen in women with pelvic floor hypertonicity [46]. Outlet constipation occurs when the puborectalis either paradoxically contracts during attempts to expel stool or, due to chronic hypertonicity, a failure of the pelvic floor to relax sufficiently to allow passage of stool. As with other symptoms related to levator ani dysfunction, pelvic floor physical therapy with biofeedback has become a mainstay in the treatment of defecatory dysfunction with studies showing improvement in both symptom severity and quality of life [34, 47–49].

In addition to its impact on nearly all other functions of the pelvic floor, levator ani hypertonicity can also have debilitating effects on female sexual function. Inability to adequately relax the pelvic floor muscles during sexual intercourse results in dyspareunia. As with the other sequelae of pelvic floor hypertonicity, a multidisciplinary approach involving physical and behavioral therapy as well as medical therapy when indicated has been shown to be beneficial in improving sexual function [46]. With respect to medical options, levator ani trigger point injections can be beneficial, and specifically, there is data that onabotulinumtoxinA injections reduce dyspareunia and can improve frequency of sexual activity [36, 50, 51].

Advantages in Pelvic Floor Disorders

While little systematic data has been published comparing formalized multidisciplinary care strategies to the traditional model of care for pelvic floor disorders, the concept of this approach can be traced back more than 20 years [8, 52]. The available data are largely focused on patient satisfaction or on outcomes specific to a particular diagnosis. Focusing on the patient-reported outcomes, one study of 113 patients who sought care at a multidisciplinary pelvic floor center found that 25% of patients ultimately underwent a combined surgical procedure with urogynecology and colorectal surgery and 73% of patients rated their care to be excellent/good [7]. A larger study of patients presenting to a multidisciplinary pelvic floor center found that 85% of patients had more than one concurrent diagnosis and, following treatment, nearly 20% of patients experienced complete resolution of their symptoms. Importantly, more than 80% of patients were satisfied/very satisfied with the care they received [53]. These high rates of patient satisfaction support the argument that a multidisciplinary approach to management of pelvic floor disorders is more patient-centered and can more actively engage patients in their chosen care strategy.

There are also logistical advantages for a patient's experience that may be driving some of the enhanced satisfaction demonstrated. Ease of referrals, reduction in duplicative paperwork, and familiarity with physical space and staff may be some features that patients find advantageous. Coordination of collaborative surgical care is also a benefit; on one series, 25% of patients evaluated at a multidisciplinary pelvic floor center underwent surgery by surgeons from more than one specialty [7, 8].

Finally, there may be academic advantages to a multidisciplinary pelvic floor care center. Clinical, patient-centered collaboration will allow for each specialty's interests and experience to guide and enhance each other's. Much like the parable of the blind men describing the disparate features of the part of the elephant to which they each happen to be nearest, there is a very interesting discussion that occurs when radiology, gastroenterology, colorectal surgery, physical therapy, and urogynecology/urology/gynecology discuss the diagnosis and treatments for posterior compartment vaginal prolapse. This multidisciplinary input is likely to improve understanding, mechanistic modeling, and terminology and to guide more sophisticated research hypothesis development. Meanwhile, the logistical advantages and patient concentration in a multidisciplinary setting can optimize patient education, recruitment, and retention, which is highly beneficial in itself.

Commentary

Jason Kim

In this chapter, the authors present a challenging case of a woman with multiple pelvic floor disorders (PFDs) who continues to experience significant symptoms which may be coexistent and/or resultant from her previous treatment. As suggested by the authors, this patient would benefit from evaluation by multiple specialties including urology, gynecology, gastroenterology, colorectal surgery, pelvic floor physical therapy, and female pelvic medicine and reconstructive surgery. The authors discuss the multiple benefits of a multidisciplinary approach including accuracy of diagnosis, efficiency of workup, appropriateness of interventions, patient quality of life, and patient satisfaction. Multidisciplinary care has been successfully implemented for conditions including cancer, breast care, wound care, and diabetes. PFDs would be an ideal target for multidisciplinary care as patients often suffer complex dysfunction of multiple organ systems.

The ideal setting to care for these patients would be a single center incorporating the multiple specialties listed above. Creating a "home" for PFD patients would increase patient access to multiple specialists. Patients with multiple PFDs often have difficulty navigating their treatment in the traditional compartmentalized "silo" approach. Previous studies have demonstrated that patients' health literacy for PFDs is limited, and our institution has previously shown that patient follow-up rates for OAB (a representative PFD) treatment are poor. Patients often get lost in the shuffle and may be offered incomplete treatment by a single specialist in the traditional model.

Despite the multiple advantages of collaboration, very few of these centers exist nationally. Madjar et al. [54] previously reported that 55.4% of gynecologists and 29.4% of urologists never collaborate in the OR for anti-incontinence or pelvic floor reconstructive procedures. Often there is competition, and turf battles among the different specialties and collaborative care may lead to perceived loss of control for the physician. Physicians must realize that multidisciplinary input is essential for optimal patient care. In Madjar's study cited above, two thirds of gynecologists and one third of urologists who did not collaborate in the OR believed they possessed sufficient expertise all by themselves.

A study of collaboration in clinical practice reported that providers' collaboration across all contexts was hampered by organizational and individual factors, including differences in professional power, knowledge bases, and professional culture [55]. The lack of appropriate collaboration between providers impeded clinical work. Specialists in PFDs represent a diverse field of specialists and are no exceptions to these issues. As healthcare shifts toward value-based medicine and accountable care organizations, collaboration will become more critical, and PFD specialists should be cognizant of the issues impeding collaboration. In the end, patient care and satisfaction should improve with increased collaboration.

References

1. Dieter AA, Wilkins MF, Wu JM. Epidemiological trends and future care needs for pelvic floor disorders. Curr Opin Obstet Gynecol. 2015;27(5):380–4.
2. Nygaard I, et al. Prevalence of symptomatic pelvic floor disorders in US women. JAMA. 2008;300(11):1311–6.
3. Wu JM, et al. Prevalence and trends of symptomatic pelvic floor disorders in U.S. women. Obstet Gynecol. 2014;123(1):141–8.
4. Bump RC, et al. The standardization of terminology of female pelvic organ prolapse and pelvic floor dysfunction. Am J Obstet Gynecol. 1996;175(1):10–7.
5. Swash M, Snooks SJ, Henry MM. Unifying concept of pelvic floor disorders and incontinence. J R Soc Med. 1985;78(11):906–11.
6. Gonzalez-Argente FX, et al. Prevalence and severity of urinary incontinence and pelvic genital prolapse in females with anal incontinence or rectal prolapse. Dis Colon Rectum. 2001;44(7):920–6.
7. Kapoor DS, et al. Management of complex pelvic floor disorders in a multidisciplinary pelvic floor clinic. Colorectal Dis. 2008;10(2):118–23.
8. Nager CW, et al. Management of pelvic floor dysfunction. Lancet. 1997;350(9093):1751.
9. Spence-Jones C, et al. Bowel dysfunction: a pathogenic factor in uterovaginal prolapse and urinary stress incontinence. Br J Obstet Gynaecol. 1994;101(2):147–52.
10. Zeleke BM, et al. Symptomatic pelvic floor disorders in community-dwelling older Australian women. Maturitas. 2016;85:34–41.
11. Whitcomb EL, et al. Prevalence of defecatory dysfunction in women with and without pelvic floor disorders. Female Pelvic Med Reconstr Surg. 2009;15(4):179–87.
12. Denton E, Conron M. Improving outcomes in lung cancer: the value of the multidisciplinary health care team. J Multidiscip Healthc. 2016;9:137–44.
13. Cancer, A.C.o.S.C.o. Cancer program standards: ensuring patient-centered care. 2016. https://www.facs.org/quality-programs/cancer/coc/standards.
14. Ellerkmann RM, et al. Correlation of symptoms with location and severity of pelvic organ prolapse. Am J Obstet Gynecol. 2001;185(6):1332–7; discussion 1337–8.
15. Jelovsek JE, et al. Functional bowel and anorectal disorders in patients with pelvic organ prolapse and incontinence. Am J Obstet Gynecol. 2005;193(6):2105–11.
16. Raza-Khan F, et al. Prevalence of bowel symptoms in women with pelvic floor disorders. Int Urogynecol J. 2010;21(8):933–8.
17. Jackson SL, et al. Fecal incontinence in women with urinary incontinence and pelvic organ prolapse. Obstet Gynecol. 1997;89(3):423–7.
18. Cundiff GW, Fenner D. Evaluation and treatment of women with rectocele: focus on associated defecatory and sexual dysfunction. Obstet Gynecol. 2004;104(6):1403–21.
19. Grimes CL, Lukacz ES. Posterior vaginal compartment prolapse and defecatory dysfunction: are they related? Int Urogynecol J. 2012;23(5):537–51.
20. Edenfield AL, et al. Is postoperative bowel function related to posterior compartment prolapse repair? Female Pelvic Med Reconstr Surg. 2014;20(2):90–4.
21. Arunachalam D, Hale DS, Heit MH. Posterior compartment surgery provides no differential benefit for defecatory symptoms before or after concomitant mesh-augmented apical suspension. Female Pelvic Med Reconstr Surg. 2018;24(2):183–7.
22. Grimes CL, et al. What happens to the posterior compartment and bowel symptoms after sacrocolpopexy? Evaluation of 5-year outcomes from E-CARE. Female Pelvic Med Reconstr Surg. 2014;20(5):261–6.
23. Grimes CL, et al. Measuring the impact of a posterior compartment procedure on symptoms of obstructed defecation and posterior vaginal compartment anatomy. Int Urogynecol J. 2016;27(12):1817–23.
24. Sung VW, et al. Changes in bowel symptoms 1 year after rectocele repair. Am J Obstet Gynecol. 2012;207(5):423.e1–5.
25. Richardson ML, Elliot CS, Sokol ER. Posterior compartment prolapse: a urogynecology perspective. Urol Clin North Am. 2012;39(3):361–9.
26. Gustilo-Ashby AM, et al. Bowel symptoms 1 year after surgery for prolapse: further analysis of a randomized trial of rectocele repair. Am J Obstet Gynecol. 2007;197(1):76.e1–5.
27. Paraiso MF, et al. Rectocele repair: a randomized trial of three surgical techniques including graft augmentation. Am J Obstet Gynecol. 2006;195(6):1762–71.
28. Chiarioni G, Asteria C, Whitehead WE. Chronic proctalgia and chronic pelvic pain syndromes: new etiologic insights and treatment options. World J Gastroenterol. 2011;17(40):4447–55.
29. Wald A, Bharucha A, Rao SSC, et al. In: Drossman DA CE, Talley NJ, et al., editors. Functional anorectal disorders, in Rome III: the functional gastrointestinal disorders. McLean: Degnon Associates; 2006. p. 639–85.
30. Faubion SS, Shuster LT, Bharucha AE. Recognition and management of nonrelaxing pelvic floor dysfunction. Mayo Clin Proc. 2012;87(2):187–93.

31. Clemens JQ. Male and female pelvic pain disorders--is it all in their heads? J Urol. 2008;179(3):813–4.
32. Rao SS, et al. Functional anorectal disorders. Gastroenterology. 2016;150:1430–42.
33. Butrick CW. Pathophysiology of pelvic floor hypertonic disorders. Obstet Gynecol Clin North Am. 2009;36(3):699–705.
34. Chiarioni G, et al. Biofeedback is superior to electrogalvanic stimulation and massage for treatment of levator ani syndrome. Gastroenterology. 2010;138(4):1321–9.
35. Tu FF, As-Sanie S, Steege JF. Musculoskeletal causes of chronic pelvic pain: a systematic review of existing therapies: part II. Obstet Gynecol Surv. 2005;60(7):474–83.
36. Jarvis SK, et al. Pilot study of botulinum toxin type A in the treatment of chronic pelvic pain associated with spasm of the levator ani muscles. Aust N Z J Obstet Gynaecol. 2004;44(1):46–50.
37. Morrissey D, et al. Botulinum toxin a injections into pelvic floor muscles under electromyographic guidance for women with refractory high-tone pelvic floor dysfunction: a 6-month prospective pilot study. Female Pelvic Med Reconstr Surg. 2015;21(5):277–82.
38. Thomson AJ, et al. The use of botulinum toxin type A (BOTOX) as treatment for intractable chronic pelvic pain associated with spasm of the levator ani muscles. BJOG. 2005;112(2):247–9.
39. Aw HC, et al. Overactive pelvic floor muscles (OPFM): improving diagnostic accuracy with clinical examination and functional studies. Transl Androl Urol. 2017;6(Suppl 2):S64–7.
40. Butrick CW, et al. Chronic pelvic pain syndromes: clinical, urodynamic, and urothelial observations. Int Urogynecol J Pelvic Floor Dysfunct. 2009;20(9):1047–53.
41. Abrams P, et al. The standardisation of terminology in lower urinary tract function: report from the standardisation sub-committee of the International Continence Society. Urology. 2003;61(1):37–49.
42. Kuo TL, Ng LG, Chapple CR. Pelvic floor spasm as a cause of voiding dysfunction. Curr Opin Urol. 2015;25(4):311–6.
43. Minardi D, et al. The role of uroflowmetry biofeedback and biofeedback training of the pelvic floor muscles in the treatment of recurrent urinary tract infections in women with dysfunctional voiding: a randomized controlled prospective study. Urology. 2010;75(6):1299–304.
44. Oyama IA, et al. Modified Thiele massage as therapeutic intervention for female patients with interstitial cystitis and high-tone pelvic floor dysfunction. Urology. 2004;64(5):862–5.
45. Schmitt JJ, et al. Prospective outcomes of a pelvic floor rehabilitation program including vaginal electrogalvanic stimulation for urinary, defecatory, and pelvic pain symptoms. Female Pelvic Med Reconstr Surg. 2017;23(2):108–13.
46. Butrick CW. Pelvic floor hypertonic disorders: identification and management. Obstet Gynecol Clin North Am. 2009;36(3):707–22.
47. Lewicky-Gaupp C, et al. Successful physical therapy for constipation related to puborectalis dyssynergia improves symptom severity and quality of life. Dis Colon Rectum. 2008;51(11):1686–91.
48. Heymen S, et al. Randomized, controlled trial shows biofeedback to be superior to alternative treatments for patients with pelvic floor dyssynergia-type constipation. Dis Colon Rectum. 2007;50(4):428–41.
49. Palsson OS, Heymen S, Whitehead WE. Biofeedback treatment for functional anorectal disorders: a comprehensive efficacy review. Appl Psychophysiol Biofeedback. 2004;29(3):153–74.
50. Abbott JA, et al. Botulinum toxin type A for chronic pain and pelvic floor spasm in women: a randomized controlled trial. Obstet Gynecol. 2006;108(4):915–23.
51. Bertolasi L, et al. Botulinum neurotoxin type A injections for vaginismus secondary to vulvar vestibulitis syndrome. Obstet Gynecol. 2009;114(5):1008–16.
52. Wall LL, DeLancey JO. The politics of prolapse: a revisionist approach to disorders of the pelvic floor in women. Perspect Biol Med. 1991;34(4):486–96.
53. Vrijens DM, et al. Patient-reported outcome after treatment of urinary incontinence in a multidisciplinary pelvic care clinic. Int J Urol. 2015;22(11):1051–7.
54. Madjar S, Evans D, Duncan R, Gousse. Collaboration and practice patterns among urologists and gynecologists in the treatment of urinary incontinence and pelvic floor prolapse: A survey of International Continence Society Members. Neurourol Urodynam. 2001;20:3–11.
55. Steihaug S, Johannessen AK, Ådnanes M, Paulsen B, Mannion R. Challenges in achieving collaboration in clinical practice: the case of norwegian health care. Int J Integr Care. 2016;16(3):3.

Part II

Treatment: Urinary Incontinence

Overview of Treatment of Urinary Incontinence

7

David Alan Ginsberg and Christine Jeanne Horton

Overview of Treatment of Urinary Incontinence

Case Scenario

A 45-year-old G2P2 obese woman with type 2 diabetes, hypertension, sleep apnea, and prior hysterectomy presents with urinary incontinence. She states her friend was cured with surgery, and she desires the same. She notes that her primary care provider had given her a medication that "didn't work" to reduce her leakage.

Our job as healthcare providers is to determine incontinence type and severity and then counsel on treatment modalities and expected outcomes. This chapter follows the outline below to consider the management options for the above patient.

Urinary Incontinence Types

The International Urogynecological Association (IUGA) and International Continence Society (ICS) proposed terminology to describe female pelvic floor dysfunction [1]. This terminology includes chronic urinary retention and coital, continuous, and extraurethral urinary incontinence to name a few. For the purposes of this chapter, we will predominantly focus on the most common causes of urinary incontinence, stress and urgency, and their treatments.

Quantifying Incontinence and Treatment Response

Treatment for urinary incontinence can be challenging as the fundamental etiology may be unclear, the diagnosis may be complex, and a definitive cure may not be available. The key to treatment is first to elicit a proper history, perform a detailed physical examination, perform further evaluations as needed, and then formulate a treatment plan or care pathway with the patient. There are a variety of tools (e.g., questionnaires) that have been developed to facilitate subjective patient reporting of not only the quantity of urinary incontinence episodes but also how it affects their quality of life. These tools can be used to help the provider and the patient identify the scope of the problem and monitor

Commentary by John P. Lavelle, Veterans Affairs Palo Alto Health Care System, Department of Surgical Service, Urology Section, Palo Alto, CA, USA

D. A. Ginsberg (✉) · C. J. Horton
Keck School of Medicine USC, Department of Urology, Los Angeles, CA, USA
e-mail: Ginsberg@med.usc.edu

K. C. Kobashi, S. D. Wexner (eds.), *Female Pelvic Medicine*,
https://doi.org/10.1007/978-3-030-54839-1_7

progress with treatment. Additionally, there are objective measures that providers can use in the initial and subsequent evaluations to delineate incontinence type, tailor treatments, and assess efficacy.

While obtaining a history, is it imperative to keep in mind the possible differential diagnoses and exacerbating factors that can lead to or impact urinary incontinence (see Table 7.1) [2–4]. In addition, there can be complicating factors associ-

Table 7.1 Differential diagnosis and exacerbating factors of urinary incontinence

System	Disorder
Neurologic	Multiple sclerosis Parkinson's disease Spinal cord injury Disc disease Cerebral vascular accident Dementia
Endocrinologic/metabolic	Diabetes mellitus Diabetes insipidus
Functional	Limited mobility Polydipsia
Psychiatric	Psychogenic polydipsia Cognitive impairment
Gastrointestinal	Constipation Fecal impaction
Infectious	Urinary tract infection Vaginitis
Congenital	Epispadias Ectopic ureter
Gynecologic	Atrophic vaginitis

Genitourinary	Nephrolithiasis
	Urethral diverticulum
	Fistula
	  Vesicovaginal
	  Ureterovaginal
	  Ureterouterine
	  Vesicouterine
	  Urethral vaginal
	Reduced bladder compliance
	Obstruction
	Overflow incontinence
	Stress urinary incontinence
	Urinary retention
	Impaired contractility
	Ectopic ureter
	Painful bladder syndrome/interstitial cystitis

Pharmacologic/exacerbating agents	Diuretics Caffeine Alcohol Narcotic analgesic Anticholinergic medications Antihistamines Psychotropic medications Alpha-adrenergic blockers Alpha-adrenergic agonists Calcium channel blockers
Neoplasm	Bladder cancer Abdominal bulk contributing to reduced bladder capacity
Others	Lack of pelvic muscle coordination Idiopathic OAB/UUI

ated with incontinence, such as pain, hematuria, recurrent urinary tract infection, history of radiation therapy, radical pelvic surgery, and/or fistula which may trigger additional evaluation such as imaging [5]. As some treatments for incontinence have significant adverse events, mitigating possible exacerbating factors, such as poorly controlled diabetes, may improve symptoms of incontinence and optimize response to therapy.

Most information can be found through patient interview. Below is an outline of a typical history of present illness that should be obtained in a patient interview for a complaint of urinary incontinence.

- For incontinence: onset, duration, frequency, severity, quantity and type of pad or other garment use, level of bother, and prior treatments. In addition, it is important to delineate why incontinence occurs and if it is associated with urgency and stress-related maneuvers, without knowledge/sensation, etc.
- Storage voiding symptoms such as urgency
- Typical daily fluid intake including volume of intake, timing of fluid intake, and exacerbating agents such as caffeine or alcohol
- Emptying: feeling of incomplete emptying, dysuria, slow stream, hesitancy, strain or splint to void
- Frequency of voids during day and time between voids
- Frequency of voids at night and presence of nighttime enuresis
- Patient goals, level of bother, and expectations of treatment [5]

Potential exacerbating factors may include obesity, chronic pulmonary disease such as asthma, constipation, sleep apnea, tobacco use, depression, certain medications, and dementia. Optimization of these factors may greatly reduce patient symptoms [4].

What Is Normal?

Most studies evaluating normal fluid intake, urinary output, and frequency are based upon cohorts of individuals without genitourinary dysfunction who have voluntarily completed a 24-hour diary. The median number of voids in a 24-hour period is 8 with a range of 4–18 and a frequency of voiding every 3–4 hours [6]. Normal intake varies by individual, environment, excursion, and fluids within food. That being said, the typical person requires approximately 24 cc/kg of fluid intake per day which equates to approximately 1.68 L per day for a 154 pound person [7]. Most guidelines will suggest no more than 2 L of fluid per day [3, 4]. This can be a rough guideline when counseling patients on normal daily fluid intake. When evaluating patients with urinary incontinence, it is important to remember that many patients believe they need to consume more fluids, which may actually exacerbate their lower urinary tract symptoms.

Subjective Measures

Validated questionnaires can be used as an adjunct to the history obtained at the time of the initial office evaluation. In addition, these questionnaires can then be used at subsequent visits to assess progression of the problem and/or treatment response. More recently, attention in research has turned from not only quantifying incontinence and/or urinary episodes but also assessing level of patient satisfaction. Table 7.2 includes a list of commonly used questionnaires based on patient response that address urinary incontinence.

Objective Measures

There are a variety of objective tools which can be used to evaluate patients with urinary incontinence (Table 7.3). This includes tools which can be completed by the patient (bladder diary, pad test, 24-hour urine collection) as well as measures done in the office. Office measurements include components of a physical examination (Q-tip test, cough stress test), a variety of urodynamic measurements, and cystoscopic evaluation. These measures may be combined in the

Table 7.2 Questionnaires for subjective reporting

Questionnaire	Defecatory dysfunction	POP	Quantification of voids	Quantification of UI	Level of bother	Quality-of-life measure	Sexual function	Pain
International Consultation on Incontinence Questionnaire – Short Form (ICIQ-SF) [8][a]				x	x			
Urogenital Distress Inventory-6 (UDI-6) and Incontinence Impact Questionnaire-7 (IIQ-7) [9]					x	x		x
Incontinence Quality of Life (I-QOL) Instrument [10]						x	x	
Pelvic Floor Distress Inventory – Short Form 20 [11]	x	x			x			x
Pelvic Floor Impact Questionnaire – Short Form 7 [11]					x	x		
Pelvic Organ Prolapse/Urinary Incontinence Sexual Function Questionnaire (PISQ-12) [12]		x					x	x
Questionnaire for Urinary Incontinence Diagnosis (QUID) [13]				x				
Incontinence Severity Index (ISI) [14]				x				

Abbreviations: *POP* pelvic organ prolapse, *UI* urinary incontinence
[a]Recommended use by the International Continence Society [5]

Table 7.3 Objective quantification and evaluation of urinary incontinence [1, 3, 15, 16]

Evaluation technique	
Postvoid residual	Routine component of office visit; via straight catheterization or bladder ultrasound scan soon after void. Normal values vary
Urinalysis	Routine component of office visit; via clean midstream sample or straight catheterization
Cough stress test	Routine component of office visit; to evaluate for SUI done with the patient coughing with a comfortably full bladder in lithotomy or standing position
Q-tip test	In-office evaluation for urethral hypermobility (defined as greater than 30 degrees from horizontal plane). Alternatives include visualization or palpation
Cystometry	Adjunctive evaluation to assess bladder sensation, capacity, compliance, and stability during filling
Uroflowmetry and pressure-flow studies	Adjunctive evaluation to assess urine flow rate and bladder emptying
Measure of urethral function	Adjunctive evaluation during urodynamic testing that can include urethral pressure profilometry, Valsalva leak point pressure, and abdominal leak point pressure. Utility has been contended
Electromyography	Generally performed during urodynamic testing to assess pelvic muscle coordination of the external urinary sphincter
Video- or fluoroscopic-assisted urodynamic studies	May be used in addition to routine urodynamic studies
Cystourethroscopy	Performed in office or operating room with a rigid or flexible cystoscope to assess the bladder and urethra for evaluation of hematuria, recurrent UTI, and atypical presentations of incontinence
Weighted pad tests: 3 and 24 hours	Completed by patients. Typically used in studies to assess level of urinary loss throughout a specified time period
24-hour urine collection	Completed by patient for assessment of total urine output
Bladder diary: 1, 3, and 7 days	Completed by patient and can include amount and timing of fluid input, pad usage, number of incontinence episodes, activities associated with incontinence, and amount of urine output

evaluation of the incontinent patient. For example, urodynamics are the most invasive and often most helpful tool we use to evaluate patients with urinary incontinence. However, if the study does not reproduce the patient's typical symptoms at home, the study is not helpful; this is where the diary is helpful as it allows the healthcare provider to determine if the symptoms experienced on a daily basis are consistent with what is represented in the urodynamic study.

In addition, a bladder diary can be a useful tool to monitor responses to treatment. According to practice guidelines, the bladder diary includes a voiding frequency-volume chart for a minimum of 24 hours though it is thought that diaries of at least 3-day duration are more useful [3]. Additional information can include fluid intake, pad usage, number of incontinence episodes, and degree of incontinence.

Physical Examination

A general physical examination should be performed with particular focus on the following: mental status and possible functional status limitations, presence of edema, flank examination, and decreased sensory or motor function including sacral nerve root reflexes such as anal wink and bulbocavernosus reflex. For genitourinary examination, external examination should first be done to assess for mass, lesion, and atrophy. Internal vaginal examination can be performed visually with a speculum or digitally if the caliber of the vagina is unable to accommodate a speculum.

Internal vaginal examination includes assessment for lesions, presence of pelvic organ prolapse (POP) including identification of affected compartment(s) and staging of the POP, cough stress test (with POP reduction if necessary), gross evidence of fistula, or urethral diverticulum. If feasible, a bimanual examination should be done to assess for pelvic floor coordination and strength as well as for any identifiable pelvic masses. Lastly, rectal examination can provide valuable information such as presence of fecal impaction, mass, hemorrhoids, fissure, prolapse, or fistula as well as sphincter tone and strength which, if abnormal, could suggest a neurologic issue.

Once an accurate history and physical exam have been obtained, the healthcare provider can more easily identify the pathologic process and form a treatment plan with the patient. Prior to any intervention, patients should be informed of correct use of absorbent products such as pads or vaginal inserts. Additionally, if mobility is an issue, having toileting devices readily accessible can be extremely helpful. When these techniques are used correctly, patients may note an increase in quality-of-life measures while dealing with urinary incontinence [17].

Stress Urinary Incontinence

Definition

Stress urinary incontinence (SUI) is defined as the "involuntary urinary leakage on effort or exertion, or on sneezing and coughing" [5]. SUI can be considered an issue of anatomy with loss of supportive structures of the urethra that contributes to coaptation or an issue of urethral closure at the time of increased abdominal pressure leading to loss of urine. The presenting symptom could include leakage associated with positional change, walking, jumping, coughing, sneezing, laughing, and sexual activity with vaginal penetration. Risk factors fall into two categories resulting in pelvic floor weakness: (1) pelvic floor disruption from an acute event such as vaginal childbirth and (2) sustained elevations of intra-abdominal pressure from chronic stressors such as obesity or chronic constipation. Treatment focuses on strengthening or reinforcing the urethral outlet.

Diagnosis

During office examination, the goal is to visualize patient leakage with stress maneuvers. Ideally, the patient has presented with a comfortably full bladder to perform a cough stress test (CST). CST confirms the urethral inability to coapt with increased abdominal pressure. However, it is also important to assess the level of urethral hypermobility as this may impact the type of treatment intervention. Lastly, it is important to perform a postvoid residual (PVR) as an elevated PVR may also suggest voiding dysfunction which would impact further evaluation and treatment options.

In cases of uncomplicated SUI (meaning a positive CST, evidence of urethral hypermobility, and a normal PVR), one can proceed through treatment modalities without further testing [18]. For more complicated cases, complex multichannel urodynamic testing may be performed to further elucidate bladder filling, compliance, and capacity. During filling cystometrogram, a patient is asked to Valsalva, and if there is direct visualized leakage, that is considered a confirmatory test for SUI [15].

Recently, there has been debate on the utility of the midurethral closure pressure (MUCP) and Valsalva leak point pressure measurements as a test within multichannel urodynamic testing. These measurements can be used to assess for intrinsic sphincter deficiency. Although there is not a formal objective definition of intrinsic sphincter deficiency (ISD), most studies use a leak point pressure of less than 60 cm H2O or a maximal urethral closure pressure less than 20 cm H2O [19–22]. Once diagnosed with SUI, factors such as prior surgery, severity of leakage, and urethral hypermobility may play a role in treatment decision-making.

Treatment

Care pathways are increasingly being utilized and can be modified to fit an office practice. Care pathways delineate the available treatment options and a rough framework for escalating care if needed for the patient condition. One can consider the primary levels of treatment to be the most conservative measures with little to no risk and each successive level, although more efficacious, with more associated risk.

Lifestyle Modification

Lifestyle modification can include dietary modification, monitoring fluid intake, and smoking cessation. If there is not an altered thirst mechanism, then patients may taper fluid intake to thirst (i.e., only drinking when thirsty). Additionally, they may attempt timed voids during the day to avoid having a full bladder, as often patients may only leak when the bladder is approaching capacity [23]. Although these techniques may be more beneficial for treatment of urgency incontinence, there have been studies showing benefit in SUI as well [2].

Bladder Training

Bladder training is generally used for urgency urinary incontinence (see below for further description) but has been helpful in SUI as well. Although there is no published standard, the goal is to increase times between voids. Typical instruction would include voiding prior to the urge to void and then extending time to longer periods with the use of a combination of techniques including distraction, mindfulness, and pelvic floor exercises. Bladder training holds little to no risk and can be used as an adjunct to any additional therapy provided [24].

Pelvic Floor Muscle Exercises (PFME)

Pelvic floor muscle exercises (PFME) include patients individually performing recruitment and relaxation of the pelvic floor with three sets of ten per day, not during urination [4]. Results vary across numerous studies of PFME. However, most patients note an improvement in symptoms and greater satisfaction when pelvic floor muscle exercises are used alone or in conjunction with other therapies [25]. Patients may be instructed with written education information and physical instruction with biofeedback or by a pelvic floor physical therapist. Pelvic floor physical therapy is a specialized form of physical therapy that may include a multimodal approach including use of biofeedback and vaginal cones and further discussion of behavioral modifications. Results for response to physical therapy vary but have been quoted to have a cure rate at 1 year up to 58% [26].

Weight Loss

One of the known risk factors for developing SUI is obesity (odds ratio 4.2) [3]. Several studies have looked at the effects of weight loss on urinary incontinence; many studies were adjuncts to larger population studies. In a 6-month structured weight loss program with approximately 8% weight loss, patients had a 47% decrease in symptoms with that decrease being more prominent for SUI symptoms as compared to urgency urinary incontinence (UUI) symptoms [27]. Given the many benefits to weight loss, if patients have obesity, weight loss counseling should be performed as part of the visit.

Medications

At this time, medical management of stress urinary incontinence is not considered standard therapy in the United States, and there are no FDA-approved medications for use [4]. However, transvaginal topical hormonal therapy has been shown to improve both SUI and UUI symptoms. Interestingly, oral hormonal therapy has been found to worsen incontinence in women [28, 29]. Additionally, duloxetine, a serotonin and norepinephrine reuptake inhibitor, has been studied and is approved for use in Europe. Duloxetine showed promise in decreasing SUI symptoms by 50% compared to the 27% placebo at 12 weeks; however, there was a noted high discontinuation rate [30].

Incontinence Pessary

The incontinence pessary is an object made of inert material, typically silicone, that is inserted vaginally. The theory is that with increased abdominal pressure, the knob is thrust toward the urethra and therefore provides occlusion. It is inserted vaginally, and there is a knob that sits below the urethra. There are also pessaries that combine concomitant prolapse support if necessary. Although not necessarily dry, when given an incontinence pessary, approximately 50% of patients noted improved symptoms, and 75% were satisfied with therapy after 12 months [31]. This is generally a temporizing measure as most patients will progress to additional therapies.

Treatment: Operative Interventions

There are no operative modalities that guarantee that a patient is dry (i.e., without any incontinence after intervention). When treating SUI surgically, potential adverse events include voiding dysfunction such as retention, incomplete voiding, increased or de novo urgency, and urinary tract infection in addition to routine adverse events from a general surgical procedure. This needs to be part of patient counseling and consent prior to proceeding with operative intervention.

Vaginal/Urethral Laser

Recent investigations include effects of laser therapy, most commonly the CO2 laser, on atrophic vaginitis and postmenopausal syndrome [32]. This has spread to research on treatment for SUI but is not approved by FDA for this indication at this time [33].

Urethral Bulking Agents

There have been several bulking agents used in the past. Ideally, the substance is non-allergenic, remains in situ, and is durable. There are presently three FDA-approved, commercially available substances in the United States: pyrolytic carbon-coated beads (Durasphere® EXP), calcium hydroxylapatite (Coaptite™), polydimethylsilaxone (Macroplastique®), and a hydrogel of water and polyacrylamide (Bulkamid®). Placement can be in the clinic or operating room setting. The mechanism of action is to place an inert substance into the midurethral submucosal region to increase coaptation. This may be better suited for those who need a minimally invasive procedure due to multiple comorbidities, have limited urethral mobility, or are less likely to have successful treatment with a midurethral sling procedure [34].

Failure rates are higher than that of other operative interventions with 25–37% of patients noting improvement at 12 months [26]. There are currently no head-to-head trials comparing the efficacy of bulking agents with other currently available modalities such as slings. Patients may require repeat injections to maintain efficacy.

Complications include transient urinary retention, hematuria, de novo urgency incontinence, urinary tract infection, immune reaction, granuloma formation, and rarely periurethral abscess and migration of material [35].

Urethropexy/Bladder Neck Suspensions

Historically, there were several operative interventions used to affix the urethra to surrounding fascia and ligamentous or bone structures. These include the Marshall-Marchetti-Krantz operation, Kelly plication, bladder neck needle suspensions (Pereyra, Raz, and Stamey techniques), and Burch urethropexy. Of the listed procedures, the Burch urethropexy, also known as retropubic suspension, is the most commonly used today; however, its rate of use continues to decline [36].

The Burch urethropexy can be performed open or laparoscopically. The goal is to tent the vagina by creating a suture bridge between the periurethral tissue and Cooper's ligament bilaterally. Success rates vary and range from 57% to 85% at 6 months to 24–70% at 5 years depending on the study [37, 38]. The SISTEr trial found autologous fascial slings (AFS) to be superior to Burch in regard to objective and subjective success rates; however, autologous slings also had a higher rate of complications related to obstruction including prolonged postoperative catheter use, voiding dysfunction, UTI (urinary tract infection), and need for surgical reintervention [39, 40]. Presently, a Burch urethropexy is often used at times of known abdominal surgical intervention during a concomitant case or for patients who do not desire a sling procedure [41].

Mesh Midurethral Sling

This is the most common anti-incontinence procedure performed for SUI with several companies offering either retropubic, transobturator, or single-incision slings [36]. The mesh used in a midurethral sling (MUS) is a type 1 polypropylene macroporous mesh which is known to be associated with fewer infections and exposures as compared to other mesh types [42]. The goal of therapy is to place mesh into a region where it will be integrated to create adequate urethral support and reduce urethral hypermobility. The two major locations that slings are anchored from the midurethra are the retropubic and transobturator spaces.

For retropubic slings, there are two modes of placement: "top-bottom" and "bottom-top." The "bottom-top" route appears to have a higher subjective and objective cure rate with fewer bladder perforations and vaginal tape erosions [43].

For transobturator slings, there are two approaches to placement: "outside-in" and "inside-out." When these approaches were compared, there seemed to be no difference in subjective and objective cure rates. The "inside-out" approach had a higher rate of voiding dysfunction, and the "outside-in" technique had higher rate of vaginal perforation and groin pain. There was no difference of mesh erosion [21, 22].

Success rates vary by timing of reporting and the definition of success. According to a large review assessing cure rates of different incontinence therapies, retropubic slings had an objective cure rate ranging from 53% to 90% at 12 months, and transobturator slings had a range from 76% to 94% [26]. A randomized equivalence trial was performed that compared retropubic versus transobturator slings. At 1 year, there was an approximately 80% composite objective success rate and approximately 90% composite subjective success without a statistically significant difference in method of mesh placement. However, at 5 years, the subjective success rates dropped to 51% for the retropubic and 43% for the transobturator placement that was statistically significantly different [44]. There is little data beyond 5 years, but what has been reported notes approximately a 67% subjective and 76% cure for transobturator slings compared to 70% subjective and 83% objective of those receiving the retropubic approach [45].

A systematic review compared retropubic versus transobturator placement and found a slightly higher rate of success at 1 year with the retropubic group, but these results were not statistically significant [40]. Lastly, when comparing efficacy for patients with intrinsic sphincter deficiency, the retropubic group had fewer requests for retreatment of SUI compared to the transobturator group [22].

Retropubic slings had a higher adverse event rate in regard to bladder perforation, major vascular/visceral injury, mean operating time, blood loss, voiding dysfunction, suprapubic pain, and length of hospital stay. Neurologic symptoms, such as groin pain and leg numbness, and reoperation were higher in the transobturator group. Mesh complications of all midurethral slings, including mesh erosion, vary from <1% to 5% depending on what study is [4, 20, 21].

Risk factors for failure included prior surgery for urinary incontinence, a negative Q-tip test defined as <30 degrees from parallel, older age, higher scoring on patient-answered questionnaires regarding subjective measures (indicating wore symptomatology at baseline), a higher pad weight on pad tests, and concomitant surgery [34]. When compared to pubovaginal slings, midurethral slings have a higher subjective cure rate with fewer side effects; however, there is the incurred risk associated with mesh [40].

The lesser studied and newer generation of mesh slings is the single-incision sling with mesh only placed in the midurethral portion and affixed to the obturator muscles. They do not continue into the retropubic or transobturator space. Success rates vary but have consistently been reported as lower objective cure rates at 1 year as compared to full-length mesh slings. Theoretically, there would be fewer complications including reduced blood loss and pain postoperatively. Some people have opted to have this performed in office and argue there is a substantial cost difference as there is no operating room cost. At this time, there is little longitudinal data to report compared to the traditional mesh midurethral sling [40, 46].

Pubovaginal Slings

Pubovaginal slings can be made of autologous fascia, xenographic materials, cadaveric materials, suture, and mesh. The most typical is autologous fascia harvested from either the fascia lata or rectus fascia [22, 40]. The sling is placed under the bladder neck or midurethra and tunneled through the retropubic space and secured above the rectus fascia. Candidates include those with or without urethral hypermobility and individuals who are not candidates for mesh slings (compromised urethra such as diverticulum, prior mesh complication in region, or concomitant urethral procedure) or who want to avoid the use of vaginally placed mesh [40, 47]. Success rates vary, but a long-term follow-up of a cohort at 5 years noted that greater than 80% of patients were satisfied with their procedure and approximately 30% reported complete continence [37].

Artificial Urinary Sphincters

Artificial urinary sphincters (AUS) are used most commonly for men after radical prostatectomy for prostate cancer. Historically, the AUS has rarely been used in the female patient and is not presently considered a standard therapy for women with stress urinary incontinence; however, this may be considered in rare cases that are refractory to other modalities [22]. The resent use of robotic placement may open the door for the more widespread use of this technique in the future. At the present time, the majority of these procedures are done in specialized centers with experienced surgeons in regards to robotic AUS placement.

Occult Stress Urinary Incontinence

Occult stress urinary incontinence is a "stress urinary incontinence that is observed only after the reduction of coexistent pelvic organ prolapse" [1]. Repair of pelvic organ prolapse, particularly the anterior compartment, is a risk factor for developing SUI [48]. Several studies using randomized controlled trials showed a lower rate of stress urinary incontinence postoperatively for those who receive a concomitant prophylactic anti-incontinence procedure such as Burch urethropexy or midurethral sling [49]. This emphasizes the importance of performing a reduction cough stress test to aid in proper counseling on treatment intervention for patients affected by pelvic organ prolapse.

Urgency Urinary Incontinence

Definition

UUI, according to the International Continence Society, is "the complaint of involuntary leakage accompanied by or immediately preceded by urgency" [5]. Overactive bladder (OAB) is an umbrella term that has symptoms of urgency with or without associated incontinence. Idiopathic detrusor overactivity (DO) is a urodynamic term use to describe detrusor contractions that occur during the filling phase of urodynamic testing defined as "overactivity when there is no clear cause" [5]. It is important to clarify that OAB is a clinical diagnosis based on patient symptoms and detrusor overactivity is a urodynamic term. For the purposes of this chapter, the focus will be UUI and/or idiopathic, non-neurogenic detrusor overactivity.

Diagnosis

UUI may be part of a mixed urinary incontinence picture with patients also reporting SUI symptoms. Additionally, patients may have exacerbation of painful bladder syndrome, also known as interstitial cystitis, and have increased frequency and urgency in an attempt to decrease their bladder discomfort. The typical history of a patient with UUI is an individual who is unable to make it to the bathroom in time and has urinary leakage after having the sensation of urgency. They can have partial or complete loss of the contents of their bladder.

Physical examination is as described above with particular attention to the differential diagnosis. One must evaluate for urinary tract infection as this can cause or contribute to symptoms. The examination process is similar with focus on the neurologic examination that includes assessing patient sensation to assess for neuropathy. Urodynamic testing can be performed in order to assess for detrusor overactivity but is often not required prior to starting therapy for most patients with OAB or UUI. In addition, it is important to note that lack of DO during urodynamics does not negate the diagnosis of UUI or OAB.

Treatment

Treatment for UUI may involve counseling as results for therapy can vary by patient and can be less immediate than what is seen after surgical intervention for SUI. The goal of therapy is to reduce inadvertent bladder contractions for reduction of symptom burden. Care pathways that include a "three-tier approach" (explained below) can be given to and explained to the patient [3, 16, 50]. Care pathways not only describe the treatment modalities but give a time frame for escalating care, if necessary. These care pathways are considered a rough framework as a provider can opt to advance beyond first-line modalities on initial patient encounter in more severe cases [16]. Most therapies will likely reduce incontinence episodes, but a patient may not necessarily be dry. A bladder diary is highly beneficial for evaluation and discussion with the patient [1].

Despite success with a therapy, the effect may wane overtime, a phenomenon that is less likely due to the body adapting to medications and more likely a reflection of disease progression. Therefore, it is important that patients are encouraged to follow up with providers if their previously stable symptoms worsen despite treatment.

Behavioral Therapy 8–12 Weeks (First Line)

Behavioral therapy consists of tapering to thirst (aka fluid management), lifestyle modifications, timed voids, or delayed or double voids as part of bladder training, bladder control strategies, distraction, self-assertion, biofeedback, and pelvic floor muscle training [1–3, 15, 26, 51]. Additionally, if there is bothersome leakage at night, having patients taper fluid intake prior to bedtime may be helpful. If there is evidence of lower extremity edema, patients may benefit from raising their legs 1 hour prior to going to bed in order to redistribute the fluid prior to sleep. There is little to no risk with these therapies, which can supplement other treatment modalities. Success rates vary but range from a 50% to 80% reduction in symptoms. There is no single modality that seems to have a higher rate of success compared to others.

Bladder training, including a scheduled voiding regimen with adjusted intervals to prolong voiding intervals, should increase capacity and reduce incontinence. Patients can combine this with timed voiding. Timed voiding is particularly successful with patients who cannot toilet independently. Weight loss is also considered beneficial with up to a 42% decrease in UUI noted after approximately an 8% weight reduction [27].

There can be overlap between painful bladder syndrome and OAB symptoms; patients may increase voiding episodes and have exacerbation of incontinence in attempts to avoid irritative voiding symptoms [52]. This subset of patients may benefit from dietary modifications to avoid bladder "irritants" such as caffeinated beverages and artificial sweeteners [2]. Although there is no data showing a significant benefit with dietary modification for patient with UUI, there is little harm in using this as an adjunctive therapy.

Medications 4–8 Weeks (Second Line)

There are two major drug classes for treatment of UUI: antimuscarinics and beta-3 agonists.

Antimuscarinic Therapy

Antimuscarinic therapy is administered either orally or topically by transdermal patch or gel. There are six FDA-approved agents that are available for use in the United States. The agents differ in muscarinic receptor selectivity and drug permeability. The mechanism of action is targeted blockade of muscarinic type 2 and 3 receptors to reduce or block involuntary detrusor contractions. There are few longitudinal comparative effectiveness trials and no proof that one drug within the class outperforms another; however, the AUA/SUFU OAB guidelines do recommend use of once-daily, extended-release drugs that are titratable, if available [53]. A list of oral agents, their dosages, and efficacy are in Table 7.4.

Efficacy varies, and clinical success in studies is often defined as a 50% reduction in incontinence episodes over a 12-week duration. In addition, long-term efficacy is an issue.

Table 7.4 Antimuscarinic and beta agonist medications for treatment of OAB Medications versus placebo for UUI

Generic name	Year of FDA approval	Dosages[a]	% reduction in incontinence episodes/day[b]	% with constipation[c]	% with dry mouth[c]
Antimuscarinic therapy					
Oxybutynin oral	IR: 1975	IR: 5 mg		IR: 15	IR: 71
	ER: 1999	ER: 5, 10, 15 mg	ER: 80	10 mg ER: 9	10 mg ER: 35
Oxybutynin transdermal	Patch: 2003	Patch: 3.9 mg/d	Patch: 62	Patch: 3	Patch: 9
	Gel: 2011	Gel: 1 g/d	Gel: 56	Gel: 1	Gel: 8
Tolterodine	IR: 1998	IR: 2 and 4 mg	53		
	ER: 2000	ER: 2 and 4 mg		4 mg ER: 6	4 mg ER: 23
Solifenacin ER	2004	5 mg	54	5 mg: 5	5 mg: 11
		10 mg		10 mg: 13	10 mg: 28
Darifenacin ER	2004	7.5 mg	64	7.5 mg: 15	7.5 mg: 20
		15 mg		15 mg: 21	15 mg: 35
Trospium chloride	IR: 2004	IR: 20 mg	59	9 (60)	11 (60)
	ER: 2007	ER: 60 mg			
Fesoterodine ER	2008	4 mg	62	4 mg: 4	4 mg: 19
		8 mg		8 mg: 6	8 mg: 35
ß-Adrenergic therapy					
Mirabegron ER	2012	25 and 50 mg	54	2.2 (50)	2.8 (50)
Placebo					
	Not applicable	Not applicable	30–47	0–4.8	0–8

Table adapted from Lukacz et al. [4]

Abbreviations: *AE* adverse events, *CNS* central nervous system, *ER* extended-release once-daily dosing, *FDA* Food and Drug Administration, *IR* immediate release

[a]See full package inserts for prescribing data. Data are based on mean results of regulatory studies used for FDA approval and do not represent true between-drug comparisons

[b]Reported efficacy from average reductions from baseline across FDA trials reported in package inserts of maximum-dose, extended-release preparations, except where noted

[c]Common adverse effects for extended-release preparations, except where noted. Discontinuation rates are less than 5% for these adverse effects

Despite studies that show clinical improvement in trials that typically lasted 3 months, high discontinuation rates are seen with only 20–40% of patients remaining on antimuscarinic therapy after 12 months and only 16% at 3 years [54]. If the patient has a poor response, one can consider dose escalation or changing to an alternative agent within or outside the drug class.

Antimuscarinic use is contraindicated for uncontrolled tachyarrhythmia, myasthenia gravis, gastric retention, and narrow-angle glaucoma unless otherwise approved. In addition, anticholinergics should be used with caution in patients with impaired gastric emptying, dementia, and urinary retention or on other anticholinergic agents. Antimuscarinics as a drug class are on the Beers criteria medication list created to list drugs to avoid or adjust dosages in the older adult [55]. Consequently, consensus statements have been released in terms of limiting antimuscarinic use in the elderly patient due to risk of mild cognitive impairment and/or clinical decline [56, 57]. Although not well studied, drugs such as darifenacin and trospium (see Table 7.4) would theoretically be less likely to have central nervous system symptoms due to their molecular structure [55].

Common side effects include constipation, dry mouth, drowsiness, tachycardia, and blurred vision for near objects. If patients are gaining a response but have bothersome side effects, focus should turn to reducing side effect burden with strategies such as placing patients on a bowel regimen to lessen constipation. Consensus statements encourage the use of the lowest possible dose to achieve effectiveness and, if available, use of the extended-release dose to mitigate side effects [3, 4, 16]. From a practical standpoint, cost should also be considered when formulating a treatment plan and may dictate the choice of medication.

Beta-Agonist

Mirabegron is currently the only FDA-approved beta-agonist for treatment of OAB (see Table 7.4 for mode and dosing). The medication targets the beta-3 receptor to downregulate detrusor contractions. Success rates are considered similar to antimuscarinic therapy without the noted common side effects of constipation and dry mouth. There are currently no head-to-head trials comparing the efficacy of mirabegron with antimuscarinic agents. There does seem to be a higher rate of continuing with therapy compared to antimuscarinic therapy; however, long-term persistence is not optimal with this drug either [58].

Contraindications are poorly controlled severe hypertension, end-stage renal disease, and severe liver impairment. Common side effects are tachycardia, headache, and diarrhea, the rates of which were similar to those noted with placebo.

Studies show promise for combined therapy with mirabegron and antimuscarinic therapy with greater symptom reduction compared to monotherapy of either modality alone. With this modality, there is a higher risk of urinary retention [59, 60].

Third-Line Therapy

According to most care pathways, third-line therapies are procedures that can be performed for UUI if oral therapy fails. This includes either direct injections of onabotulinumtoxinA into the detrusor muscle or two forms of neuromodulation as described below.

Percutaneous/Peripheral Tibial Nerve Stimulation (PTNS)

Percutaneous tibial nerve stimulation (PTNS) involves stimulation of the posterior tibial nerve just superior and posterior to the medial malleolus. PTNS was approved for treatment of OAB in 2010, and there are several models available. The physiology of action is not completely understood; however, the theory is that the electrical signal provides neurostimulation via the S3 nerve root that then downregulates bladder contractions. Current therapy is 12-weekly 30-minute treatments followed by monthly maintenance therapy if effective. Patients can expect up to a 60% subjective improvement after a 12-week course with studies noting continued benefit up to 24 months [26, 61]. Research is ongoing for implantable devices that could be patient controlled and thus require fewer office visits.

Intradetrusor onabotulinumtoxinA

The FDA approved the use of 100 units of onabotulinumtoxinA for use in UUI patients in 2013 [4]. The mechanism of action is to block presynaptic acetylcholine release at the neuromuscular junction, thus decreasing muscarinic receptor activation and resulting in decreased detrusor contractions. A phase 3, randomized, double-blind, placebo-controlled trial assessed the efficacy of 100 U of onabotulinumtoxinA for idiopathic OAB. Patient eligibility included eight or more UUI episodes on a 3-day bladder diary in patients that were no longer candidates for antimuscarinic therapy either due to lack of response or side effects. The group in the treatment arm received 20 injections of 0.5 ml onabotulinumtoxinA 1 cm apart and 2 mm deep into the detrusor, and the placebo group received normal saline. At 12 weeks, 58% versus 29% of patients had a 50% reduction in symptoms, and 23% versus 7% reported continence in the treatment and placebo arms, respectively. There was a mean of 2.65 fewer incontinence episodes per day versus 0.87 fewer episodes for placebo [62].

Repeat injection is recommended no sooner than 12 weeks from the last treatment, but in a longitudinal prospective cohort, median time of effect is typically just over 7 months with a third of patients actually noting an effect for up to a year. Follow-up after 3.5 years of use has shown no difference in efficacy nor increase in adverse effects [63]. It is important to note that if the patient is concomitantly undergoing onabotulinumtoxinA therapy for other conditions, they should not receive more than 400 U in a 3-month period to avoid overdosing. Common risks of this procedure included urinary tract infection (18–33%) and incomplete emptying with approximately 5% of patients requiring catheterization [62, 64]. Therefore, if a patient is unable or unwilling to catheterize, another modality may be warranted.

Sacral Nerve Stimulation

Sacral nerve stimulation (SNS) is also known as sacral neuromodulation and is not only used for OAB patients with and without associated incontinence but also is FDA-approved for non-obstructive urinary retention and fecal incontinence. SNS involves placement of an implantable lead wire next to the 3rd sacral nerve root and a battery in the subcutaneous fatty tissue above the gluteus muscles. This modality was approved for UUI in 1997. The mechanism of action is not entirely understood but is believed to be via modulation of both efferent and afferent pathways [65].

There are variable programs that can be modified by both patient and provider. Prior to permanent placement of the device, a 1- to 2-week test stimulation is performed. This can be done using a non-permanent percutaneous test electrode (usually placed in the office) or a permanent lead (usually placed in the operating room) that will continue to be used if the trial is successful.

The FDA recommends implantation of the device only if the patient is considered a clinical responder, defined as at least a 50% reduction in symptoms during the test phase. The effect can last for as long as the battery life, which is typically 5 -7 years for the older, non-rechargeable systems and up to 15 years for the newer, rechargeable systems.

At 12 months, 60% of 272 patients who had a successful staged implant had at least a 50% reduction in leaks per day from baseline, and 36% had achieved continence. At 5 years, 45% of 118 patients noted at least a 50% reduction in leaks per day, and 45% noted continence. Adverse events included a 22% need for reoperation, 15% implant site pain, and 13% loss of effect. Over 5 years, 19% of patients had permanent explantation due to lack of desired response or need for an MRI [66]. MRI below the neck is currently contraindicated with older SNS devices [50]. The latest generation of SNS devices is MRI compatible.

Rare: Cystoplasty and Urinary Diversion [16]

Augmentation cystoplasty, detrusor myomectomy, or urinary diversion can be used for refractory urgency incontinence, but their use is quite rare and is now typically utilized in cases of OAB with neurogenic etiologies. Prior to the existence of the newer pharmacologic and neuromodulation therapies listed above, these procedures were more common. Risks include the morbidities from a larger surgery and malignancy. Disadvantages also include the need for continued monitoring and possible need for long-term intermittent self-catheterization to facilitate bladder emptying.

Mixed Urinary Incontinence

Mixed urinary incontinence is defined as the “complaint of involuntary leakage associated with urgency and also with effort, exertion, sneezing and coughing” [67]. Most patients note that they have a combination of stress and urgency incontinence and therefore will require a multimodal therapy. Focus is generally on the most bothersome condition initially (see Chap. 8 for more details on mixed urinary incontinence) [5].

Incontinence as a Result of Non-neurogenic Chronic Urinary Retention

Chronic urinary retention (CUR) is defined as PVR >300 cc that has persisted for at least 6 months [68]. Poor bladder emptying can result from either bladder outlet obstruction or detrusor underactivity. If obstruction is the main etiology, relief from the obstruction can remedy the issue. Possible causes of outlet obstruction in women include high-grade pelvic organ prolapse or an obstructing sling. In these cases, prolapse repair or sling release, respectively, may be considered. Medications such as alpha blockers are more successful in male than female patients. The cholinergic agonist bethanechol has been used for detrusor underactivity, but studies have generally not shown this to be clinically successful. The initiation of regular catheterizations should be considered if incomplete emptying results in symptoms or if the upper tracts are threatened [68]. Given that SNS is FDA-approved for non-obstructive urinary retention, this would be an option to consider for patients with detrusor areflexia or underactivity [69].

Upcoming/Experimental Therapies

Treatment modalities are ever-changing. There are a variety of therapies that have been evaluated but have yet to show clinical efficacy. These therapies, which include acupuncture for SUI and UUI, stem cell therapy for SUI, treatment of the urinary microbiome, beta-2 agonists for SUI, and newer neuromodulation techniques for SUI and UUI, are considered experimental and should only be used in the context of clinical trials.

Discussion of Clinical Case

Returning to the case at the beginning of the chapter, there are several issues to evaluate and address. These include optimization of her pre-existing conditions, determination of the type and severity of her incontinence, and performance of physical examination prior to proceeding with intervention. It may be that she has mixed urinary incontinence, and ultimately a combination of the above-listed therapies will mitigate her symptoms without ever requiring operative intervention that she initially requested. Additionally, patient counseling is of paramount importance in creating a treatment plan and monitoring response. Lastly, patients may opt to defer treatment all together after hearing of all their options. On balance, if there is no chronic urinary obstruction threatening the upper genitourinary tract, after thorough counseling, a patient may choose to opt out of treatment since there is little long-term health risk.

Resources for Patients

Several downloadable pamphlets and websites are available as tools to assist in patient education and counseling. Links are available in the References section [70–72].

Commentary

John P. Lavelle

This is a very interesting case.

"A 45-year-old G2P2 obese woman with type 2 diabetes, hypertension, sleep apnea, and prior hysterectomy presents with urinary incontinence. She states her friend was cured with surgery, and she desires the same. She notes that her primary care provider had given her a medication that 'didn't work' to reduce her leakage."

The chapter presents a very thorough method for considering the problem of urinary incontinence and the treatment options for this lady. Importantly, the history, and physical exam as it pertains to incontinence, is carefully explained. Many of the various options for treatment of female incontinence are explained. However, when considering this particular case, a number of medical options need to be considered. The problem is that the case is very complex and multifaceted and that one or more factors need to be considered and each one needs to be eliminated or minimized to come to an acceptable treatment plan, which may take many months to execute completely, leading to an acceptable outcome for the patient.

One of the problems is that the lady in the case assumes that her incontinence has the same cause as her friend's, and thus the procedure should fix her incontinence. This problem requires a lot of patience and education from the physician after a thorough evaluation to determine the precise cause(s) of this patient's incontinence, with evaluation of her contributing factors, and thus realign her expectations with what is possible, and how she can be helped, and why her expectation of an operation may or may not work for her.

If one, at the outset, considers from the history:

Obesity: Is this severe? Does it contribute to metabolic syndrome? Is there a hormonal problem? Is it related to stress and overeating due to an anxiety disorder or prior psychological or physical trauma? It can add to stress incontinence if present on physical examination. Did she have Sheehan's syndrome during childbirth, and is she now having problems with the treatment? Is what appears to be obesity really ascites or perhaps some large abdominal mass such as an ovarian cyst causing mass effect in the pelvis?

Diabetes: Is it well controlled? Does she have polyuria? Does she have peripheral neuropathy? Nephropathy with polyuria? Diabetic cystopathy? Are we assuming diabetes mellitus, where in fact she has diabetes insipidus due to lithium use for depression, which might be partly related to her incontinence? Is this diabetes insipidus contributing to her incontinence due to polyuria with urgency and inability to make it to the bathroom?

Hypertension: Is this being treated with diuretics? If so, the drug-induced increase in urine output can exacerbate her urgency and incontinence secondary to a more rapid filling of her bladder.

Sleep apnea: Is her incontinence nocturnal, thus related to untreated sleep apnea, with potential cardiac arrhythmias, and diuresis from ANF release?

G2P2: Was the bladder or pelvic floor injured during childbirth, and is there pudendal neuropathy or prolapse? The possibility of STDs with herpes lesions affecting bladder function might also be considered.

Prior hysterectomy: Is there subsequent prolapse contributing to incontinence, and is there neuropathy of the bladder due to interference with the pelvic nerves on the lateral fornixes innervating the bladder? Have there been other prior anti-incontinence procedures performed concurrently or subsequent to the hysterectomy? Is there a possible vesicovaginal fistula?

Medication that did not work: Was this something for overactive bladder or something different? Was it expected to work? Importantly, why did the medication "not work"? This would need to be explained to her.

In the background: With diabetes, obesity, and hypertension, and being female, is she at risk of serious cardiac event from a surgical procedure? Does she have adequate pulmonary status to manage anesthesia?

In the background: Does she potentially have spinal disorder, due to her obesity, and exacerbating degenerative disc disease, contributing to incontinence?

During the examination, many of these items can be assessed, but ultimately you have to decide whether the problem is related to polyuria, stress, urge, and mixed, overflow, or fistula incontinence or a combination. Each particular problem has to be addressed as a separate entity and treated as such. Ultimately this should be based on objective data and examination. Importantly as pointed out in this chapter, the use of urodynamics should explain the symptoms by the findings and not fit the findings to the symptoms.

This chapter is a great summary of available options to medically or surgically correct urinary incontinence which primarily impact patient's quality of life. Did we write this section? I do not recall seeing this in the original chapter. So, with Dr. Lavelle also as an author, I am wondering if he was asked to write a summary of the chapter at the end (since he was otherwise not a co-author)? If so, ask him to work on this section. If not, please let me know and I will rewrite as it needs work. We must respect the patient's rights to autonomy, self-determination, and freedom of will, to decide if and when they do or do not want any or all of these proposed or recommended procedures. However, this should be done in the circumstance of a full, frank, and open discussion(s) of the indications, nature of the treatment(s), and the risks, benefits, alternatives, and consequences of, and of not, performing each procedure as none are ideal. While we strive as physicians to make better options for our patients, they ultimately have to live with the consequences of these decisions. This is best if the patients can go into the procedure(s) "eyes wide open," fully prepared, and comfortable with their decision, with the full support of their medical and caregiver teams. This is the final most important point of this chapter, where in the discussion of the case, the authors acknowledge the patient's right to decline treatment.

References

1. Haylen BT, de Ridder D, Freeman RM, Swift SE, Berghmans B, Lee J, et al. An International Urogynecological Association (IUGA)/International Continence Society (ICS) joint report on the terminology for female pelvic floor dysfunction. NeurourolUrodyn. 2010;29(1):4–20.
2. Gleason JL, Richter HE, Redden DT, Goode PS, Burgio KL, Markland AD. Caffeine and urinary incontinence in US women. Int Urogynecol J. 2013;24:295–302.
3. Kenton K. Urinary incontinence in women. Practice bulletin no. 155. American College of Obstetricians and Gynecologists. Obs Gynecol [Internet]. 2015 [cited 2018 Aug 22];126:e66–81. Available from: www.niddk.nih.gov/.
4. Lukacz ES, Santiago-Lastra Y, Albo ME, Brubaker L. Urinary incontinence in women a review. JAMA. 2017;318(16):1592–604.
5. Abrams P, Andersson KE, Birder L, Brubaker L, Cardozo L, Chapple C, et al. Fourth International Consultation on Incontinence Recommendations of the International Scientific Committee: evaluation and treatment of urinary incontinence, pelvic organ prolapse, and fecal incontinence. Neurourol Urodyn [Internet]. 2010 [cited 2018 Sep 29];29:213–40. Available from: www.interscience.wiley.com.
6. Fitzgerald M, Stablein C, Brubaker L. Urinary habits among asymptomatic women. AJOG. 2002;187:1384–8.
7. Hashim H, Mousa R. Management of fluid intake in patients with overactive bladder. Curr Urol Rep. 2009;10:428–33.
8. Avery K, Donovan J, Peters TJ, et al. ICIQ: a brief and robust measure for evaluating the symptoms and impact of urinary incontinence. NeurourolUrodyn. 2004;23:322.
9. Ubersax JS, Wyman JF, Shumaker SA, et al. Short forms to assess life quality and symptom distress for urinary incontinence in women: the Incontinence Impact Questionnaire and the Urogenital Distress Inventory. NeurourolUrodyn. 1995;14:131.
10. Patrick DL, Martin ML, Bushnell DM, et al. Quality of life of women with urinary incontinence: further development of the incontinence quality of life instrument [I-QOL]. Urology. 1999;53:71.
11. Barber MD, Bump RCWM. Short forms of two condition-specific quality of life questionnaires for women with pelvic floor disorders. Am J Obstet Gynecol. 2005;193:103.
12. Rogers RG, Coates KW, Kammerer-Doak D, et al. A short form of the pelvic organ prolapse/urinary incontinence sexual questionnaire [PISQ-12]. Int Urogynecol J. 2003;14:164.
13. Bradley C, Rahn D, Nygaard I, Barber M, Nager C, Kenton KS. The questionnaire for urinary incontinence diagnosis (QUID): validity and responsiveness to change in women undergoing non-surgical therapies for treatment of stress predominant urinary incontinence. NeurourolUrodyn. 2010;29:727–34.
14. Sandvik H, Seim A, Vanvik A, Hunskaar S. A severity index for epidemiological surveys of female urinary incontinence: comparison with 48-hour pad-weighing tests. NeurourolUrodyn. 2000;19:137–45.
15. Winters JC, Dmochowski RR, Goldman HB, Herndon CDA, Kobashi KC, Kraus SR, et al. Urodynamic studies in adults: AUA/SUFU guideline. J Urol [Internet]. Elsevier Inc. 2012 [cited 2014 Feb 20];188(6 Suppl):2464–72. Available from: http://www.ncbi.nlm.nih.gov/pubmed/23098783.
16. Gormley EA, Lightner DJ, Faraday M, Vasavada SP. Diagnosis and treatment of overactive bladder (non-neurogenic) in adults: AUA/SUFU guideline amendment. J Urol [Internet]. Elsevier. 2015 [cited 2018 Sep 30];193(5):1572–80. Available from: https://www-sciencedirect-com.libproxy1.usc.edu/science/article/pii/S0022534715001779.
17. Fader M, Cottenden AM, Getliffe K. Absorbent products for moderate-heavy urinary and/or faecal incontinence in women and men. Cochrane Database Syst Rev [Internet]. John Wiley & Sons, Ltd. 2008 [cited 2018 Sep 30];(4). Available from: https://doi.org/10.1002/14651858.CD007408.
18. van Leijsen SAL, Kluivers KB, Mol BWJ, Milani AL, Roovers J-PWR, et al. Value of urodynamics before stress urinary incontinence surgery: a randomized controlled trial. Obstet Gynecol [Internet]. 2013 [cited 2014 Feb 17];121(5):999–1008. Available from: http://www.ncbi.nlm.nih.gov/pubmed/23635736.
19. Haylen BT, Freeman RM, Swift SE, Cosson M, Davila GW, Deprest J, et al. An International Urogynecological Association (IUGA)/ International Continence Society (ICS) joint terminology and classification of the complications related directly to the insertion of prostheses (meshes, implants, tapes) & grafts in female pelvic [Internet]. 2010 [cited 2018 Sep 29]. Available from: https://outlook.office.com/owa/?realm=med.usc.edu&path=/attachmentlightbox.
20. Kenton K, Norton PA, Sirls LT, Kraus SR, Chai TC, Lemack GE, et al. Retropubic versus transobturator

midurethral slings for stress incontinence. N Engl J Med [Internet]. Massachusetts Medical Society. 2010;362(22):2066–76. Available from: https://doi.org/10.1056/NEJMoa0912658.

21. Ford A, Rogerson L, Cody J, Ogah J. Mid-urethral sling operations for stress urinary incontinence in women. Cochrane Database Syst Rev [Internet]. 2015;CD006375(7):1–287. Available from: www.cochranelibrary.com.
22. Cameron AP, Haraway AM. The treatment of female stress urinary incontinence: an evidenced-based review. Open access J Urol [Internet]. Dove Press. 2011 [cited 2018 Sep 30];3:109–20. Available from: http://www.ncbi.nlm.nih.gov/pubmed/24198643.
23. Ostaszkiewicz J, Johnston L, Roe B. Timed voiding for the management of urinary incontinence in adults. Cochrane Database Syst Rev [Internet]. John Wiley & Sons, Ltd. 2004 [cited 2018 Sep 30];(1). Available from: https://doi.org/10.1002/14651858.CD002802.pub2.
24. Wallace SA, Roe B, Williams K, Palmer M. Bladder training for urinary incontinence in adults. Cochrane Database Syst Rev [Internet]. John Wiley & Sons, Ltd. 2004 [cited 2018 Sep 30];(1). Available from: https://doi.org/10.1002/14651858.CD001308.pub2.
25. Dumoulin C, Hay-Smith EJC, Mac Habée-Séguin G. Pelvic floor muscle training versus no treatment, or inactive control treatments, for urinary incontinence in women. Cochrane Database Syst Rev [Internet]. 2014 [cited 2018 Sep 30]. Available from: www.cochranelibrary.com.
26. Riemsma R, Hagen S, Kirschner-Hermanns R, Norton C, Wijk H, Andersson K-E, et al. Can incontinence be cured? A systematic review of cure rates. [cited 2018 Sep 29]. Available from: https://bmcmedicine.biomedcentral.com/track/pdf/10.1186/s12916-017-0828-2.
27. Subak LL, Wing R, West DS, Franklin F, Vittinghoff E, Creasman JM, et al. Weight loss to treat urinary incontinence in overweight and obese women. PRIDE Investigators. N Engl J Med. 2009;360:481–90.
28. Hendrix SL, Cochrane BB, Nygaard IE, Handa VL, Barnabei VM, Iglesia C, et al. Effects of estrogen with and without progestin on urinary incontinence. JAMA [Internet]. American Medical Association; 2005 [cited 2018 Sep 30];293(8):935. Available from: http://jama.jamanetwork.com/article.aspx?doi=10.1001/jama.293.8.935.
29. Cody JD, Jacobs ML, Richardson K, Moehrer B, Hextall A. Oestrogen therapy for urinary incontinence in post-menopausal women. Cochrane Database Syst Rev [Internet]. John Wiley & Sons, Ltd. 2012 [cited 2018 Sep 30];(10). Available from: https://doi.org/10.1002/14651858.CD001405.pub3.
30. Dmochowski RR, Miklos JR, Norton PA, Zinner NR, Yalcin I, Bump RC. Duloxetine versus placebo for the treatment of North American women with stress urinary incontinence. J Urol [Internet]. Elsevier. 2003 [cited 2018 Sep 30];170(4):1259–63. Available from: https://www-sciencedirect-com.libproxy2.usc.edu/science/article/pii/S0022534705631412.
31. Richter HE, Burgio KL, Brubaker L, Nygaard IE, Ye W, Weidner A, et al. Continence pessary compared with behavioral therapy or combined therapy for stress incontinence. Obstet Gynecol [Internet]. 2010 [cited 2018 Sep 29];115(3):609–17. Available from: http://content.wkhealth.com/linkback/openurl?sid=WKPTLP:landingpage&an=00006250-201003000-00020.
32. Samuels JB, Garcia MA. Treatment to external labia and vaginal canal with CO2 laser for symptoms of vulvovaginal atrophy in postmenopausal women. Aesthetic Surg J [Internet]. 2018 [cited 2018 Sep 30]. Available from: https://academic.oup.com/asj/advance-article/doi/10.1093/asj/sjy087/4992010.
33. Walter J, Larochelle A. No. 358-intravaginal laser for genitourinary syndrome of menopause and stress urinary incontinence- clinical key. JOGC [Internet]. 2018 [cited 2018 Sep 30];40(4):503–11. Available from: https://www-clinicalkey-com.libproxy2.usc.edu/#!/content/playContent/1-s2.0-S1701216317312082?returnurl=null&referrer=null.
34. Nager CW, Sirls L, Litman HJ, Richter H, Nygaard I, Chai T, et al. Baseline urodynamic predictors of treatment failure 1 year after mid urethral sling surgery. J Urol [Internet]. American Urological Association Education and Research, Inc. 2011;186(2):597–603. Available from: https://doi.org/10.1016/j.juro.2011.03.105.
35. Mamut A, Carlson KV. Periurethral bulking agents for female stress urinary incontinence in Canada. Can Urol Assoc J [Internet]. Canadian Urological Association. 2017 [cited 2018 Sep 30];11(6S2):152. Available from: http://www.cuaj.ca/index.php/journal/article/view/4612.
36. Jonsson Funk M, Levin PJ, Wu JM. Trends in the surgical management of stress urinary incontinence. Obstet Gynecol [Internet]. NIH Public Access. 2012 [cited 2018 Sep 30];119(4):845–51. Available from: http://www.ncbi.nlm.nih.gov/pubmed/22433349.
37. Brubaker L, Richter HE, Norton PA, Albo M, Zyczynski HM, Chai TC, et al. 5-year continence rates, satisfaction and adverse events of burch urethropexy and fascial sling surgery for urinary incontinence. J Urol [Internet]. NIH Public Access. 2012 [cited 2018 Sep 30];187(4):1324–30. Available from: http://www.ncbi.nlm.nih.gov/pubmed/22341290.
38. Lapitan MCM, Cody JD, Mashayekhi A. Open retropubic colposuspension for urinary incontinence in women. Cochrane Database Syst Rev [Internet]. John Wiley & Sons, Ltd. 2017 [cited 2018 Oct 17];(7). Available from: https://doi.org/10.1002/14651858.CD002912.pub7.
39. Michael A, Richter H, Brubaker L, Norton P, Kraus S, Philippe Z, Chai T, Zyczynski H, Diokno A, Tennstedt S. Burch colposuspension versus fascial sling to reduce urinary stress incontinence. N Engl J Med. 2007;356(21):2143–54.
40. Schimpf MO, Rahn DD, Wheeler TL, Patel M, White AB, Orejuela FJ, et al. Sling surgery for stress urinary incontinence in women: a systematic review and metaanalysis. Am J Obstet Gynecol [Internet].

Mosby. 2014 [cited 2018 Sep 30];211(1):71.e1–71.e27. Available from: https://www.sciencedirect.com/science/article/pii/S0002937814000593.

41. Brubaker L, Cundiff GW, Fine P, Nygaard I, Richter HE, Visco AG, et al. Abdominal sacrocolpopexy with burch colposuspension to reduce urinary stress incontinence [Internet]. N Engl J Med. 2006 [cited 2018 Sep 30]. 354. Available from: www.nejm.org.
42. Patel H, Ostergard DR, Sternschuss G. Polypropylene mesh and the host response. [cited 2018 Sep 29]. Available from: http://2015.iuga.org/wp-content/uploads/workshops/ws29_literature1.pdf.
43. Ogah J, Cody JD, Rogerson L. Minimally invasive synthetic suburethral sling operations for stress urinary incontinence in women. In: Ogah J, editor. Cochrane Database of Systematic Reviews [Internet]. Chichester, UK: John Wiley & Sons, Ltd. 2009 [cited 2018 Sep 30]:CD006375. Available from: http://www.ncbi.nlm.nih.gov/pubmed/19821363.
44. Kenton K, Stoddard AM, Zyczynski HM, Albo ME, Rickey L, Norton PA, et al. 5-year longitudinal follow-up after retropubic and transobturator midurethral slings. J Urol. 2015;193(1):203–10.
45. Ford AA, Rogerson L, Cody JD, Aluko P, Ogah JA. Mid-urethral sling operations for stress urinary incontinence in women. Cochrane Database Syst Rev [Internet]. John Wiley & Sons, Ltd. 2017 [cited 2018 Oct 17],(7). Available from: https://doi.org/10.1002/14651858.CD006375.pub4.
46. Nambiar A, Cody JD, Jeffery ST, Aluko P. Single-incision sling operations for urinary incontinence in women. Cochrane Database Syst Rev [Internet]. John Wiley & Sons, Ltd. 2017 [cited 2018 Sep 30];(7). Available from: https://doi.org/10.1002/14651858.CD008709.pub3.
47. McCoy O, Vaughan T, Nickles SW, Ashley M, MacLachlan LS, Ginsberg D, et al. Outcomes of autologous fascia pubovaginal sling for patients with transvaginal mesh related complications requiring mesh removal. J Urol [Internet]. Elsevier. 2016 [cited 2018 Sep 30];196(2):484–9. Available from: https://www-sciencedirect-com.libproxy2.usc.edu/science/article/pii/S0022534716034649.
48. Weber AM. Pelvic organ prolapse. Obstet Gynecol. 2005;106(3):615–34.
49. Brubaker L, Cundiff G, Fine P, Nygaard I, Richter H, Visco A, et al. A randomized trial of colpopexy and urinary reduction efforts (CARE): design and methods. Control Clin Trials. 2003;24(5):629–42.
50. Kirby AC, Kellogg ES. Trends in utilization of third-line therapies for non-neurogenic overactive bladder: sacral neuromodulation, peripheral tibial nerve stimulation, and intradetrusor onabotulinumtoxinA. 2018 [cited 2018 Sep 30];13:25–30. Available from: https://doi.org/10.1007/s11884-018-0462-7.
51. Gormley EA, Lightner DJ, Faraday M, Vasavada SP, American Urological Association, Society of Urodynamics, Female Pelvic Medicine. Diagnosis and treatment of overactive bladder (non-neurogenic) in adults: AUA/SUFU guideline amendment. J Urol [Internet]. 2015 [cited 2018 Oct 1];193(5):1572–80. Available from: http://www.ncbi.nlm.nih.gov/pubmed/25623739.
52. Ackerman AL, Lai HH, Parameshwar PS, Eilber KS, Anger JT. Symptomatic overlap in overactive bladder and interstitial cystitis/painful bladder syndrome - development of a new algorithm. BJU Int [Internet]. 2018 [cited 2018 Oct 1]. Available from: http://www.ncbi.nlm.nih.gov/pubmed/30253040.
53. Reynolds WS, McPheeters M, Blume J, Surawicz T, Worley K, Wang L, et al. Comparative effectiveness of anticholinergic therapy for overactive bladder in women. Obstet Gynecol [Internet]. 2015 [cited 2018 Sep 30];125(6):1423–32. Available from: http://insights.ovid.com/crossref?an=00006250-201506000-00022.
54. Brostrom S, Hallas J. Persistence of antimuscarinic drug use. Eur J Clin Pharmacol [Internet]. 2009 [cited 2018 Sep 29];65:309–14. Available from: https://search-proquest-com.libproxy2.usc.edu/docview/214487128?accountid=14749.
55. American Geriatrics Society 2015 updated beers criteria for potentially inappropriate medication use in older adults. J Am Geriatr Soc [Internet]. Wiley/Blackwell (10.1111). 2015 [cited 2018 Sep 30];63(11):2227–46. Available from: https://doi.org/10.1111/jgs.13702.
56. American Urogynecologic Society (AUGS) Guidelines Committee, Thomas T, Walter M. AUGS consensus statement: association of anticholinergic medication use and cognition in women with overactive bladder. Female Pelvic Med Reconstr Surg [Internet]. 2017;23(3):177–8. Available from: http://www.ncbi.nlm.nih.gov/pubmed/28441276.
57. Risacher SL, McDonald BC, Tallman EF, West JD, Farlow MR, Unverzagt FW, et al. Association between anticholinergic medication use and cognition, brain metabolism, and brain atrophy in cognitively normal older adults. JAMA Neurol [Internet]. 2016 [cited 2018 Sep 30];73(6):721. Available from: http://www.ncbi.nlm.nih.gov/pubmed/27088965.
58. Chapple CR, Nazir J, Hakimi Z, Bowditch S, Fatoye F, Guelfucci F, et al. Persistence and adherence with mirabegron versus antimuscarinic agents in patients with overactive bladder: a retrospective observational study in UK clinical practice. Eur Urol [Internet]. Elsevier. 2017 [cited 2018 Sep 30];72(3):389–99. Available from: https://www-sciencedirect-com.libproxy1.usc.edu/science/article/pii/S0302283817300623.
59. Abrams P, Kelleher C, Staskin D, Kay R, Martan A, Mincik I, et al. Combination treatment with mirabegron and solifenacin in patients with overactive bladder: exploratory responder analyses of efficacy and evaluation of patient-reported outcomes from a randomized, double-blind, factorial, dose-ranging, Phase II study (SYMPHONY). World J Urol [Internet]. 2017 [cited 2018 Oct 1];35(5):827–38. Available from: https://doi.org/10.1007/s00345-016-1908-1.
60. Drake MJ, Chapple C, Esen AA, Athanasiou S, Cambronero J, Mitcheson D, et al. Efficacy and safety

of mirabegron add-on therapy to solifenacin in incontinent overactive bladder patients with an inadequate response to initial 4-week solifenacin monotherapy: a randomised double-blind multicentre phase 3B study (BESIDE). Eur Urol [Internet]. 2016 [cited 2018 Oct 1];70(1):136–45. Available from: https://linkinghub.elsevier.com/retrieve/pii/S0302283816002074.
61. Del Río-Gonzalez S, Aragon IM, Castillo E, Milla-España F, Galacho A, Machuca J, et al. Percutaneous tibial nerve stimulation therapy for overactive bladder syndrome: clinical effectiveness, urodynamic, and durability evaluation. Urology [Internet]. 2017 [cited 2018 Oct 1];108:52–8. Available from: https://linkinghub.elsevier.com/retrieve/pii/S0090429517306969.
62. Nitti VW, Dmochowski R, Herschorn S, Sand P, Thompson C, Nardo C, et al. OnabotulinumtoxinA for the treatment of patients with overactive bladder and urinary incontinence: results of a phase 3, randomized, placebo controlled trial. J Urol. 2017;197(2):S216–23.
63. Nitti VW, Ginsberg D, Sievert K-D, Sussman D, Radomski S, Sand P, et al. Durable efficacy and safety of long-term onabotulinumtoxinA treatment in patients with overactive bladder syndrome: final results of a 3.5-year study. J Urol [Internet]. Elsevier. 2016 [cited 2018 Sep 30];196(3):791–800. Available from: https://www-sciencedirect-com.libproxy2.usc.edu/science/article/pii/S0022534716300945.
64. Sun Y, Luo D, Tang C, Yang L, Shen H. The safety and efficiency of onabotulinumtoxinA for the treatment of overactive bladder: a systematic review and meta-analysis. Int Urol Nephrol [Internet]. 2015 [cited 2018 Sep 30];3:1779–88. Available from: https://search-proquest-com.libproxy2.usc.edu/docview/1728359169?accountid=14749.
65. Yamanishi T, Kaga K, Fuse M, Shibata C, Uchiyama T. Neuromodulation for the treatment of lower urinary tract symptoms. LUTS Low Urin Tract Symptoms. 2015;7(3):121–32.
66. Siegel S, Noblett K, Mangel J, Bennett J, Griebling TL, Sutherland SE, et al. Five-year follow-up results of a prospective, multicenter study of patients with overactive bladder treated with sacral neuromodulation. J Urol [Internet]. Elsevier Ltd. 2018;199(1):229–36. Available from: https://doi.org/10.1016/j.juro.2017.07.010.
67. Abrams P, Cardozo L, Fall M, Gri D, Rosier P, Ulmsten U, et al. The standardisation of terminology of lower urinary tract function: report from the Standardisation Sub-committee of the International Continence Society. Neurourol Urodyn. 2002;178:167–78.
68. Stoffel J, Lightner D, Peterson A, Sandhu J, Suskind A, Wei J. Non-neurogenic chronic urinary retention: consensus definition, management strategies, and future opportunities [Internet]. 2016 [cited 2018 Oct 1]. Available from: https://www.auanet.org/guidelines/chronic-urinary-retention.
69. Gross C, Habli M, Lindsell C, Al E. Sacral neuromodulation for nonobstructive urinary retention: a meta-analysis. Female Pelvic Med Reconstr Surg. 2010;16:249.
70. Patient resources — incontinence causes and treatments | National Association for Continence [Internet]. [cited 2018 Oct 1]. Available from: https://www.nafc.org/resource-center/.
71. Home - your pelvic floor [Internet]. [cited 2018 Oct 1]. Available from: https://www.yourpelvicfloor.org/.
72. Urinary incontinence - ACOG [Internet]. [cited 2018 Oct 1]. Available from: https://www.acog.org/Patients/FAQs/Urinary-Incontinence.

8 Mixed Urinary Incontinence: Strategic Approach

Steven J. Weissbart and Ariana L. Smith

Case Scenario

A 62-year-old woman complains of multiple daily episodes of urinary incontinence that occur with preceding urgency as well as during exertion. She finds the incontinence bothersome. Her examination is within normal limits, and she has not been previously treated for incontinence.

Introduction

Mixed urinary incontinence (MUI) is defined by the International Continence Society (ICS) as "the complaint of involuntary leakage associated with urgency and also with exertion, effort, sneezing or coughing" [1]. MUI can also be defined by the presence of both detrusor overactivity (DO) and stress urinary incontinence (SUI) on urodynamics. Data from the Nurses' Health Study demonstrated that among women with incontinence, 22% experience MUI, 51% experience SUI, and 27% experience urgency urinary incontinence (UUI) [2]. The prevalence of MUI has been shown to increase with age, and clinicians will likely care for more women with MUI as the population ages [3, 4]. MUI can cause a considerable impact on health-care-related quality of life, and research has indicated that women with MUI are actually more bothered by their incontinence compared to women with pure SUI or pure UUI [5, 6].

Management of MUI can be challenging for numerous reasons. Women with MUI represent a heterogeneous population and may have stress-predominant symptoms, urgency-predominant symptoms, or equal stress- and urgency-predominant symptoms. In fact, it is hard to universally characterize patients with MUI, and patients may be labeled differently according to the definition of MUI used [7, 8]. Additionally, women with MUI may have varying treatment goals and different comorbidities, such as pelvic organ prolapse, that may complicate management. Furthermore, the pathophysiology of MUI is unclear [9–11], and treating one component of MUI (i.e., the urgency component or the stress component) may potentially improve or worsen the other component of the incontinence. Lastly, in comparison to women with either pure SUI or pure UUI, women with MUI appear to have higher rates of surgical treatment failure [12]. For these reasons, MUI patients have often been

Commentary by Marcio A. Averbeck, Neuro-urology, Video-urodynamics Unit, Moinhos De Vento Hospital, Department of Urology, Porto Allegre, Brazil

S. J. Weissbart
Stony Brook University Hospital, Department of Urology, Stony Brook, NY, USA

A. L. Smith (✉)
Pelvic Medicine & Reconstructive Surgery, University of Pennsylvania Health System, Philadelphia, PA, USA
e-mail: ariana.smith@uphs.upenn.edu

K. C. Kobashi, S. D. Wexner (eds.), *Female Pelvic Medicine*, https://doi.org/10.1007/978-3-030-54839-1_8

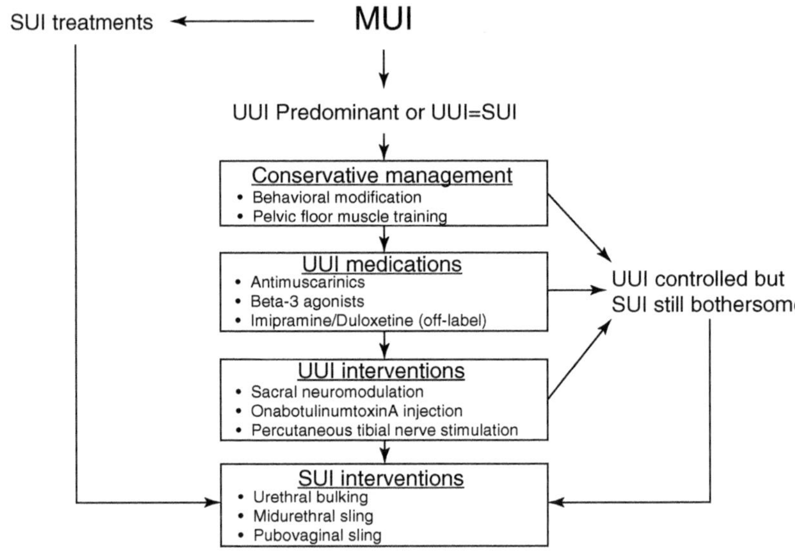

Fig. 8.1 Mixed urinary incontinence treatment algorithm from [76]. (Reused with permission © Springer Nature)

excluded from treatment trials for SUI- and UUI-directed therapies further limiting the information on therapy effects in the MUI population. Therefore, management of women with MUI is typically performed on a case-by-case basis, with several reasonable treatment strategies available (Fig. 8.1). In this chapter, we review the management of MUI.

How to Approach (Order of Addressing Components)

An appropriate history and physical examination are important first steps in the evaluation of women with MUI. While the evaluation of women with pelvic floor dysfunction was discussed in Chap. 1, as a review, the patient history of women with MUI should capture the timing of incontinence episodes and the degree of bother associated with the incontinence. Specifically, women should be asked whether the incontinence episodes occur during exertional activities, such as laughing or coughing, or are preceded by urgency. Women should also be asked about any incontinence episodes that may occur without awareness (i.e., insensible incontinence) [13]. A thorough history on the situation and triggers of incontinence is critical in this population as many patients find it challenging to differentiate stress and urgency symptoms. Clinicians should ask about the use of protective pads and how many, if any, are used throughout the day. The presence of associated urinary symptoms, such as hematuria, dysuria, and obstructive voiding symptoms, should also be assessed as well as the presence of vaginal bulge/prolapse symptoms and bowel symptoms, such as fecal incontinence. Clinicians should ask about prior treatment history, such as prior midurethral sling placement and/or prolapse repair (and if mesh was used). A bladder diary can be very useful in assessing patients with MUI, and several validated urinary symptom questionnaires, such as the Medical, Epidemiological, and Social Aspects of Aging (MESA), Questionnaire for Urinary Incontinence Diagnosis (QUID), Urinary Distress Inventory-6 (UDI-6), and 3 Incontinence Questions (3IQ), are available that may help assess patients with MUI.

Physical examination should include both a pelvic and focused neurologic exam. During pelvic examination, the clinician should assess for urethral hypermobility or scarring (i.e., fixed urethra), as well as assess for the presence of pelvic organ prolapse, vaginal atrophy, or other concomitant pelvic pathology. A cough stress test with a full bladder can help clinicians demonstrate SUI. Specifically, leakage associated with hypermobility, leakage in the absence of hypermobility, or cough-induced urgency with delayed leakage may be demonstrated. Urine analysis should be conducted to assess for infection. Measurement of post-void residual (PVR) urine volume is important to assess for the presence of incomplete emptying, which may worsen urinary incontinence.

Ultimately, after the history and physical exam are completed, an attempt should be made to categorize the patient as having stress-predominant MUI, urgency-predominant MUI, or equal stress- and urgency-predominant MUI. Additionally, the clinician should determine which component of incontinence is most bothersome to the patient. Unfortunately, in women with MUI, there is no Level 1 evidence available to guide clinicians in deciding whether to first treat the stress component or the urgency component of MUI [14]; one randomized trial investigating the best first treatment of MUI (surgical versus non-surgical therapy) was stopped prematurely in March 2009 due to poor enrollment (MIMOSA) [15], and a second randomized trial *E*ffects of *S*urgical *T*reatment *E*nhanced with *E*xercise for *M*ixed Urinary Incontinence (ESTEEM) was completed, but analyses are not yet available [16]. Therefore, we typically begin treatment by counseling patients with MUI on available treatment options and encouraging them to begin treatment with the most conservative therapy for the component of incontinence that is most bothersome to them.

Conservative treatment for women with MUI includes fluid modification, weight loss, pelvic floor muscle training, and pessary placement. Research has demonstrated that fluid reduction can improve urinary frequency and incontinence episodes [17]. Although it may be difficult for patients to reduce their fluid intake by large volumes, patients may experience a benefit from a 25% reduction in fluid intake [18]. Pelvic floor muscle training is another efficacious treatment for MUI [19] as a Cochrane review specifically demonstrated that pelvic floor muscle training was an effective first-line therapy for all forms of incontinence [20]. Appropriate education from a nurse, the addition of biofeedback, and even virtual reality may be helpful when performing pelvic floor muscle training for women with MUI [21–23]. Weight loss is another conservative management option for women with MUI. Subak et al. randomized 338 women with urinary incontinence to a 6-month weight loss program (including diet and exercise along with behavioral modification) or to a structured education program and found that a higher proportion of women assigned to the weight loss program had a clinically relevant reduction in both SUI and UUI episodes [24]. Pessary placement is also a reasonable first-line therapy for women with MUI. Donnelly et al. reviewed the efficacy of a pessary for 239 women with SUI or MUI and found that half of the women fitted with a pessary continued to use it at 6 months [25]. The Ambulatory Treatments for Leakage Associated with Stress Incontinence (ATLAS) trial was a three-arm randomized trial comparing a pessary, behavioral therapy, and combination therapy (pessary and behavioral therapy) for women with SUI (although 54% of women in the trial had MUI). At 12 months of follow-up, 50% of women assigned to the pessary arm were satisfied with the treatment [26].

Pharmacotherapies can also be an effective treatment for women with MUI [27]. For women with MUI who have bothersome urgency, anticholinergic and/or beta-3 agonist therapy can be initiated. Staskin and Te investigated the efficacy of solifenacin in patients with MUI and found a reduction in incontinence episodes in patients taking solifenacin compared to placebo with over 40% of patients taking solifenacin regaining continence after 12 weeks of therapy [28]. Kelleher et al. investigated the efficacy of solifenacin in women with MUI and found that once-daily solifenacin was as effective and as tolerated in women with MUI as compared to pure UUI [29]. This finding was similar to that of a previous trial by Kreder et al. that found that tolterodine was as effective in reducing incontinence episodes in patients with MUI as compared to patients with pure UUI [30]. The MERIT (Mixed Incontinence Effectiveness Research Investigating Tolterodine) trial demonstrated that women with MUI taking tolterodine experienced a considerable improvement in UUI episodes (−12.3) compared to placebo (−8) [31]. Interestingly, data suggests that the presence of SUI does not appear to diminish the efficacy of anticholinergics in patients with overactive bladder (OAB) unless there is more severe SUI [32], and it has been reported that women with MUI taking anticholinergics may overall experience an approximately 50–60% reduction in the urgency component of their incontinence [10].

A trial of vaginal estrogen may be helpful for women with MUI, though research has provided conflicting evidence on the use of vaginal estrogen. One meta-analysis suggested that vaginal estrogen was efficacious for SUI [33], while a different review suggested efficacy for the symptoms of urinary urgency and frequency [34]. Duloxetine is a serotonin-norepinephrine reuptake inhibitor that may be an attractive pharmacotherapy for the treatment of MUI as it has been shown to improve bladder relaxation and also increase outlet resistance. Bent et al. randomized 588 women with MUI to either duloxetine or placebo and found women receiving duloxetine had a larger median reduction in incontinence episode frequency (60% versus 47%) compared to women receiving placebo [35]. It should be noted that duloxetine is not FDA approved for urinary incontinence treatment. Aside from duloxetine, the tricyclic antidepressant, imipramine, is another medication that have been used for MUI treatment but is not FDA approved for this indication [36].

Unfortunately, many patients with MUI may experience bothersome incontinence that is refractory to conservative and oral pharmacotherapies. After the above treatments have been discussed/attempted and more advanced options such as surgery are being considered, it must be decided whether to proceed with treating the stress component of MUI versus the urgency component of MUI. For women with MUI who are mostly bothered by SUI symptoms, surgical therapy using synthetic midurethral sling placement or autologous fascial sling placement appears to be a reasonable treatment option (as discussed below) [37]. Urethral bulking agents also appear to be a reasonable treatment options for women with MUI who have bothersome SUI symptoms and are frail and/or decline urethral sling placement [38]. For women with MUI who are more bothered by refractory urgency and UUI, we discuss all third-line OAB treatment options as described by the AUA OAB guideline including onabotulinumtoxinA, sacral neuromodulation (SNM), and tibial nerve stimulation [39]. In women with equally bothersome stress and urgency symptoms, it can be difficult to determine which component to treat first. We counsel these patients extensively on the goals of each treatment modality and present the advantages and disadvantages of each. We also consider other factors, such as urodynamic findings (as described below), in determining a treatment plan.

Pros and Cons of Each Approach

Treating the Stress Component First

After conservative therapies have been exhausted, addressing the stress component of MUI first is advantageous for several reasons. Research has suggested that stress incontinence events may lead to urgency incontinence events, and, thus, treating SUI may actually improve UUI. In a rat model, Jung et al. showed that urethral perfusion modulated the micturition reflex and suggested that SUI can induce DO [40]. In examining 30-day bladder diary data among 35 women with MUI, Minassian et al. found that a stress activity preceded 52.5% of UUI episodes and that 69% of women reported stress-induced UUI [41]. Therefore, initially treating SUI may potentially help to resolve urgency and UUI in patients with MUI in addition to SUI symptoms.

Numerous trials have demonstrated that SUI surgery is efficacious in women with MUI as it can treat both the SUI and urgency symptoms. Duckett and Tamilselvi reported on 51 women with urodynamic evidence of both DO and SUI who underwent tension-free vaginal tape (TVT) placement and found that 47% were objectively cured of DO, 63% reported subjective cure of urgency symptoms, and SUI was cured in 92% [42]. Abdel-Fattah et al. analyzed data from 83 women with stress-predominant MUI who underwent transobturator tension-free vaginal tape (TOT) placement and found a patient-reported success rate of 75% and an objective cure rate of 90% [43]. Of note, urgency and UUI resolved after TOT placement in over 50% of women in their study. Jain et al. conducted a systematic review examining the effectiveness of midurethral slings specifically in women with MUI [37]. Among the seven prospective studies included in their review, they found an overall subjective cure of 56.4% at 35 months of follow-up. Following midurethral sling placement, they also found an overall cure of urgency and UUI ranging from 30% to 85% and a cure rate of SUI ranging from 85% to 97%. More recently, Zyczynski et al. conducted a secondary analysis of three large multicenter urinary incontinence treatment trials (the Stress Incontinence Surgical Treatment Efficacy Trial, SISTEr; the Trial of Midurethral Slings, TOMUS; and the Value of Urodynamic Evaluations trial, ValUE) in women with stress-predominant MUI who underwent surgical therapy for SUI and found that 50–71% experienced an improvement in OAB symptoms [44].

Burch colposuspension and pubovaginal sling may also effectively treat MUI. Osman performed Burch colposuspensions in 24 women with MUI (with a VLPP of ≥90 cm H_2O) and found that 87% of women became completely dry postoperatively [45]. Fulford et al. performed rectus fascial pubovaginal sings in 85 women with SUI and found that 97% were symptomatically cured of SUI and that 69% also experienced resolution of urgency [46]. Interestingly, they conjectured that resolution of urgency was attributable to appropriately tensioning the sling to achieve bladder neck closure.

Treatment of the stress component of MUI using a bulking agent is another reasonable option in women with MUI and may be especially useful in women who decline or are not ideal candidates for midurethral sling placement (e.g., are frail, have underwent prior pelvic radiotherapy, and failed prior midurethral sling placement). Mohr et al. studied periurethral Bulkamid in women with MUI and found considerable improvements for all domains of the King's Health Questionnaire, pad weights, and visual analogue scores. Complications were low (13%) with the majority being urinary tract infections [38]. Poon and Zimmern also found significant improvement in urinary symptoms (as measured by UDI-6 question scores) in women with MUI who underwent periurethral collagen injection [47]. A Cochrane review however found limited evidence for urethral bulking agents for SUI [48].

Unfortunately, SUI surgery may fail to resolve or even worsen urinary urgency and UUI, and this may be especially problematic for women with MUI who are initially bothered by urgency at baseline. Early studies on SUI therapy suggested higher rates of de novo urgency and worsening urgency and may be related to procedures being performed at the bladder neck rather than the midurethra. Among 754 women with MUI, Lee et al. found that 40% and 32% of women had persistent urgency and UUI, respectively, after midurethral sling placement [49]. Urgency is recognized as a common reason for dissatisfaction after midurethral sling placement [50], and thus, a main disadvantage of treating the SUI component first in women with MUI is the possibility of worsening urgency after anti-incontinence surgery. Needless to say, disadvantages of treating MUI with SUI surgery also include the usual surgical risks of treatment [51].

Treating the Urgency Component First

There are several advantages of treating the urgency component of MUI first in women with MUI. Urgency has been reported to be one of the most bothersome urinary symptoms [52], and, thus, by first treating urgency, one may improve quality of life and eliminate the need for other treatments. In women who fail treatment with an anticholinergic or beta-3 agonist, third-line OAB therapies, including sacral neuromodulation (SNM), tibial nerve stimulation, and onabotulinumtoxinA, can be effective in women with OAB and UUI [39]. Additionally, treatment of urinary urgency with neuromodulation or onabotulinumtoxinA may pose fewer and more reversible surgical complications compared to SUI surgery. Therefore, a patient with MUI and bothersome urgency may opt to try a third-line OAB therapy before proceeding with SUI surgery and consider SUI surgery only if symptoms are not controlled with a third-line OAB therapy.

While third-line OAB therapies have not been extensively studied in women with MUI, they have been demonstrated to improve urgency/urgency incontinence symptoms. In terms of tibial nerve stimulation, the SUmiT trial randomized 220 adults to either percutaneous tibial nerve stimulation or sham treatment for 12 weeks and found that 54% of subjects in the active treatment group reported moderate or marked improvement in bladder symptoms compared to 21% of subjects in the sham group [53]. Numerous studies have supported the efficacy of onabotulinumtoxinA for women with OAB [54]. Recently, Herschorn et al. randomized patients with overactive bladder and urinary incontinence to onabotulinumtoxinA 100 U, solifenacin 5 mg, or placebo and found that both onabotulinumtoxinA 100 U and solifenacin 5 mg were more efficacious than placebo, with a third of patients receiving onabotulinumtoxinA experiencing a 100% reduction in incontinence [55]. Siegel et al. randomized 147 subjects to SNM versus standard medical therapy for OAB and found greater therapeutic success in the SNM group compared to the standard medical therapy group (61% versus 42%) [56]. In the Refractory Overactive Bladder: Sacral Neuromodulation vs Botulinum Toxin Assessment (ROSETTA) trial, which was a randomized trial comparing onabotulinumtoxinA 200 U to sacral neuromodulation in women with UUI, there was a reduction of 3.9 and 3.3 incontinence episodes per day after 6 months in women receiving onabotulinumtoxinA 200 U and SNM, respectively [57].

What Directs Decisions

Multiple factors should be considered when deciding how to treat MUI, including the type of MUI (i.e., stress-predominant MUI, urgency-predominant MUI, and equal stress- and urgency-predominant MUI), patient preferences/goals, physical exam findings (e.g., concomitant prolapse), comorbidities, and urodynamic findings. Of these factors, the role of urodynamics (UDS) in the evaluation of MUI has been widely studied in the literature. Specifically, research has investigated both the correlation between urodynamic findings and urinary symptoms and the urodynamic predictors of success and/or failure after midurethral sling placement in patients with MUI in order to determine what role urodynamics plays in directing MUI treatment.

It is debatable how well urodynamic findings correlate with patient-reported symptoms, and it is, therefore, unclear to what extent urodynamic findings should factor into the treatment approach (i.e., whether to first treat SUI versus UUI) for each patient. For example, many women who report the symptom of urinary urgency, or SUI, do not demonstrate SUI or DO on UDS. A systematic review including 23 studies attempting to classify patients by incontinence type found a poor level of agreement between clinical evaluation and urodynamics [58]. Interestingly, this study found that the reclassification rate of incontinence type was highest among patients with MUI; 46% of patients with a clinical diagnosis of MUI had SUI on UDS, while 21% had DO on UDS. On the other hand, Digesu et al. examined urodynamic findings of 1626 women with MUI symptoms and found reasonable correlation between UDS findings and urinary symptoms [59]. Among women with stress-predominant MUI, 82% demonstrated urodynamic SUI, and among those with urgency-predominant MUI, 64% had DO on UDS. Among women with equal stress- and urgency-predominant MUI, 46% had DO, and 54% demonstrated SUI. Lewis et al. examined the records of 99 women with MUI and also found urodynamic differences that correlated with symptoms [60]. In their study, 100% of women with stress-predominant MUI demonstrated SUI on UDS compared to 61% of women with urgency-predominant MUI, and 70% of women with urgency-predominant MUI demonstrated DO on UDS compared to 26% of women with stress-predominant MUI.

Overall, as the reported correlation between patient symptoms and urodynamic findings has varied in the literature, we rely on the patient history to categorize a patient's type of MUI (i.e., stress-predominant, urgency-predominant, and equal stress- and urgency-predominant MUI) and consider UDS when the clinical picture is unclear and/or in women who have undergone prior surgery. Additionally, UDS may be advisable in women with MUI prior to surgical intervention [14]. According to AUA guidelines, urodynamics may be performed prior to SUI surgery in women with MUI [61] as well as before any potentially morbid treatment is considered [61]. Additionally, according to AUA guidelines, the absence of DO on UDS in patients with MUI does not exclude it as an etiology for urgency [62].

Several studies have also investigated the role of UDS in predicting midurethral sling or third-line OAB therapy outcomes that may, therefore, be used to help direct decision-making in treating patients with MUI. In women with MUI, Panayi et al. found that the opening detrusor pressure was predicative of postoperative DO after TVT placement [63], and Lee et al. found that preoperative DO was predictive of postoperative urgency after midurethral sling placement [49]. Other studies have found that low maximum urethral closure pressure [64] and low maximum cystometric capacity [65] were associated with persistent urgency and/or detrusor overactivity after midurethral sling placement. Unfortunately, in patients undergoing treatment for urgency and UUI, Cohen et al. did not find any relationship between urodynamic variables and clinical response to onabotulinumtoxinA [66], and Nobrega et al. did not find any relationship between urodynamic variables and SNM outcomes [67].

Patient characteristics may also factor into the decision-making for MUI treatment. Among patient characteristics, the severity of baseline urgency appears to be an important risk factor for poor surgical outcomes after midurethral sling placement in women with MUI. In a study by Kulseng-Hanssen et al., 1113 women with MUI were stratified into 3 groups according to their type of MUI (stress-predominant incontinence group, urgency-predominant incontinence group, and an equal stress- and urgency-predominant incontinence group) [68]. At 38 months of follow-up, objective cure results were 64.2%, 45.2, and 51.3% for women with stress-predominant MUI, urgency-predominant MUI, and equal stress- and urgency-predominant MUI, respectively. Thus, women with stress-predominant MUI symptoms appear to have better outcomes compared to women with urgency-predominant MUI. Preoperative anticholinergic use is another patient characteristic that can be a risk factor for persistent urgency after anti-incontinence surgery and may be useful for patient counseling and decision-making. Kenton et al. investigated risk factors associated with bothersome UUI after Burch colposuspension or midurethral sling placement and found that patients with prior anticholinergic use, preoperative urgency, or DO were more likely to have postoperative UUI [69]. Barber et al. also found that preoperative anticholinergic medication use was associated with recurrent urinary incontinence after midurethral sling placement [70]. Age is another important factor that can be considered in the treatment of MUI, as older women may be at increased risk for urgency after midurethral sling placement. Among 103 women with MUI who underwent TOT, Yoo and Kim found that older women were at high risk of using anticholinergics postoperatively [71].

Choosing the type of midurethral sling is another important decision for patients with MUI who elect to undergo SUI surgery. While overall there does not appear to be a difference in efficacy between retropubic and TOT midurethral slings [72], some data has suggested that TOT slings may have a lower rate of de novo urgency, while retropubic slings may be more efficacious in women with intrinsic sphincter deficiency (ISD). Botros et al. studied 257 women with SUI or MUI who underwent retropubic or TOT slings and found lower rates of de novo UUI in women undergoing TOT (8%) compared to women undergoing retropubic slings (33%) [73]. However, they did not find a difference in resolution of DO, UUI, and de novo DO between the groups. Of note, among patients with preoperative UUI, only 6% who underwent TOT had worsening UUI compared to 14–16% who underwent a retropubic sling placement. Schierlitz et al. compared retropubic sling outcomes to TOT midurethral sling outcomes in women with ISD and found a higher rate of persistent stress urinary incontinence in the TOT group (45%) compared to the retropubic sling group (21%) [74]. Conversely, a meta-analysis examining midurethral sling outcomes for women with MUI found that the odds of overall subjective cure were similar between retropubic and TOT slings [37].

Important Caveats of Counseling

Patients being treated for MUI require extensive counseling. Goals of care should be discussed as this appears to be a major determinant of satisfaction in women undergoing pelvic floor surgery [75]. When considering midurethral sling placement in women with MUI, women should be informed that urgency may not improve and may even potentially worsen after surgery. Mallet et al. found that patients undergoing SUI surgery expect improvement in storage symptoms [76, 77], and in a study by Aigmueller, urgency was reported to be a common reason for dissatisfaction after TVT in women with MUI [50]. Interestingly, a different study found that women with persistent UUI are dissatisfied by midurethral sling placement even if their SUI improves [46]. Additionally, women with MUI undergoing midurethral sling placement should also be counseled that they may be at higher risk of surgical failure compared to women with pure SUI [12] and that they may need combination treatment for their urinary incontinence. The ESTEEM trial, which is being conducted by the Pelvic Floor Disorders Network, is randomizing women with MUI to either midurethral sling placement alone or to midurethral sling placement with perioperative behavioral therapy to see if the addition of pelvic floor muscle therapy will improve MUI (primary aim) and SUI and/or urgency/UUI (secondary aims) symptoms after midurethral sling placement [16]. Pending the results of this trial, women may be counseled on the role of perioperative pelvic floor therapy in addition to midurethral sling placement for the treatment of MUI and the potential role of combination therapy.

Summary

MUI is a very common form of urinary incontinence that can be challenging to treat. Women with MUI should be classified according to the type of their incontinence (i.e., stress-predominant, urgency-predominant, and equal stress- and urgency-predominant MUI), and initial treatment can be targeted to the most bothersome component of their incontinence. Numerous conservative therapies and pharmacotherapies are available to treat MUI, and midurethral sling placement as well as third-line OAB therapies can be effective treatment options for women who have refractory symptoms. Urodynamic factors and patient characteristics may help guide the initial treatment approach, and research has demonstrated that treating one component of MUI may improve or worsen the other component. Women with MUI should be extensively counseled regarding all treatment options and informed that they may require multiple treatments to improve their incontinence.

Commentary

Marcio A. Averbeck

The chapter entitled "Mixed Urinary Incontinence: Strategic Approach" deals with a highly relevant subject in the clinical practice. Dr. Steven J. Weissbart and Dr. Ariana L. Smith adeptly described the strategic approach to mixed incontinence, in a comprehensive fashion, starting with the importance of diagnostic workup and then addressing the pros and cons of treatment options, including conservative measures and minimally invasive procedures for refractory cases.

Medical history and physical examination remain the cornerstones of medical assessment of women with mixed urinary incontinence (MUI). As mentioned by the authors, conservative treatments comprise fluid modification, weight loss, pelvic floor muscle training, and pessary placement. Despite the lack of high level evidence to propose specific regimens, conservative treatment should always be offered to the patients, since minimally invasive procedures may be associated with inherent complications. Thus, precise guidance on the risks and benefits of all available treatments is truly important to effectively manage patients' expectations and avoid future frustrations. Retrieving clear information on the most bothersome component of female urinary incontinence may be challenging sometimes. In this context, urodynamics (UDS) represent a valid tool to reproduce the patients' urinary complaints. The authors described honestly the role of UDS in predicting midurethral sling or third-line OAB therapy outcomes for those patients refractory to behavioral and medical treatments. Although UDS should not be seen as a panacea in the assessment of such difficult cases, this method sheds a light toward decision-making.

This chapter certainly brings valuable insights not only to the initial management but also to the third-line treatments of refractory MUI patients.

References

1. Abrams P, Cardozo L, Fall M, Griffiths D, Rosier P, Ulmsten U, et al. The standardisation of terminology of lower urinary tract function: report from the Standardisation Sub-committee of the International Continence Society. Am J Obstet Gynecol. 2002;187(1):116–26.
2. Minassian VA, Devore E, Hagan K, Grodstein F. Severity of urinary incontinence and effect on quality of life in women, by incontinence type. Obstet Gynecol. 2013;121(5):1083.
3. Lifford KL, Townsend MK, Curhan GC, Resnick NM, Grodstein F. The epidemiology of urinary incontinence in older women: incidence, progression, and remission. J Am Geriatr Soc. 2008;56(7):1191–8.
4. Hannestad YS, Rortveit G, Sandvik H, Hunskaar S. A community-based epidemiological survey of female urinary incontinence: the Norwegian EPINCONT study. J Clin Epidemiol. 2000;53(11):1150–7.
5. Frick AC, Huang AJ, Van Den Eeden SK, Knight SK, Creasman JM, Yang J, et al. Mixed urinary incontinence: greater impact on quality of life. J Urol. 2009;182(2):596–600.
6. Dooley Y, Lowenstein L, Kenton K, FitzGerald M, Brubaker L. Mixed incontinence is more bothersome than pure incontinence subtypes. Int Urogynecol J. 2008;19(10):1359–62.
7. Brubaker L, Stoddard A, Richter H, Zimmern P, Moalli P, Kraus SR, et al. Mixed incontinence: comparing definitions in women having stress incontinence surgery. Neurourol Urodyn. 2009;28(4):268–73.
8. Brubaker L, Lukacz ES, Burgio K, Zimmern P, Norton P, Leng W, et al. Mixed incontinence: comparing definitions in non surgical patients. Neurourol Urodyn. 2011;30(1):47–51.
9. Myers DL. Female mixed urinary incontinence: a clinical review. JAMA. 2014;311(19):2007–14.
10. Bandukwala NQ, Gousse AE. Mixed urinary incontinence: what first? Curr Urol Rep. 2015;16(3):9.
11. Lai HH, Simon M, Boone TB. The impact of detrusor overactivity on the management of stress urinary incontinence in women. Curr Urol Rep. 2006;7(5):354–62.
12. Gleason JL, Parden AM, Jauk V, Ballard A, Sung V, Richter HE. Outcomes of midurethral sling procedures in women with mixed urinary incontinence. Int Urogynecol J. 2015;26(5):715–20.
13. Haylen BT, de Ridder D, Freeman RM, Swift SE, Berghmans B, Lee J, et al. An International Urogynecological Association (IUGA)/International Continence Society (ICS) joint report on the terminology for female pelvic floor dysfunction. J Assoc Chart Physiother Women Health. 2012;110:33.
14. Kammerer-Doak D, Rizk DE, Sorinola O, Agur W, Ismail S, Bazi T. Mixed urinary incontinence: international urogynecological association research and development committee opinion. Int Urogynecol J. 2014;25(10):1303–12.
15. Brubaker L, Moalli P, Richter HE, Albo M, Sirls L, Chai T, et al. Challenges in designing a pragmatic clinical trial: the mixed incontinence—medical or surgical approach (MIMOSA) trial experience. Clin Trials. 2009;6(4):355–64.
16. Sung VW, Borello-France D, Dunivan G, Gantz M, Lukacz ES, Moalli P, et al. Methods for a multicenter randomized trial for mixed urinary incontinence: rationale and patient-centeredness of the ESTEEM trial. Int Urogynecol J. 2016;27(10):1479–90.
17. Swithinbank L, Hashim H, Abrams P. The effect of fluid intake on urinary symptoms in women. J Urol. 2005;174(1):187–9.
18. Hashim H, Abrams P. How should patients with an overactive bladder manipulate their fluid intake? BJU Int. 2008;102(1):62–6.
19. Sar D, Khorshid L. The effects of pelvic floor muscle training on stress and mixed urinary incontinence and quality of life. J Wound Ostomy Cont Nurs. 2009;36(4):429–35.
20. Dumoulin C, Hay-Smith J. Pelvic floor muscle training versus no treatment, or inactive control treatments, for urinary incontinence in women. Cochrane Database Syst Rev. 2010;1(1):CD005654.
21. Ng S-C, Lin T-L, Chang S-J, Tai H-L, Hu S-W, Chen G-D. Nursing intervention to enhance efficacy of home practice of pelvic floor muscle exercises in treating mixed urinary incontinence. Int Urogynecol J. 2008;19(5):637–42.
22. Herderschee R, Hay Smith EJC, Herbison GP, Roovers JP, Heineman MJ. Feedback or biofeedback to augment pelvic floor muscle training for urinary incontinence in women. Cochrane Library. 2011.

23. Elliott V, de Bruin ED, Dumoulin C. Virtual reality rehabilitation as a treatment approach for older women with mixed urinary incontinence: a feasibility study. Neurourol Urodyn. 2015;34(3):236–43.
24. Subak LL, Wing R, West DS, Franklin F, Vittinghoff E, Creasman JM, et al. Weight loss to treat urinary incontinence in overweight and obese women. N Engl J Med. 2009;360(5):481–90.
25. Donnelly MJ, Powell-Morgan S, Olsen AL, Nygaard IE. Vaginal pessaries for the management of stress and mixed urinary incontinence. Int Urogynecol J. 2004;15(5):302–7.
26. Richter HE, Burgio KL, Brubaker L, Nygaard IE, Ye W, Weidner A, et al. Continence pessary compared with behavioral therapy or combined therapy for stress incontinence: a randomized controlled trial. Obstet Gynecol. 2010;115(3):609–17.
27. Hashim H, Abrams P. Pharmacological management of women with mixed urinary incontinence. Drugs. 2006;66(5):591–606.
28. Staskin DR, Te AE. Short- and long-term efficacy of solifenacin treatment in patients with symptoms of mixed urinary incontinence. BJU Int. 2006;97(6):1256–61.
29. Kelleher C, Cardozo L, Kobashi K, Lucente V. Solifenacin: as effective in mixed urinary incontinence as in urge urinary incontinence. Int Urogynecol J. 2006;17(4):382–8.
30. Kreder K, Brubaker L, Mainprize T. Tolterodine is equally effective in patients with mixed incontinence and those with urge incontinence alone. BJU Int. 2003;92(4):418–21.
31. Khullar V, Hill S, Laval K-U, Schiøtz HA, Jonas U, Versi E. Treatment of urge-predominant mixed urinary incontinence with tolterodine extended release: a randomized, placebo-controlled trial. Urology. 2004;64(2):269–74.
32. Michel MC, de la Rosette JJ, Piro M, Goepel M. Does concomitant stress incontinence alter the efficacy of tolterodine in patients with overactive bladder? J Urol. 2004;172(2):601–4.
33. Fantl JA, Cardozo L, McClish DK. Estrogen therapy in the management of urinary incontinence in postmenopausal women: a meta-analysis. First report of the Hormones and Urogenital Therapy Committee. Obstet Gynecol. 1994;83:12–8.
34. Sultana CJ, Walters MD. Estrogen and urinary incontinence in women. Maturitas. 1994;20(2–3):129–38.
35. Bent AE, Gousse AE, Hendrix SL, Susan L, Klutke CG, Monga AK, et al. Duloxetine compared with placebo for the treatment of women with mixed urinary incontinence. Neurourol Urodyn. 2008;27(3):212–21.
36. Hunsballe J, Djurhuus JC. Clinical options for imipramine in the management of urinary incontinence. Urol Res. 2001;29(2):118–25.
37. Jain P, Jirschele K, Botros SM, Latthe PM. Effectiveness of midurethral slings in mixed urinary incontinence: a systematic review and meta-analysis. Int Urogynecol J. 2011;22(8):923–32.
38. Mohr S, Marthaler C, Imboden S, Monga A, Mueller MD, Kuhn A. Bulkamid (PAHG) in mixed urinary incontinence: what is the outcome? Int Urogynecol J. 2017;28(11):1657–61.
39. Gormley EA, Lightner DJ, Burgio KL, Chai TC, Clemens JQ, Culkin DJ, et al. Diagnosis and treatment of overactive bladder (non-neurogenic) in adults: AUA/SUFU guideline. J Urol. 2012;188(6):2455–63.
40. Jung SY, Fraser MO, Ozawa H, Yokoyama O, Yoshiyama M, De Groat WC, et al. Urethral afferent nerve activity affects the micturition reflex; implication for the relationship between stress incontinence and detrusor instability. J Urol. 1999;162(1):204–12.
41. Minassian VA, Yan XS, Pitcavage J, Stewart WF. Mixed incontinence masked as stress induced urgency urinary incontinence. J Urol. 2016;196(4):1190–5.
42. Duckett JR, Tamilselvi A. Urogynaecology: effect of tension-free vaginal tape in women with a urodynamic diagnosis of idiopathic detrusor overactivity and stress incontinence. BJOG. 2006;113(1):30–3.
43. Abdel-Fattah M, Mostafa A, Young D, Ramsay I. Evaluation of transobturator tension-free vaginal tapes in the management of women with mixed urinary incontinence: one-year outcomes. Am J Obstet Gynecol. 2011;205(2):150.e1–6.
44. Zyczynski HM, Albo ME, Goldman HB, Wai CY, Sirls LT, Brubaker L, et al. Change in overactive bladder symptoms after surgery for stress urinary incontinence in women. Obstet Gynecol. 2015;126(2):423.
45. Osman T. Stress incontinence surgery for patients presenting with mixed incontinence and a normal cystometrogram. BJU Int. 2003;92(9):964–8.
46. Fulford S, Flynn R, Barrington J, Appanna T, Stephenson T. An assessment of the surgical outcome and urodynamic effects of the pubovaginal sling for stress incontinence and the associated urge syndrome. J Urol. 1999;162(1):135–7.
47. Poon CI, Zimmern PE. Is there a role for periurethral collagen injection in the management of urodynamically proven mixed urinary incontinence? Urology. 2006;67(4):725–9.
48. Kirchin V, Page T, Keegan PE, Atiemo K, Cody JD, McClinton S. Urethral injection therapy for urinary incontinence in women. Cochrane Library. 2012.
49. Lee JS, Dwyer P, Rosamilia A, Lim Y, Polyakov A, Stav K. Persistence of urgency and urge urinary incontinence in women with mixed urinary symptoms after midurethral slings: a multivariate analysis. BJOG. 2011;118(7):798–805.
50. Aigmueller T, Bjelic-Radisic V, Kargl J, Hinterholzer S, Laky R, Trutnovsky G, et al. Reasons for dissatisfaction ten years after TVT procedure. Int Urogynecol J. 2014;25(2):213–7.
51. Herschorn S. Midurethral sling complications. Can Urol Assoc J. 2017;11(6Suppl2):S141.
52. Agarwal A, Eryuzlu LN, Cartwright R, Thorlund K, Tammela TL, Guyatt GH, et al. What is the most bothersome lower urinary tract symptom? Individual- and population-level perspectives for both men and women. Eur Urol. 2014;65(6):1211–7.

53. Peters KM, Carrico DJ, Perez-Marrero RA, Khan AU, Wooldridge LS, Davis GL, et al. Randomized trial of percutaneous tibial nerve stimulation versus Sham efficacy in the treatment of overactive bladder syndrome: results from the SUmiT trial. J Urol. 2010;183(4):1438–43.
54. Anger JT, Weinberg A, Suttorp MJ, Litwin MS, Shekelle PG. Outcomes of intravesical botulinum toxin for idiopathic overactive bladder symptoms: a systematic review of the literature. J Urol. 2010;183(6):2258–64.
55. Herschorn S, Kohan A, Aliotta P, McCammon K, Sriram R, Abrams S, et al. The efficacy and safety of onabotulinumtoxinA or solifenacin compared with placebo in solifenacin naïve patients with refractory overactive bladder: results from a multicenter, randomized, double-blind phase 3b trial. J Urol. 2017;198(1):167–75.
56. Siegel S, Noblett K, Mangel J, Griebling TL, Sutherland SE, Bird ET, et al. Results of a prospective, randomized, multicenter study evaluating sacral neuromodulation with InterStim therapy compared to standard medical therapy at 6-months in subjects with mild symptoms of overactive bladder. Neurourol Urodyn. 2015;34(3):224–30.
57. Amundsen CL, Richter HE, Menefee SA, Komesu YM, Arya LA, Gregory WT, et al. OnabotulinumtoxinA vs sacral neuromodulation on refractory urgency urinary incontinence in women: a randomized clinical trial. JAMA. 2016;316(13):1366–74.
58. van Leijsen SA, Evert JS, Mol BWJ, Vierhout ME, Milani AL, Heesakkers JP, et al. The correlation between clinical and urodynamic diagnosis in classifying the type of urinary incontinence in women. A systematic review of the literature. Neurourol Urodyn. 2011;30(4):495–502.
59. Digesu GA, Salvatore S, Fernando R, Khullar V. Mixed urinary symptoms: what are the urodynamic findings? Neurourol Urodyn. 2008;27(5):372–5.
60. Lewis JB, Ng AV, O'Connor RC, Guralnick ML. Are there differences between women with urge predominant and stress predominant mixed urinary incontinence? Neurourol Urodyn. 2007;26(2):204–7.
61. Kobashi KC, Albo ME, Dmochowski RR, Ginsberg DA, Goldman HB, Gomelsky A, et al. Surgical treatment of female stress urinary incontinence: AUA/SUFU guideline. J Urol. 2017;198(4):875–83.
62. Winters JC, Dmochowski RR, Goldman HB, Herndon CA, Kobashi KC, Kraus SR, et al. Urodynamic studies in adults: AUA/SUFU guideline. J Urol. 2012;188(6):2464–72.
63. Panayi D, Duckett J, Digesu G, Camarata M, Basu M, Khullar V. Pre operative opening detrusor pressure is predictive of detrusor overactivity following TVT in patients with pre operative mixed urinary incontinence. Neurourol Urodyn. 2009;28(1):82–5.
64. Paick J-S, Ku JH, Kim SW, Oh S-J, Son H, Shin JW. Tension-free vaginal tape procedure for the treatment of mixed urinary incontinence: significance of maximal urethral closure pressure. J Urol. 2004;172(3):1001–5.
65. Gamble TL, Botros SM, Beaumont JL, Goldberg RP, Miller J-JR, Adeyanju O, et al. Predictors of persistent detrusor overactivity after transvaginal sling procedures. Am J Obstet Gynecol. 2008;199(6):696.e1–7.
66. Cohen BL, Caruso DJ, Kanagarajah P, Gousse AE. Predictors of response to intradetrusor botulinum toxin-A injections in patients with idiopathic overactive bladder. Adv Urol. 2009;2009:328364.
67. Nobrega RP, Solomon E, Jenks J, Greenwell T, Ockrim J. Predicting a successful outcome in sacral neuromodulation testing: are urodynamic parameters prognostic? Neurourol Urodyn. 2018;37:1007–10.
68. Kulseng-Hanssen S, Husby H, Schiøtz HA. Follow-up of TVT operations in 1,113 women with mixed urinary incontinence at 7 and 38 months. Int Urogynecol J. 2008;19(3):391–6.
69. Kenton K, Richter H, Litman H, Lukacz E, Leng W, Lemack G, et al. Risk factors associated with urge incontinence after continence surgery. J Urol. 2009;182(6):2805–9.
70. Barber MD, Kleeman S, Karram MM, Paraiso MFR, Ellerkmann M, Vasavada S, et al. Risk factors associated with failure 1 year after retropubic or transobturator midurethral slings. Am J Obstet Gynecol. 2008;199(6):666.e1–7.
71. Yoo E-H, Kim D. Predictors of postoperative antimuscarinics in women with mixed urinary incontinence after transobturator surgery. Int Urogynecol J. 2013;24(3):401–6.
72. Ford AA, Rogerson L, Cody JD, Aluko P, Ogah JA. Mid urethral sling operations for stress urinary incontinence in women. Cochrane Library. 2017.
73. Botros SM, Miller JJR, Goldberg RP, Gandhi S, Akl M, Beaumont JL, et al. Detrusor overactivity and urge urinary incontinence following trans obturator versus midurethral slings. Neurourol Urodyn. 2007;26(1):42–5.
74. Schierlitz L, Dwyer PL, Rosamilia A, Murray C, Thomas E, De Souza A, et al. Effectiveness of tension-free vaginal tape compared with transobturator tape in women with stress urinary incontinence and intrinsic sphincter deficiency: a randomized controlled trial. Obstet Gynecol. 2008;112(6):1253–61.
75. Elkadry EA, Kenton KS, FitzGerald MP, Shott S, Brubaker L. Patient-selected goals: a new perspective on surgical outcome. Am J Obstet Gynecol. 2003;189(6):1551–7.
76. Mallett VT, Brubaker L, Stoddard AM, Borello-France D, Tennstedt S, Hall L, et al. The expectations of patients who undergo surgery for stress incontinence. Am J Obstet Gynecol. 2008;198(3):308.e1–6.
77. Lee EW, Kobashi KC. Mixed incontinence: what takes precedence in its management? Curr Urol Rep. 2014;15(12):461.

Complex Cases of SUI

9

Victor W. Nitti and Rachael D. Sussman

Introduction

In this chapter, we present five patients with complicated cases of stress urinary incontinence. For each case, we discuss the various treatment options in an effort to elucidate the nuances of decision-making in a complex patient.

Treatment Options

The treatment options for stress urinary incontinence (SUI) have been discussed in detail in Chap. 4. To review, treatment options include nonsurgical management (behavioral modifications, pelvic floor exercises, physical therapy, and anti-incontinence pessary), urethral bulking agents, and surgical intervention. Surgical intervention is most often with either a synthetic midurethral sling (MUS) via a retropubic (RP) or transobturator (TO) approach or an autologous fascia pubovaginal sling (AF-PVS). Burch retropubic colposuspension has been shown to be a safe and effective treatment for SUI; however, today this procedure is done less frequently, usually for a patient who is undergoing a laparotomy or laparoscopy for a concomitant abdominal surgery that cannot be performed vaginally and where there is limited vaginal access or via a laparoscopic approach or via a laparoscopic approach.

Guidance on Treatment Options and Counseling: A Case-Based Approach

Case Scenario 1

A 57-year-old woman complains of stress-predominant mixed urinary incontinence. She complains mostly of leakage with exercise, bending, and lifting and has urgency and frequency with rare leakage which is less bothersome. She has failed behavioral therapy and is not interested in taking a medication daily. She desires treatment of her incontinence. Bladder diaries indicated a relatively small functional bladder capacity with 1200 ml urine output/24 hours. On physical exam, she has a positive cough test with urethral hypermobility. Urodynamic testing (UDS) demonstrated detrusor overactivity (DO) without incontinence and evidence of SUI with an ALPP of 90 cm H_2O.

Commentary by E. Ann Gormley, Geisel School of Medicine at Dartmouth, Hanover, NH, USA
Dartmouth-Hitchcock Medical Center, Section of Urology, Department of Surgery, Lebanon, NH, USA

V. W. Nitti (✉) · R. D. Sussman
Department of Urology Georgetown University, Female Pelvic Medicine and Reconstructive Surgery, New York University, Department of Urology, New York, NY, USA
e-mail: vnitti@mednet.ucla.edu

K. C. Kobashi, S. D. Wexner (eds.), *Female Pelvic Medicine*,
https://doi.org/10.1007/978-3-030-54839-1_9

Patients with mixed urinary incontinence can be challenging to treat and are often more bothered by their symptoms than those patients with pure SUI [1]. When the history is not straightforward and patients either do not have demonstrable SUI on physical exam or have a history of mixed incontinence with significant urgency and/or urgency urinary incontinence (UUI), UDS can be very helpful to guide treatment decisions. Similarly, the American Urological Association guidelines on the surgical treatment of SUI recommend further evaluation in these patients [2].

In this patient, UDS demonstrated significant SUI along with DO but no urgency urinary incontinence (UUI). Assuming that the patient has significant bother from the SUI, it is reasonable to focus treatment on SUI based on UDS. It would be reasonable to start her an anticholinergic or beta-3 agonist to help with her overactive bladder (OAB) symptoms if she were interested, but this patient was mostly bothered by leakage associated with stress maneuvers and not interested in taking a daily medication. Occasionally patients with similar complaints will show significant UUI with no or minimal SUI, and these patients are best treated with therapies for OAB before surgical treatment for SUI.

Up to 50% of patients with SUI may have concomitant DO and UUI [3]. In this particular case, the patient was less bothered by urgency and frequency but more bothered by leakage of urine, which was clearly demonstrated with stress maneuvers on UDS. Thus, in this case, surgery for SUI would be offered to the patient with the understanding that OAB symptoms and urgency incontinence may persist postoperatively even if the SUI is cured.

Several studies have evaluated the effect of transvaginal sling placement for SUI on pre-existing urgency and UUI. Generally speaking, OAB symptoms will resolve postoperatively in 50–74% of patients, while 16–40% will have persistent or worsening of their OAB and UUI [4–8]. It is important that patients be well counseled in the preoperative period to set realistic expectations since patients with persistent OAB symptoms have decreased patient satisfaction after surgery [9].

Data on resolution of DO and UUI postoperatively by sling type are mixed. Some studies favor the TO MUS as this sling type has been associated with the least amount of persistent DO and UUI postoperatively [10, 11]. Other studies have found no difference in resolution of DO/UUI between RP and TO slings [7]. It is conceivable that the RP sling may be more obstructive compared to the TO, which could theoretically lead to a higher rate of OAB symptoms postoperatively.

A study of 305 women who underwent sling procedures for SUI found the TO sling to be least associated with persistence of DO on postoperative UDS. More clinically valuable, this same study looked at subjective data and found TO to have the lowest rate of postoperative UUI when compared to transvaginal tape (TVT), suprapubic arc sling (SPARC), and AF-PVS; however, this finding was only statistically significant for AF-PVS (odds ratio 4.06; 95% confidence interval 2.32–7.08) [11]. If the theory that obstruction may lead to persistence of OAB symptoms postoperatively holds, this finding makes sense, as AF-PVS are thought to be the most obstructive.

While long-term data is lacking, there is some suggestion that RP slings may be associated with better long-term results when compared to TO slings. This comes out of a randomized controlled trial by Schierlitz et al. [12], which found that women undergoing a TO sling were 15 times more likely (95% confidence interval 2–13) to fail when compared to those undergoing a RP sling. Similarly a meta-analysis by Ford et al. [13] found that while there was a limited long-term data to inform the need for repeat incontinence surgery, it was more likely in patients with a TO than RP sling (relative risk 8.79, 95% confidence interval 3.36–23.00).

Many advocates of the TO sling cite the TOMUS (Trial of Midurethral Sling) data, which showed that the overall number of serious adverse events was higher in the RP sling group than the TO sling group [14]. Most of this difference was attributed to the higher number of mesh exposures, voiding dysfunction requiring surgical intervention, and bladder perforation associated with the RP. While it is certainly important to inform patients undergoing sling placement of this data, bladder perforation, which, when recognized intraoperatively, causes minimal harm to the patient, accounted for 35% of those serious adverse events seen with RP slings in the TOMUS trial. Routine cystoscopy is done for the sole purpose of identifying such an injury, and if present, the trocar is simply re-passed. Even after a cystotomy during RP sing placement, the majority of patients can be successfully discharged home without catheter drainage [15]. Meanwhile, patients in the TO group were more likely to report neurologic symptoms, such as leg weakness and groin numbness, which, while rare, can be devastating for patients.

In patients such as this one, once the decision has been made to proceed with a MUS, the physician and patient must weigh the potential for increased postoperative urinary urgency with or without urgency incontinence following a RP sling, a potential for lower long-term efficacy with a TO sling, and the complication profile of both slings. After a prolonged discussion of risks and benefits associated with each sling type, this patient chose to proceed with a RP sling. Postoperatively she was dry with stable urgency and frequency of urination. She later expressed interest in trying a medication to help with these symptoms and was started on an anticholinergic medication. She is currently dry with minimal urgency and frequency.

Case Scenario 2

A 48-year-old obese woman with body mass index (BMI) of 35 and history of isolated stress urinary incontinence requiring six pads per day. On exam with a relatively empty bladder, the patient was found to have little urethral mobility (Q-tip test showing 10 degrees of deflection with Valsalva), and SUI was demonstrated. She comes with a report of urodynamics performed by an outside urologist which demonstrated isolated stress urinary incontinence with ALPP of 32. The patient has tried multiple diets and weight loss programs unsuccessfully.

It is not uncommon to see obese patients with complaints of SUI, as obesity itself manifests increased intra-abdominal pressures, which adversely stresses the pelvic floor and may contribute to the development of SUI [16]. In fact, epidemiological studies show a clear dose-response effect of weight on urinary incontinence with each 5-unit increase in BMI associated with about a 20–70% increase in risk for urinary incontinence [17]. Weight loss itself should be recommended for a patient's general health and may lead to improvement in SUI [18]. A randomized trial comparing a 6-month weight loss program with a structured education program in overweight and obese women with urinary incontinence showed that a mean weight loss of only 7.8 kg (8% of baseline weight) in the intervention group leads to a significant reduction in incontinence episodes (47% vs 28%, respectively) [19]. While weight loss itself may help, in a patient who is significantly bothered by symptoms and in whom weight loss is not realistic or who has attempted to lose weight unsuccessfully, definitive treatment should be offered.

There are two generally accepted mechanisms for the development of SUI in women: weakness of suburethral support resulting in urethral hypermobility and a defective urethral sphincter mechanism also known as intrinsic sphincter deficiency (ISD). Classically, patients with ISD have been described as having a "pipe-stem" or fixed urethra. It is important to realize that urethral hypermobility and ISD are not dichotomous and many patients may have features of both [20].

While there is not a consistent definition of ISD based on UDS parameters in the literature, most pelvic floor surgeons accept a maximum urethral closure pressure (MUCP) below 20 cm H_2O [21] or an ALPP below 60 cm H_2O to be suggestive of ISD [22]. Unfortunately, the rather arbitrary application of ALPP to the definition of ISD has been less than scientific. However, in this case, the very low ALPP of 32 cm H_2O (essentially gravitational incontinence) and the relative lack of urethral mobility are highly suggestive, if not diagnostic, of significant ISD.

While this patient came with a UDS report from an outside urologist corroborating the diagnosis of ISD, when SUI is seen on exam, UDS is not always necessary prior to offering treatment. The American Urological Association guideline on the surgical treatment of SUI [2] state that physicians may omit UDS when SUI is clearly demonstrated on exam in an uncomplicated patient. This guideline is supported by the Value of Urodynamic Evaluation (ValUE) trial which found that among women with uncomplicated demonstrable stress incontinence when compared to office evaluation alone, the addition of UDS showed no difference in outcomes as measured by clinical reduction in complaints [23]. Given this patient's elevated BMI, fixed urethra, and severity of incontinence, her clinical scenario would not be considered "uncomplicated," and therefore it is reasonable to offer UDS.

While it would be reasonable to offer this patient a RP sling or bulking agent, the gold standard for treatment for ISD is an AF-PVS. In this particular patient, one must specifically consider the patient's BMI, which increases surgical morbidity, and her expectations from the treatment.

The use of a midurethral sling (MUS) for the treatment of SUI theoretically works by correcting a weakness in the suburethral tissues by causing a dynamic kinking of the urethra with increases in abdominal pressure. Some argue that in cases of a fixed urethra, a MUS is not advised since additional tension may be needed to obtain the desired result, and this should be avoided when using mesh slings. Wlazlak et al. [24] looked at 109 women with urodynamically determined ISD who underwent TVT insertion and found that while there was an overall 6-month success rate of 81.6% in ISD patients, the reduced cure rates when compared to the entire SUI population were due to the subgroup with a hypomobile urethra. In cases of a true fixed urethra, we would not recommend treatment with an MUS; however, in patients with a low ALPP and a mobile urethra, RP slings have been shown to have success.

Treatment with a bulking agent may be appealing as it can be done under local anesthesia and avoids the risks associated with general anesthesia, which may be higher in an obese patient. A prospective study by Maher et al. [25] compared urethral bulking with Macroplastique to PVS in patients with ISD. When compared to PVS, Macroplastique was associated with a higher cost but reduced operative time, blood loss, hospital stay, and a quicker return to normal activity. While, in the short term, subjective cure rates were similar between Macroplastique and PVS (77% vs 90%, respectively, $p = 0.41$), objective cure rates at 6 months were significantly worse (9% vs 81%, $p < 0.001$), and at 5-year follow-up, the PVS group had reported higher continence and satisfaction rates compared to the Macroplastique group (69% vs 21% and 69 vs 29%, $p = 0.057$, respectively). In a patient who would like to avoid anesthesia, or who is motivated to lose a significant amount of weight and desires a short-term solution, treatment with a urethral bulking agent is a good option with the understanding that durable results are unlikely.

The gold standard for the treatment of all SUI caused by ISD associated with a fixed urethra is an AF-PVS. The modern-day PVS was popularized by McGuire and Lytton in 1978 [26]. Allografts, xenografts, and synthetic materials have been tried in an effort to decrease operative time, morbidity, pain, and hospital stay [27]. Woodruff et al. [28] performed a histological comparison of PVS materials (ten synthetic, five autologous, five allograft, and four xenograft) and found that the greatest degree of host fibroblast infiltration and neovascularization with minimal inflammatory or foreign body reaction was in autologous materials, which remains the gold standard.

Fascia lata harvested from the thigh has very similar properties to rectus fascia and can be used with comparable success rates [29]. Fascia lata harvest may have improved recovery time and unlike rectus fascia does not put the patient at risk for abdominal hernia formation. Disadvantages of this approach include intraoperative repositioning of the patient, which may increase operative time, and operating in an area that is less familiar to most pelvic surgeons [30]. While there are not any published studies directly comparing the complication profile and outcomes of rectus fascia to fascia lata, in our experience, we have found obese patients tend to have fewer complications with fascia lata given their increased risk of postoperative seroma and hernia formation with rectus fascia harvest. An exception to this is if a patient desires simultaneous abdominoplasty during which the rectus fascia can be harvested.

The above patient underwent an uncomplicated PVS with fascia lata harvest. She was observed overnight without complication and discharged the next day after her catheter was removed and she voided without difficulty. She was seen in the office for her 2-week follow-up appointment, at which point she denied any pain or urinary leakage.

Case Scenario 3

An 87-year-old female with a long-standing history of SUI requiring two to three pads per day that causes her significant perineal skin irritation. She reports leakage is most often with cough and worsens with exacerbations of her chronic obstructive pulmonary disease (COPD). Exam demonstrates severe vaginal atrophy with vulvar inflammation and erythema and a positive cough stress test. In addition to COPD, her past medical history includes severe arthritis, coronary artery disease, and atrial fibrillation, for which she is on anticoagulation.

While elderly patients comprise a large proportion of those presenting with urinary incontinence, there is a paucity of Level 1 evidence for interventions in the frail and elderly, and there is a systemic failure to include older people in clinical trials [31]. In any patient, prolonged contact of urine with the skin may lead to altered elasticity and blood flow causing incontinence-associated dermatitis [32]. This may be exacerbated in elderly patients who may have functional and dexterity limitations leading to less frequent pad changes. In addition to a barrier cream to prevent skin irritation, this patient would benefit from a topical vaginal estrogen cream to help with her atrophy and vulvar irritation. It should be noted that atrophic vaginitis by itself does not cause SUI and should not be treated solely for the purpose of decreasing incontinence [33].

In an elderly patient who is on anticoagulation and at a higher risk of complications from surgery, a less invasive treatment option is preferred. For cognitively intact frail persons, lifestyle changes, bladder training, and pelvic muscle exercises may be considered, but they have not been well studied in this population [33]. In patients with persistent and bothersome leakage, an incontinence pessary and a bulking agent are excellent next options.

While there are no comparative or direct observational studies concerning the use of incontinence pessaries to other treatments, these are low-risk devices and may be a good option for women looking for a noninvasive option, particularly those with very predictable leakage or poor surgical candidates. Robert et al. [34] studied the 1-year use of the incontinence ring pessary in women with urodynamically proven SUI and found that only 6 of 38 women (16%) continued to use the pessary at 1 year, with reasons for discontinuation being no benefit in 69% and inability to retain the pessary in 16% [34]. An additional barrier to pessary use in this patient is her limited dexterity, which would preclude her from doing self-pessary care and require regular visits for pessary maintenance and monitoring of tissue quality.

MUS may be offered to geriatric patients (defined as 65 years old or older in most studies); however, they should be counseled that they have a lower likelihood of successful clinical outcomes compared with younger patients [2]. Given the increased surgical risk in this patient due to her age, coronary artery disease, and need for anticoagulation, a urethral bulking agent is an excellent option. This can be done in the office and avoids the risk associated with general anesthesia. While there are no published studies looking at the safety of urethral bulking agents in patients on anticoagulation, it has been our experience that this can be done safely in patients in whom stopping is not deemed safe. As discussed above, urethral bulking agents do have limited success in the long term; however, this is less of a concern in an elderly patient with a shorter life expectancy than it may be in a younger patient looking for a long-term durable result.

This patient underwent an in-office urethral injection with calcium hydroxylapatite (Coaptite™) without stopping her warfarin. She had some mild hematuria postoperatively which resolved within 1 week. She voided without difficulty and while not completely dry now leaks only occasionally with a full bladder and wears one pad per day.

Case Scenario 4

A 55-year-old woman with SUI requiring four pads per day. She has a history of spina bifida and has been on clean intermittent catheterization (CIC) since childhood with no spontaneous voiding. She has been on anticholinergic medications to help with leakage but is not currently taking them, as she has not found them to be of benefit.

Adult patients with spina bifida have high incontinence rates with approximately 45–75% reporting some degree of urinary leakage [35]. In school-aged children with spina bifida, 68% have SUI [36]. SUI in patients with spina bifida and other neurologic conditions represents a different entity than SUI affecting neurologically intact patients and occurs due to a different pathophysiology. Malfunction of the pudendal nerve in these patients can result in an open fixed bladder neck and can prevent reflex contraction of the striated sphincter fibers during stress [37].

Patients with spina bifida and other spinal cord lesions may suffer from the other sequelae of neurogenic bladder including decreased bladder capacity, low compliance, and neuropathic overactivity. McGuire first associated a detrusor leak point pressure >40 cm H_2O with deterioration of renal function in children with myelomeningocele, and it is this number that most urologists use as a threshold to alter or escalate treatment [38]. When discussing treatment options of SUI in patients with neurogenic bladder, of utmost importance is maintaining bladder pressures at acceptable levels (<40 cm H_2O) to protect kidney function. Roth et al. [39] found that among 47 children with neurogenic bladder undergoing artificial urinary sphincters (AUS), 7 patients (15%) had a persistent physiologic alteration of detrusor dynamics consisting of a rigid, noncompliant bladder, which highlights the importance of follow-up UDS after a procedure to increase outlet resistance.

Prior to any surgical intervention in a patient with neurogenic bladder, we recommend obtaining baseline urodynamic testing to evaluate bladder function, specifically compliance, and ensure low filling pressures [2]. In this patient, we performed urodynamics which showed a bladder capacity of 400 mL with an end filling detrusor pressure of 9 cm H_2O, no detrusor overactivity, and SUI with an ALPP of 92 cm H_2O. As expected, she was unable to void during the study. While not an issue in this patient, in patients with detrusor overactivity and especially in those with significantly impaired compliance, it is important to optimize their bladder pressures (e.g., with anticholinergics, intradetrusor botulinum toxin injections, or in some cases bladder augmentation) prior to treatment of SUI.

The goal of surgical intervention in a patient who self-catheterizes is different than that of routine MUS placement. Because these patients rely on CIC to empty, the goal of anti-incontinence surgery in this population is simply to increase outlet resistance to prevent leakage in between catheterizations. An AF-PVS is ideal in this scenario as it is obstructive and can be tensioned appropriately with less concern for erosion or other mesh-related complications when compared with a synthetic sling [40]. Athanasopoulos et al. [41] looked at AF-PVS in women with SUI and neuropathic bladder and found success rates of 90.9%. Similarly, Gormley et al. [42] looked at AF-PVS in adolescent women with neurogenic bladder and found an overall continence rate of 92%.

Primary treatment of neurogenic SUI with bulking agent injections into an incompetent bladder neck may sound appealing because of its minimally invasive nature but has been shown to be of limited value. Halachmi et al. [43] found that endoscopic injection of a bulking agent in 33 patients with neurogenic SUI resulted in no cure and only 42% of patient reported any symptom improvement at a mean follow-up of 13 months. Similarly a recent study of 89 patients with neurogenic bladder and persistent incontinence after an AF-PVS found bladder neck injection to be of limited value, with repeat injections yielding no additional benefit [44].

In a patient with neurogenic bladder who does not rely on CIC, one may consider a synthetic MUS as this may have a lower rate of voiding dysfunction and urinary retention postoperatively. A recent prospective study of women with pathology at or below S2 looked at 40 women with neurogenic bladder undergoing either TVT or PVS and found cure rates (defined as a negative cough stress test at 250 mL) to be 80 and 85%, respectively, and found that while postoperative CIC was needed in all patients after PVS, de novo postoperative CIC could be avoided in 50% of patients after TVT [37].

The artificial urinary sphincter has also been used in women with neurogenic SUI in both women who void and those dependent on CIC. A recent series of 26 patients reported long-term functional outcomes after AUS and found an overall continence rate of 57.7% with a mean follow-up of 7.5 years (13.9–23.8.). In this series, survival rates without AUS revision were 75%, 51%, 51%, and 51% at 5, 10, 15, and 20 years, respectively, and survival rates without AUS explanation were 90%, 84%, 84%, and 74% at 5, 10, 15, and 20 years, respectively [45].

After baseline urodynamic testing, this patient underwent a successful AF-PVS with rectus fascia. An indwelling Foley catheter was left in place for 3 days after surgery, and after removal, the patient was able to resume CIC without difficulty. She denied any SUI in between catheterizations. In patients such as this, we recommend repeat urodynamic testing 6–12 months after sling placement to ensure low filling pressures and a follow-up renal ultrasound to ensure the absence of hydronephrosis.

This patient returned for videourodynamics 7 months after AF-PVS. At that time, she reported catheterizing every 4–6 hours for approximately 250 mL without any leakage in between. For the urodynamic study, she was filled to a capacity of 387 mL – after 300 mL, she had a slight rise in her detrusor pressure to an end filling pressure of 15 cm H_2O. Her fluoroscopic images showed no evidence of SUI and a closed bladder neck at rest. Her renal ultrasound did not show any hydronephrosis.

Case Scenario 5

A 67-year-old woman presents with recurrent SUI, dysuria, and urgency after failure of two prior midurethral slings, the first TO and the second RP. Office cystoscopy revealed a mesh erosion into the distal urethra, and urodynamics revealed no evidence of obstruction with urodynamic SUI and an abdominal leak point pressure (ALPP) of 70 cm H_2O.

An AF-PVS is ideal in this patient for two reasons. First, she has concomitant mesh erosion, and second, she has failed two prior synthetic slings.

The first step in this patient is to treat her urethral erosion with a mesh excision and urethral repair. As is outlined in the American Urological Association guidelines on the surgical treatment of SUI [2], it is not advisable to place another synthetic sling at the time of urethral reconstruction. If one were to elect a repeat synthetic sling, it would need to be done in a two-stage procedure with an initial mesh excision and urethral repair followed by a second procedure after a minimum of 3 months to allow for urethral healing. A single definitive operation to treat this patient's mesh erosion and recurrent SUI is ideal. Contrary to a synthetic sling, an AF-PVS can be placed at the same time as the initial mesh excision with similar success rates when compared to a staged procedure [46].

After failure of one synthetic sling, it would be appropriate to attempt a second synthetic sling as was initially done in this patient. In fact, a recent survey of members of the International Urogynecological Association (IUGA) found that when asked what treatment option they preferred for recurrent SUI after failed MUS, RP sling and urethral bulking agents were the most common responses offered by 81.5% and 48.6% of respondents, respectively [47]. Having failed a

TO sling, this patient underwent a repeat RP sling. While certainly reasonable, one must realize that repeat MUS have lower success rates than initial sling placement. A review of 1225 women undergoing MUS [48] found that the subjective cure rate was significantly lower in women undergoing a repeat MUS compared to those undergoing a primary MUS (62% vs 86%, $p < 0.001$). Among women undergoing a repeat MUS, the RP approach has significantly better success rates when compared to the TO approach (71% vs 48%, $P = 0.04$). Unlike synthetic slings, a recent multicenter prospective study [49] looked at women undergoing AF-PVS after MUS and found that objective and subjective cure rates did not differ significantly among women with prior MUS and those undergoing primary AF-PVS. This study did find higher rates of urinary retention requiring intermittent catheterization (8.5% vs 3.1%, $p < 0.001$) and higher re-operation rates for persistent incontinence (13.6% vs 3.5%, $p = 0.01$) in those patients with prior MUS. Another retrospective study [50] looked at women who underwent AF-PVS after failed MUS and reported a success rate of 69.7% that appeared to be durable at a mean follow-up of 14.5 months.

This patient not only has failed two MUS, but she also has a urethral erosion. That affects future treatment as much as any other factor. We would not recommend placement of another synthetic sling after a prior erosion. In a patient with a mesh erosion in the absence of recurrent SUI, it is debatable whether or not to proceed with a sling at the time of mesh removal. While there are no studies to date looking specifically at the development of recurrent SUI after sling removal for erosion, there are multiple studies looking at the need for repeat anti-incontinence procedures after sling removal for obstruction with rates ranging from 13% to 14% [51, 52]. For this reason, with urethral erosion in the absence of SUI, some may argue to treat the erosion and monitor the patient for the development of SUI prior to an additional procedure. In our experience, we have found rates of recurrent SUI to be higher when sling removal is done for erosion than obstruction. Thus, it is reasonable to consider concomitant sling placement due to the high risk of SUI after mesh removal and urethroplasty. Risks of the sling must be weighed against the risk of needing another intervention in the future. Therefore, we feel that placing an AF-PVS at the time of mesh removal and urethroplasty should be done on an individual basis with shared decision-making between the patient and the surgeon.

The patient presented here has both a urethral erosion and recurrent SUI. The risk of persistent SUI after mesh excision and urethroplasty approaches 100%, so if an AF-PVS is not done, the patient should expect a second procedure in the future if she desires to treat SUI. This patient underwent a mesh excision, urethroplasty, and AF-PVS. The eroded mesh appeared to be from the RP sling and was removed. The suburethral portions and bilateral arms of the both the RP and TO slings that were easily accessible were also removed to avoid any mesh in close proximity at the time of urethroplasty. The urethra was reconstructed, the periurethral fascia was closed, and a rectus fascia AF-PVS was placed. The patient had some difficulty urinating in the immediate postoperative period and required intermittent clean catheterization initially. She was voiding spontaneously with minimal leakage at her 2-week follow-up appointment.

Projection of What the Future Holds

While we have many excellent treatment options for women with SUI, there may be new treatments in the pipeline. In recent years, there has been a significant interest in stem cell use for treatment of SUI. Stem cells, which can be derived from a number of tissues including embryonic, adipose, muscle, bone marrow, mesenchymal, urinary, and umbilical cord tissue, are thought to improve tissue repair via multilineage differentiation and self-renewal [53].

Carr et al. [54] performed the first North American muscle-derived stem cell trials for SUI and demonstrated promising results with few adverse events and near 90% success at 1 year (defined as 50% or greater reduction in pad weight). A recent systematic review of the literature found that while to date cell therapy for SUI has been shown to be safe, it is too early to draw firm conclusions about the success of these treatments due to the small numbers of patients and the varied cell types, concentration rates, delivery methods, and numbers of doses in the current literature [55].

Pharmacologic research has been focused on drugs to increase outlet resistance. Duloxetine is a combined norepinephrine and serotonin reuptake inhibitor that has been shown to increase sphincteric activity in an animal experimental model [56]. The most recent Cochrane review on the use of duloxetine for SUI [57] found no difference in objective cure rates in patients treated with duloxetine, and while the drug may improve the quality of life for patients with SUI, it is unclear whether these benefits are sustainable. Duloxetine is currently approved in the European Union for women with moderate to severe stress incontinence and approved in the United States for the treatment of other disorders, but not currently approved for SUI.

The pelvic floor is rich in androgen receptors, and current evidence supports the use of androgens to increase pelvic floor muscle mass and strength [58]. In mice, the tissue-selective androgen receptor modulator (SARM) enobosarm has been shown to increase pelvic floor muscles in ovariectomized mice [59]. There is a current phase 2 clinical trial evaluating the use of this drug in postmenopausal women with SUI.

While not commonly used in the United States, in Europe, the artificial urinary sphincter (AUS) is considered a second-line treatment for SUI in women who have failed previous surgery or as a primary treatment in women with severe intrinsic sphincter deficiency [60, 61]. Recently robotic AUS placement has been studied and was found to be associated with decreased blood loss, complications, and hospital stay with comparable success rates [62].

The Vesair™ balloon (Solace Therapeutics, Framingham, MA) is a long-term, intravesical, polyurethane pressure-attenuating balloon that compresses during transient increases in intravesical pressure, such as a cough or a sneeze, and attenuates pressure fluctuations similar to a "shock absorber" [63]. A randomized trial evaluated the use of this balloon in women with SUI when compared to a sham procedure and found it to be safe and effective with 81% of women in the treatment arm having a 50% decrease in pad weight compared to 45% in the control group ($p = 0.0143$) and 41.6% of treatment patients with dry pad weights (<1 g) compared to 0% in the control group ($p < 0.001$) [64].

Another completely different minimally invasive balloon, Adjustable Continence Therapy (ACT™), is an adjustable continence device that consists of two silicone balloons placed on either side of the proximal urethra under the bladder neck, each attached to a titanium port buried in the labia to allow postoperative titration. In 57 women with urodynamically proven ISD who had failed prior pelvic therapy, ACT was found to decrease mean pad use from 5.6 times daily at baseline to 0.41 at 6-year follow-up [65]. While not approved in the United Sates, ACT is used in Europe in cases of women with intrinsic sphincter deficiency who have failed other therapies [66].

Summary

As highlighted in these five scenarios, not all SUI is the same. The importance of taking a careful history to elicit exactly how and when leakage happens, how urinary symptoms affect our patients lives, what patients find most bothersome, and what their treatment goals are cannot be overemphasized. In addition to a careful physical exam, voiding diaries or UDS can be useful adjuncts when the diagnosis remains unclear.

Commentary

E. Ann Gormley

Drs. Nitti and Sussman discuss five cases that illustrate the breadth and depth of decision-making in stress urinary incontinence (SUI) surgery. They discuss the details that are important to consider when deciding which procedure for which patient. The cases that they have provided are controversial, and they discuss the variety of options available to each patient, and then they justify their treatment choices.

In the introduction, they discuss the surgical options available for SUI. Although a Burch colposuspension is a safe and effective treatment option especially for the patient with limited vaginal access, in the patient who is undergoing concomitant abdominal surgery, we need to ensure that the patient understands that the outcomes with a Burch are inferior to an autologous fascia sling (AF-PVS) [67]. This is particularly important when counseling patients who seek alternatives to a synthetic. The patient who doesn't want a synthetic should be educated about the safety of midurethral slings (MUS) and if they still refuse to consider a MUS counseled about the cure rates and complications of all of their options. We need to ensure that the patient who refuses a synthetic shouldn't be offered only an inferior procedure.

The patient with stress-predominant mixed incontinence in Case Scenario 1 was offered treatment for SUI first as she was most bothered by her stress incontinence. Conversely, one may choose to try medical therapy prior to SUI surgery to ensure that the patient can take the prescribed drug. Patients with mixed incontinence may not experience much change in their incontinence on drug treatment, but after a 4- to 6-week course, they at least know that, should they require treatment for OAB post SUI treatment, there is a drug they can tolerate. Since patients with persistent OAB symptoms have decreased patient satisfaction after surgery, one can argue that it is reasonable to try patients with mixed UI on medical therapy for OAB prior to their SUI surgery. The patient who can't tolerate drugs for OAB can be forewarned that she may need third-line therapy if her OAB persists post SUI treatment.

In Case Scenario 2, the patient has a urodynamic test showing a low ALPP of 32 cm H_2O. The authors discuss that in some cases of ISD, provided that the urethra is not fixed, a MUS, typically a retropubic sling, can be used. In addition to considering ALPP and urethral mobility, another factor to consider when counseling patients about which sling to have is to consider how wet they are. In the TOMUS trial, the patients with ISD as a group were not terribly wet with relatively small pad weight tests [68]. Patients, like this patient, with large volume stress incontinence who wear six pads per day will likely do better in the long term with an AF-PVS.

Using fascia lata in the very obese patient is an excellent choice as not only should this reduce the risk of abdominal hernia, but it may also reduce the risk of abdominal wound breakdown. Wound breakdown following abdominal fascia harvest is often due to a seroma that requires that the wound be opened and then allowed to close by secondary intention. These wounds are large and deep and may require a wound vac. As the authors note, this has not been studied but it is a technique worth considering.

The patient in Case Scenario 3 is an ideal patient for an in-office urethral injection. As noted, anticoagulants don't need to be stopped; however, in many elderly patients, an upcoming procedure does provide a good opportunity to have the person prescribing the anticoagulation to re-assess the need for anticoagulation vs the ongoing risk. Although the treatment of the patient's atrophic vaginitis will not decrease her incontinence, it can be easier to inject transurethrally into healthier vs atrophic tissue. In the patient with very friable urethral mucosa, there may also be a role for a periurethral injection.

An AF-PVS is the best treatment for the patient in Case Scenario 4 with a history of spina bifida and a low-pressure, good capacity bladder. Since the patient already does CIC, many surgeons do tension slings in such patients tighter than in a patient without a neurogenic bladder. When the sling is placed at the bladder neck, there is no risk of erosion with a fascial sling. The patient will be able to easily continue to catheterize herself which may not be the case with an AUS.

The patient in Case Scenario 5 with the eroded sling, as the authors note, may also be treated in a staged manner. Although these patients often want "everything" fixed all at once, a staged approach allows one to ensure that the initial damage is fixed prior to potentially causing new complications. In this patient, I would likely have removed the portion of eroded sling prior to evaluating the leakage. I, too, generally recommend a fascial sling and not a repeat synthetic following a urethral erosion partially because the fascial sling at the bladder neck will be away from the repaired urethra. The major downside of doing everything at once is that when retention occurs post-op, the patient has to catheterize through her recently repaired urethra. There are surgeons who do a staged repair and after everything is healed offer the patient an MUS or an AF-PVS.

Drs. Nitti and Sussman finish this chapter with a review of new treatments. While our surgical treatments for SUI are very good, none are perfect. Additional treatments to our armamentarium will be welcomed by our patients.

References

1. Dooley Y, et al. Mixed incontinence is more bothersome than pure incontinence subtypes. Int Urogynecol J Pelvic Floor Dysfunct. 2008;19(10):1359–62.
2. Kobashi KC, et al. Surgical treatment of female stress urinary incontinence: AUA/SUFU guideline. J Urol. 2017;198(4):875–83.
3. Chou EC, et al. Effective treatment for mixed urinary incontinence with a pubovaginal sling. J Urol. 2003;170(2 Pt 1):494–7.
4. Wang KH, et al. Voiding dysfunction following TVT procedure. Int Urogynecol J Pelvic Floor Dysfunct. 2002;13(6):353–7; discussion 358.
5. Segal JL, et al. Prevalence of persistent and de novo overactive bladder symptoms after the tension-free vaginal tape. Obstet Gynecol. 2004;104(6):1263–9.
6. Choe JH, Choo MS, Lee KS. The impact of tension-free vaginal tape on overactive bladder symptoms in women with stress urinary incontinence: significance of detrusor overactivity. J Urol. 2008;179(1):214–9.
7. Botros SM, et al. Detrusor overactivity and urge urinary incontinence following trans obturator versus midurethral slings. NeurourolUrodyn. 2007;26(1):42–5.
8. Holmgren C, et al. Long term results with tension-free vaginal tape on mixed and stress urinary incontinence. Obstet Gynecol. 2005;106(1):38–43.
9. Mahajan ST, et al. Patient-centered surgical outcomes: the impact of goal achievement and urge incontinence on patient satisfaction one year after surgery. Am J Obstet Gynecol. 2006;194(3):722–8.
10. Lee JK, et al. Persistence of urgency and urge urinary incontinence in women with mixed urinary symptoms after midurethral slings: a multivariate analysis. BJOG. 2011;118(7):798–805.
11. Gamble TL, et al. Predictors of persistent detrusor overactivity after transvaginal sling procedures. Am J Obstet Gynecol. 2008;199(6):696.e1–7.
12. Schierlitz L, et al. Three-year follow-up of tension-free vaginal tape compared with transobturator tape in women with stress urinary incontinence and intrinsic sphincter deficiency. Obstet Gynecol. 2012;119(2 Pt 1):321–7.
13. Ford AA, et al. Mid-urethral sling operations for stress urinary incontinence in women. Cochrane Database Syst Rev. 2017;7:CD006375.
14. Richter HE, et al. Retropubic versus transobturator midurethral slings for stress incontinence. N Engl J Med. 2010;362(22):2066–76.
15. Crosby EC, et al. Expectant management of cystotomy at the time of midurethral sling placement: a retrospective case series. Int Urogynecol J. 2013;24(9):1543–6.
16. Cummings JM, Rodning CB. Urinary stress incontinence among obese women: review of pathophysiology therapy. Int Urogynecol J Pelvic Floor Dysfunct. 2000;11(1):41–4.
17. Subak LL, Richter HE, Hunskaar S. Obesity and urinary incontinence: epidemiology and clinical research update. J Urol. 2009;182(6 Suppl):S2–7.
18. Vissers D, et al. The effect of non-surgical weight loss interventions on urinary incontinence in overweight women: a systematic review and meta-analysis. Obes Rev. 2014;15(7):610–7.
19. Subak LL, et al. Weight loss to treat urinary incontinence in overweight and obese women. N Engl J Med. 2009;360(5):481–90.
20. Kayigil O, Iftekhar Ahmed S, Metin A. The coexistence of intrinsic sphincter deficiency with type II stress incontinence. J Urol. 1999;162(4):1365–6.
21. Sand PK, et al. The low pressure urethra as a factor in failed retropubic urethropexy. Obstet Gynecol. 1987;69(3 Pt 1):399–402.
22. McGuire EJ, et al. Clinical assessment of urethral sphincter function. J Urol. 1993;150(5 Pt 1):1452–4.
23. Nager CW, et al. A randomized trial of urodynamic testing before stress-incontinence surgery. N Engl J Med. 2012;366(21):1987–97.
24. Wlazlak E, et al. Role of intrinsic sphincter deficiency with and without urethral hypomobility on the outcome of tape insertion. NeurourolUrodyn. 2017;36(7):1910–6.
25. Maher CF, et al. Pubovaginal sling versus transurethral Macroplastique for stress urinary incontinence and intrinsic sphincter deficiency: a prospective randomised controlled trial. BJOG. 2005;112(6):797–801.
26. McGuire EJ, Lytton B. Pubovaginal sling procedure for stress incontinence. J Urol. 1978;119(1):82–4.
27. Niknejad K, et al. Autologous and synthetic urethral slings for female incontinence. Urol Clin North Am. 2002;29(3):597–611.
28. Woodruff AJ, et al. Histologic comparison of pubovaginal sling graft materials: a comparative study. Urology. 2008;72(1):85–9.

29. Latini JM, Lux MM, Kreder KJ. Efficacy and morbidity of autologous fascia lata sling cystourethropexy. J Urol. 2004;171(3):1180–4.
30. Govier FE, et al. Pubovaginal slings using fascia lata for the treatment of intrinsic sphincter deficiency. J Urol. 1997;157(1):117–21.
31. McMurdo ME, et al. Improving recruitment of older people to research through good practice. Age Ageing. 2011;40(6):659–65.
32. Ladha M, Wagg A, Dytoc M. An approach to urinary incontinence for dermatologists. J Cutan Med Surg. 2017;21(1):15–22.
33. Thuroff JW, et al. EAU guidelines on urinary incontinence. Eur Urol. 2011;59(3):387–400.
34. Robert M, Mainprize TC. Long-term assessment of the incontinence ring pessary for the treatment of stress incontinence. Int Urogynecol J Pelvic Floor Dysfunct. 2002;13(5):326–9.
35. Capitanucci ML, et al. Long-term urological follow-up of occult spinal dysraphism in children. Eur J Pediatr Surg. 1996;6 Suppl 1:25–6.
36. Hunt GM. Spina bifida: implications for 100 children at school. Dev Med Child Neurol. 1981;23(2):160–72.
37. El-Azab AS, El-Nashar SA. Midurethral slings versus the standard pubovaginal slings for women with neurogenic stress urinary incontinence. Int Urogynecol J. 2015;26(3):427–32.
38. McGuire EJ, et al. Prognostic value of urodynamic testing in myelodysplastic patients. J Urol. 1981;126(2):205–9.
39. Roth DR, et al. Urinary tract deterioration associated with the artificial urinary sphincter. J Urol. 1986;135(3):528–30.
40. Leach GE, et al. Female stress urinary incontinence clinical guidelines panel summary report on surgical management of female stress urinary incontinence. The American Urological Association. J Urol. 1997;158(3 Pt 1):875–80.
41. Athanasopoulos A, Gyftopoulos K, McGuire EJ. Treating stress urinary incontinence in female patients with neuropathic bladder: the value of the autologous fascia rectus sling. Int Urol Nephrol. 2012;44(5):1363–7.
42. Gormley EA, et al. Pubovaginal slings for the management of urinary incontinence in female adolescents. J Urol. 1994;152(2 Pt 2):822–5; discussion 826–7
43. Halachmi S, et al. Efficacy of polydimethylsiloxane injection to the bladder neck and leaking diverting stoma for urinary continence. J Urol. 2004;171(3):1287–90.
44. De Vocht TF, et al. Long-term results of bulking agent injection for persistent incontinence in cases of neurogenic bladder dysfunction. J Urol. 2010;183(2):719–23.
45. Phe V, et al. Stress urinary incontinence in female neurological patients: long-term functional outcomes after artificial urinary sphincter (AMS 800(TM)) implantation. NeurourolUrodyn. 2017;36(3):764–9.
46. McCoy O, et al. Outcomes of autologous fascia pubovaginal sling for patients with transvaginal mesh related complications requiring mesh removal. J Urol. 2016;196(2):484–9.
47. Giarenis I, et al. Management of recurrent stress urinary incontinence after failed midurethral sling: a survey of members of the International Urogynecological Association (IUGA). Int Urogynecol J. 2015;26(9):1285–91.
48. Stav K, et al. Repeat synthetic mid urethral sling procedure for women with recurrent stress urinary incontinence. J Urol. 2010;183(1):241–6.
49. Parker WP, Gomelsky A, Padmanabhan P. Autologous fascia pubovaginal slings after prior synthetic anti-incontinence procedures for recurrent incontinence: a multi-institutional prospective comparative analysis to de novo autologous slings assessing objective and subjective cure. NeurourolUrodyn. 2016;35(5):604–8.
50. Milose JC, et al. Success of autologous pubovaginal sling after failed synthetic mid urethral sling. J Urol. 2015;193(3):916–20.
51. Singla N, et al. Management of urinary incontinence following suburethral sling removal. J Urol. 2017;198(3):644–9.
52. Clifton MM, et al. Risk of repeat anti-incontinence surgery following sling release: a review of 93 cases. J Urol. 2014;191(3):710–4.
53. Tran C, Damaser MS. The potential role of stem cells in the treatment of urinary incontinence. Ther Adv Urol. 2015;7(1):22–40.
54. Carr LK, et al. 1-year follow-up of autologous muscle-derived stem cell injection pilot study to treat stress urinary incontinence. Int Urogynecol J Pelvic Floor Dysfunct. 2008;19(6):881–3.
55. Vinarov A, et al. Cell therapy for stress urinary incontinence: present-day frontiers. J Tissue Eng Regen Med. 2018;12:e1108–21.
56. Thor KB, Katofiasc MA. Effects of duloxetine, a combined serotonin and norepinephrine reuptake inhibitor, on central neural control of lower urinary tract function in the chloralose-anesthetized female cat. J Pharmacol Exp Ther. 1995;274(2):1014–24.
57. Mariappan P, et al. Serotonin and noradrenaline reuptake inhibitors (SNRI) for stress urinary incontinence in adults. Cochrane Database Syst Rev. 2005;3:CD004742.
58. Ho MH, Bhatia NN, Bhasin S. Anabolic effects of androgens on muscles of female pelvic floor and lower urinary tract. Curr Opin Obstet Gynecol. 2004;16(5):405–9.
59. Ponnusamy S, et al. Tissue selective androgen receptor modulators (SARMs) increase pelvic floor muscle mass in ovariectomized mice. J Cell Biochem. 2017;118(3):640–6.
60. Lucas MG, et al. EAU guidelines on surgical treatment of urinary incontinence. Actas Urol Esp. 2013;37(8):459–72.
61. Abrams P, et al. Fourth International Consultation on Incontinence Recommendations of the International Scientific Committee: evaluation and treatment of

urinary incontinence, pelvic organ prolapse, and fecal incontinence. NeurourolUrodyn. 2010;29(1):213–40.
62. Peyronnet B, et al. Artificial urinary sphincter implantation in women with stress urinary incontinence: preliminary comparison of robot-assisted and open approaches. Int Urogynecol J. 2016;27(3):475–81.
63. van Koeveringe GA, et al. Minimal device encrustation on vesair intravesical balloons in the treatment of stress urinary incontinence: analysis of balloons removed from women in the SOLECT trial. Adv Ther. 2017;34(7):1686–94.
64. Wyndaele JJ, et al. A randomized, controlled clinical trial of an intravesical pressure-attenuation balloon system for the treatment of stress urinary incontinence in females. NeurourolUrodyn. 2016;35(2):252–9.
65. Kocjancic E, et al. Adjustable continence therapy for severe intrinsic sphincter deficiency and recurrent female stress urinary incontinence: long-term experience. J Urol. 2010;184(3):1017–21.
66. Vidart A, et al. Guidelines for the treatment of non-neurological urinary incontinence in women using periurethral balloons. Prog Urol. 2010;20 Suppl 2:S150–4.
67. Brubaker L, et al. Five year continence rates, satisfaction and adverse events of burch urethropexy and fascial sling surgery for urinary incontinence. J Urol. 2012;187(4):1324–30.
68. Richter HE, et al. Retropubic versus transobturator midurethral slings for stress incontinence. N Engl J Med. 2010;362(22):2066–76.

10 Refractory Overactive Bladder

Philip E. V. Van Kerrebroeck

Case Scenario 1

A 42-year-old woman is referred by her general practitioner to the urologist because of persistent symptoms of overactive bladder (OAB) (wet) after conservative therapy (pelvic floor exercises, several antimuscarinics). The referral letter ends with the question: "What is the possible additional therapy?"

Refractory OAB

Following are the first and foremost questions:

- What is OAB (overactive bladder)?
- What is refractory OAB?

The ICS definition of OAB (reference ICS) states that it is synonymous to: "Urgency with or without urgency incontinence, usually with frequency and nocturia" [1]. Additionally, the OAB definition has been complemented by a division of the patients in two groups: the OAB-wet (patients with urgency incontinence) and the OAB-dry group (patient with the urgency frequency syndrome without urgency incontinence). This may be important as the difference in symptoms or the accumulation of symptoms may have an impact on the expectations of the patient [2]. This will influence the patient-reported outcomes (PROs), and thus, the definition of failure of conservative therapy, which accordingly defines "refractory OAB."

In the treatment of patients with OAB-wet, the treating physician may consider a decrease in pad use to suggest that a treatment is effective, but the patient might striving to be completely dry. Another important consideration regarding efficacy is the durability of the treatment. For how long should a treatment be efficacious before it can be classified as "successful," which would render any subsequent OAB symptoms to be "recurrent" rather than "refractory" to treatment? Also which additional treatments remain viable options after initial approaches have failed?

Equally important is the question: "What is the definition of failure of previous, maximal conservative treatment?"

Failure is arguably the opposite of success, but then again what is success? Successful treatment is treatment that turns a symptomatic patient into an asymptomatic individual. However, the patient's perspective may differ from that of the clinician, and the patient's perspective can be modulated by defining what can be expected from a specific treatment prior to its implementation. Consequently, it is very important for the

Commentary by David E. Rapp, University of Virginia, Department of Urology, Charlottesville, VA, USA

P. E. V. Van Kerrebroeck (✉)
Maastricht University Medical Center, Department of Urology, Maastricht, The Netherlands

K. C. Kobashi, S. D. Wexner (eds.), *Female Pelvic Medicine*,
https://doi.org/10.1007/978-3-030-54839-1_10

patient and physician to define clearly the goals of treatment. Realistic expectations are the key to success. Furthermore, as OAB is a syndrome composed of several elements, a complete disappearance of all symptoms is the optimal outcome, but a partial relief may be perceived as sufficient by the patient. Therefore, aspects of quality of life (QoL) are very important in the evaluation of patients with OAB. The impact of a treatment on QoL can be appreciated by the simple question "Are you satisfied with the treatment?" or can be evaluated with validated questionnaires, for example, (just to quote one!) the Patients Perception of Bladder Condition (PPBC). In clinical practice, the individual appreciation of the patient with OAB symptoms will determine if a treatment modality is considered successful or at least sufficient, and if the OAB must be defined as "refractory or persistent" and indeed necessitates additional treatment.

Evaluation of Treatment Success

Treatment success can be defined in various different ways [3]. Basically, we can employ either an anchor-based approach or a distribution-based approach of outcome measure. In both approaches, a predefined goal is essential, and this is the basis in the calculation of minimal important difference values for outcome questionnaires.

The Anchor-Based Approach to Treatment Success

After treatment, the patient is dry with complete urinary control as a patient-reported outcome (PRO) and objective confirmation with pad test and frequency–volume chart (FVC). In an anchor-based approach, the outcome of treatment is reported as a change of parameter value above or below a predefined cut-off point: for example, in the above example, treatment in the OAB-wet patient is considered successful if the patient is dry. As for another example of an anchor-based approach: in QoL evaluation after treatment, this could mean that the subject has achieved a score that is above the cut-off point for normals.

The Distribution-Based Approach to Treatment Success

Success of treatment can arbitrarily be defined as a 25% improvement in relevant (but is 25% clinically significant?) parameter(s) when comparing treatment with a placebo or an active comparator. In such a distribution-based approach, the outcome of treatment is reported as a change in the distribution of parameter values. Other examples are: treatment in OAB-wet patients is successful if a more than 50% decrease in leaking episodes is achieved or in QoL evaluation if a 20% improvement in score is achieved, as compared to the pretreatment level. In the latter example another question arises, namely, what does the patient consider a "relevant" or "clinically significant"improvement?

Clinical Significance

Clinical significance as perceived by clinicians is usually derived from distribution-based outcomes in RCTs and registration studies and not based on PROs. Some level of clinical efficacy of a treatment modality is not necessarily equivalent to cure or clinical relevance. Typically, however, an anchor-based approach of treatment outcome better defines the possibilities for cure of the patient and a distribution-based approach better and more easily shows some level of efficacy of the treatment.

Step-Up Approach in Refractory OAB

The fact to be confronted with refractory or persistent OAB raises the demand for a step-up algorithm (second- or third-line treatment). Such algorithms are not evidence based and, hence, clinical practice and experience (expert opinion!) will leading. Fortunately, in recent years, some progress has been made and controlled randomized series tried to guide the choice of additional treatment. However, it is not only the lack of evidence that limits the description of the "ideal" step-up algorithm, but other factors are important as well. Is such a step-up algorithm (after drug failure) identical for OAB-wet and OAB-dry patients, or are there differences in the cost-effectiveness or cost-utility equation? The expectations of the patient are as important as nonurological determinants, such as regulatory and cultural issues, access to treatment modalities, local budget restraints, and the framework of individual clinical practice (are all additional treatment modalities present in a specific environment).

Failure of conservative treatment in OAB is often due to unrealistic expectations of the patient or poor previous management based on an inadequate evaluation. Many patients that come for treatment of refractory OAB have never even completed the most basic of assessments, namely, an FVC or bladder diary. In most failures, it is therefore appropriate to just start from the beginning and recommence conservative management. Furthermore, the possible benefits of combination treatments (medication and pelvic floor rehabilitation exercises) have often not been tried and, therefore, should be considered before embarking on additional treatment modalities.

Discussion on the failure of conservative treatment should include an evaluation of other health problems. Some OAB patients seem to fail because of constipation as a side effect of anticholinergic medication. In these patients, the combination of an anticholinergic and medication for the treatment of constipation or a switch to a β3 agonist may be appropriate and more effective. Case series of women who underwent surgical repair for pelvic organ prolapse in the presence of urgency urinary incontinence have indicated that resolution of urgency urinary incontinence can be expected in one-third to two-thirds of selected (i.e., with low-pressure detrusor overactivity) patients [4].

Furthermore, many patients with refractory OAB, unlike neurogenic detrusor overactivity patients, complain of pain or hypersensitivity of the urethra and/or the bladder. This is a specific group of OAB patients in which alternative additional therapies may be indicated not directly aiming at alleviating the symptoms of OAB.

Behavioral treatment should always go hand in hand with drugs. However, the intensity of treatment needed for this type of therapy to achieve effectiveness has not been established. Furthermore, methods of long-term maintenance remain undefined.

Case Scenario 2

A 42-year-old woman is referred by her general practitioner to the urologist because of persistent symptoms of OAB (wet) after conservative therapy (pelvic floor exercises, several antimuscarinics). The referral letter ends with the question: “What is the possible additional therapy?”

After careful evaluation, idiopathic OAB-wet was confirmed, and conservative therapy (6 weeks of antimuscarinics in combination with pelvic floor exercises) was tried without any significant amelioration.

This patient is confirmed to suffer from OAB (wet) and presents with a failure of conservative therapy. However was the conservative therapy maximal or is there still room for continuation/adaptation of the conservative therapy? For example, it has been shown that increasing the dosage of the antimuscarinic solifenacin from 5 to 10 mg can further improve OAB symptoms in patients who requested a dose increase after 8 weeks of treatment with 5 mg solifenacin [5]. That study supported the view that patients with severe OAB symptoms can benefit from a higher antimuscarinic dose. However, it also has been demonstrated that consecutive trials with different antimuscarinics significantly reduce the percentage of success that can be reached. Hence, it seems questionable that multiple courses of antimuscarinic treatment should be prescribed. A new pharmacological category, the β3-agonists, have been added to our therapeutic armamentarium for the treatment of OAB. In phase III clinical trials, the β3-agonist mirabegron showed significant efficacy in treating symptoms of OAB and appeared to be well tolerated [6]. Furthermore, the efficacy of mirabegron in patients who failed antimuscarinic therapy is similar to that of treatment-naive patients. A recent review of the literature, therefore, concluded that antimuscarinic monotherapy, mirabegron monotherapy, or combination treatment with mirabegron added to the antimuscarinic agent solifenacin significantly reduces the symptoms of urgency compared with placebo [7]. The same authors state that combination therapy with mirabegron added on to solifenacin also significantly reduces the symptoms of severe urgency compared with antimuscarinic agent monotherapy. Hence, a combination therapy provides an alternative treatment in patients with OAB who respond poorly to first-line monotherapy and who may otherwise often move on to more invasive treatments.

Case Scenario 3

A 42-year-old woman is referred by her general practitioner to the urologist because of persistent symptoms of OAB (wet) after conservative therapy (pelvic floor exercises, several antimuscarinics). The referral letter ends with the question: "What is the possible additional therapy?"

After careful evaluation, idiopathic OAB-wet was confirmed and conservative therapy (6 weeks of antimuscarinics in combination with pelvic floor exercises) was tried without any significant amelioration.

The β3 agonist mirabegron was prescribed at 50 mg for 6 weeks with limited effect and later combined with solifenacin 10 mg for another 6 weeks without clinically significant amelioration. The patient returns to the urologist and asks for additional treatment.

The urologist discusses different forms of neuromodulation therapy or onabotulinum toxin A injections.

Neuromodulation

When starting the evaluation of a patient considered a potential candidate for neuromodulation as a treatment for refractory OAB, the patient should be asked about her expectations. Often, these turn out to be unrealistic, and in the mind of the patient, the centers for neuromodulation might even look more like a "pilgrimage center for refractory OAB-sufferers that is going to offer a miracle cure," than a clinical facility. Furthermore, a considerable minority suffers from psychological or even psychiatric problems that may not be obvious at first visit. Referral to a psychiatrist, when the suspicion arises, is useful but usually is not very helpful if the goal is "cure" of the psychiatric problem. Cooperation with a psychiatrist may be helpful in terms of looking for a confirmation of the suspicion of a psychiatric problem, and/or exclusion from further evaluation for neuromodulation.

Different forms of neuromodulation exist and new neuromodulation approaches are emerging. There is no clear guidance regarding which algorithm should be followed, and there is lack of uniformity in the different stimulation programs and settings that should be applied. Noninvasive forms of neuromodulation (TENS stimulation, intravaginal and intra-anal stimulation, magnetic stimulation) have been applied with variable successes [8, 9]. Even if they have become less fashionable in recent years, it still may be worthwhile in individual motivated patients. These therapies also require strong motivation from the caregivers, are laborious, and a high recurrence rate has been observed after stopping the therapy. Other forms of minimal invasive neuromodulation techniques have been developed for treatment of OAB. The most researched option that has FDA approval is the percutaneous tibial nerve stimulation (PTNS) [10]. With this technique, a needle is percutaneously placed in the neighborhood of the tibial nerve and stimulation is applied through an external stimulator at various intervals. Chronic maintenance stimulation is generally needed at 30 min/day. Recently, an implantable device has been developed that allows for permanent unilateral implantation at the level of the tibial nerve and can achieve excellent results in refractory OAB (Fig. 10.1) [11].

Sacral Nerve Stimulation

As a permanent form of neuromodulation for OAB (wet and dry), sacral nerve stimulation (SNS) has been explored and has been available for clinical application for over 25 years [12, 13].

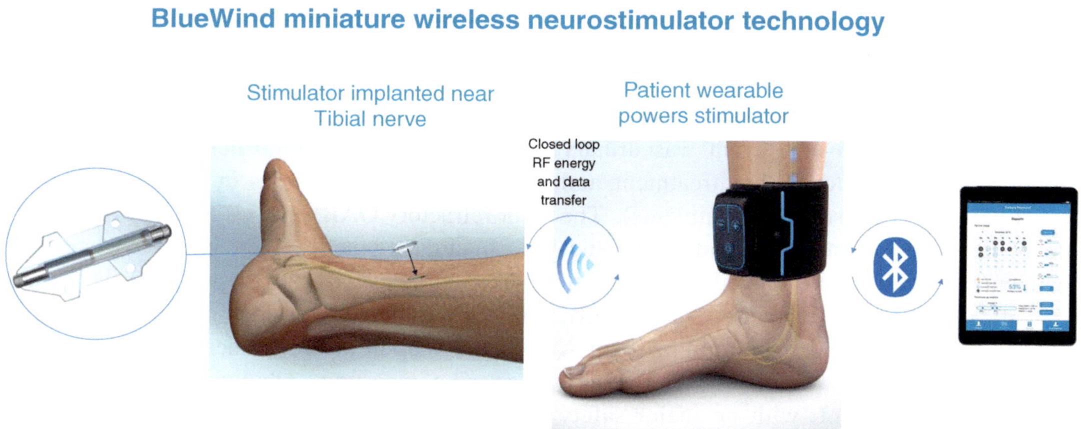

Fig. 10.1 The BlueWind RENOVA iStim™ system for permanent tibial nerve stimulation. (Reused with permission. Copyright BlueWind Medical)

Formerly, about 50% of patients passed the traditional PNE test and were candidates for implantation. After a follow-up of 5 years, 85.7% of patients that were successful at 12 months were still successful [14]. However, after the introduction of the two-stage implant technique, using the permanent electrode (tined lead), the percentage of patients that went on to a permanent implant increased to about 70–75% [15]. Recent published long-term results of OAB patients who underwent a two-stage implant with the tined lead technique have confirmed the excellent long-term results with 82% of patients still successful after 5 years [16]. These excellent results however have to be matched against the potential adverse events. In these series, the cumulative rate of adverse events that required surgical intervention was 22.4%. In total, a surgical intervention was performed in 30.9% of patients due to adverse events, and 33.5% of patients underwent an intervention for battery replacement.

Recently, a new form of sacral nerve stimulation has been developed in which a permanent sacral electrode is connected to an on-demand pulse generator that can be recharged with an external system (Fig. 10.2) [17]. This battery should have a life span of up to 25 years. In clinical research, this system is an effective treatment for patients with OAB and promises to be a more cost-effective alternative to the non-rechargeable pacemaker that needs replacement every 4–6 years.

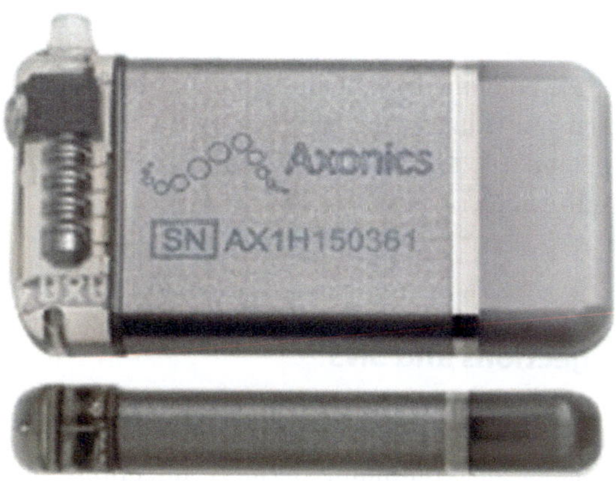

Fig. 10.2 The Axonics® rechargeable Sacral Neuromodulation (r-SNM®) system for the treatment of urinary and bowel dysfunction. (Reused with permission. Copyright John Wiley and Sons (24))

The Axonic rechargeable implant is MRI proof and since January 2020 also Medtronic introduced an MRI proof rechageable and recharge free implant.

Botulinum Toxin Injection

In both Europe and the USA, onabotulinum toxin A has been registered for treatment of nonneurogenic OAB at a dosage of 100 UI and is reimbursed in many countries. A prospective, multicenter, 3.5-year follow-up study with 100 UI onabotulinum toxin A for OAB showed consistent mean reductions in urinary incontinence, ranging from 74% following the first injection to 78.3–83.2% after subsequent treatments [18]. The median duration of effect was 7.6 months. The most common adverse event was urinary tract infection (17% after the first treatment, and 14.4–17.5% after subsequent treatments). The rate of de novo catheterization after the first treatment was 4.0%, and it ranged from 0.6% to 1.7% after subsequent treatments. Accordingly, it seems that long-term onabotulinum toxin A treatment consistently decreases OAB symptoms and improves QoL with no major safety signals.

However, in view of the potential risk of even temporary urinary retention or incomplete bladder emptying, and an increased incidence of urinary tract infections, it is advisable to discuss these potential risks with the patient beforehand, and individuals must be prepared to accept the potential need to perform intermittent self-catheterization.

Choice Between Onabotulinum Toxin Injections and SNS

Before continuing on the path of neuromodulation or onabotulinum toxin A injections in a case in which the diagnostic process has been completed elsewhere, the clinician should ensure that they are comfortable with the evaluation. Re-evaluation or completion of the evaluation at one's own institution should be performed as deemed necessary by the treating physician. The quality of the previous treatment should also be scrutinized to confirm the conclusion that a given patient is truly refractory to (maximal) conservative management and is willing to accept the pros and cons of these additional therapies.

Discussion regarding the durability of an effective treatment is also relevant. Patients on botulinum toxin will need to have repeat injections within a window of 6–12 months, and this may influence her decision to choose this treatment versus neuromodulation as a permanent therapy. However, actual pacemaker technology necessitates battery replacement surgery at regular intervals (4-6 years), although the available rechargeable systems potentially reduce the need for replacement surgey significantly. Additional follow-up studies should help to position these new treatment modalities in the final algorithm for refractory OAB.

In clinical practice, there is still a debate as to which strategy is best: to start with botulinum injections first or consider neuromodulation as the first step in third-line therapy following conservative measures. Obviously, after consideration of balanced information regarding both modalities, the patient's preference will be an important factor. Some patients are reluctant to accept implantation of a foreign body and, therefore, refuse sacral neuromodulation. Others cannot accept the eventual risk of retention and the potential need for intermittent catheterization and will therefore not choose for botulinum toxin injections.

Currently, an evidence-based choice between sacral neuromodulation and botulinum toxin remains open for discussion. The ongoing comparative trial in a large group of US women with severe urgency urinary incontinence (UUI) who received sacral neuromodulation (InterStim) (Fig. 10.3) or 200 UI of onabotulinum toxin A (Botox A) therapy at 2-year follow-up showed that both therapies had similar success in reducing UUI symptoms, and adverse events were low [19]. However, women in the Botox A group had higher satisfaction and endorsement with their

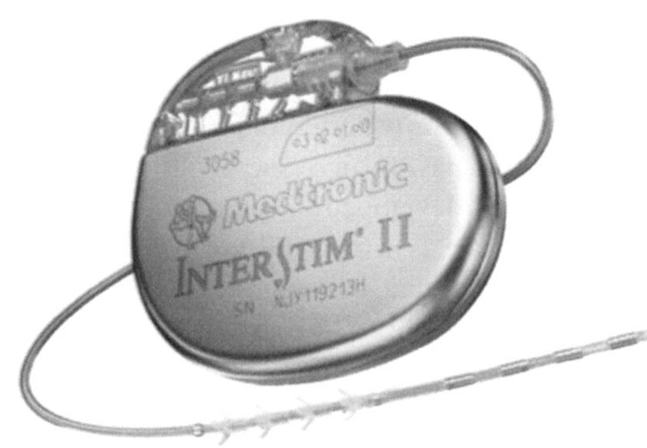

Fig. 10.3 The Medtronic InterStim II implantable pulse generator for sacral neuromodulation. (Reused with permission. Copyright Medtronic)

treatment, albeit with a higher risk of developing a urinary tract infection (24% versus 10%) and a 6% risk of needing to perform self-catheterizations after the second injection.

Case Scenario 4

A 42-year-old woman is referred by her general practitioner to the urologist because of persistent symptoms of OAB (wet) after conservative therapy (pelvic floor exercises, several antimuscarinics). The referral letter ends with the question: "What is the possible additional therapy?"

After careful evaluation, idiopathic OAB-wet was confirmed and conservative therapy (6 weeks of antimuscarinics in combination with pelvic floor exercises) was tried without any significant amelioration.

The β3 agonist mirabegron was prescribed at 50 mg for 6 weeks with limited effect and later combined with solifenacin 10 mg for another 6 weeks without clinically significant amelioration. The patient returned to the urologist and asked for additional treatment.

The urologist discussed treatment with onabotulinum toxin injections or SNS.

The patient chooses onabotulinum toxin injection treatment. Under local anesthesia, 100 UI Botox is injected, divided into 20 injections into the detrusor wall. After 6 weeks, the onabotulinum toxin injection(s) have insufficient effect.

Failure of Onabotulinum Toxin Injection(s)

Several reasons for failure of a first session of onabotulinum toxin A can be considered. The first cause could be a suboptimal dosage. The dose in nonneurogenic OAB as recognized by regulatory bodies is 100 IU, but in some patients, a higher dosage may be necessary in order to achieve sufficient effect. Of course, injection technique may play a role as inadequate injection (too deep, too superficial, incorrect location) may limit the effective dosage that reaches the intramural nerve fibers. Furthermore, as with medical therapy, the effect may be incomplete and persistent symptoms may occur. Also the efficacy may be limited in duration (less than 6 months). Increasing the dosage for a next series of injections hence may be the answer but must be balanced against the increased risk of side effects (postvoid residual, need for catheterization, recurrent urinary tract infections). Globally, lack of success can be classified into three categories: no symptomatic relief, partial response (some symptoms such as urgency urinary incontinence may disappear, while others such as abnormal voiding frequency remain), persistent symptoms with reduced intensity or frequency. Persistent symptoms can also be the consequence of a lower urinary tract infection, and therefore, urine should be checked for infection in patients with refractory OAB after onabotulinum toxin injection.

In cases of partial or complete failure, reinjection may be considered using optimal technique (a procedure under sedation or anesthesia may be considered if this facilitates injections). If no technical issues are obvious, increasing the dosage could be an option if the patient accepts the potential increased risk for side effects. In the situation of partial effects, additional therapy may be emphasized, making use of the possibilities available. This may include conservative therapy (lifestyle and behavior modification, acupuncture even hypnotherapy, pelvic floor rehabilitation, pharmacological support) as well as electrical stimulation (TENS, intravaginal, intraanal PTNS).

If failure is persistent despite multiple attempts and adaptations of technique and dosages, patient scenario 5 can be considered.

Case Scenario 5

A 42-year-old woman is referred by her general practitioner to the urologist because of persistent symptoms of OAB (wet) after conservative therapy (pelvic floor exercises, several antimuscarinics). The referral letter ends with the question: "What is the possible additional therapy?"

After careful evaluation, idiopathic OAB-wet was confirmed and conservative therapy (6 weeks of antimuscarinics in combination with pelvic floor exercises) was tried without any significant amelioration.

The β3 agonist mirabegron was prescribed at 50 mg for 6 weeks with limited effect and later combined with solifenacin 10 mg for another 6 weeks without clinically significant amelioration. The patient returned to the urologist and asked for additional treatment.

The urologist discussed treatment with botulinum toxin injections or neuromodulation therapy.

The patient chose onabotulinum toxin A injection treatment. However, either multiple injection sessions had no effect, or in spite of initial symptom relief, the efficacy was not durable, and the patient requests additional treatment. Another potential scenario may include a patient who has successful onabotulinum toxin A injection(s) but wishes to pursue a more "permanent" solution.

SNM Treatment After (Failed/Successful) Onabotulinum Toxin Injection(s)

Limited evidence is available on the effects of SNM after onabotulinum toxin A injection(s). Two studies that looked specifically at this question indicate that sacral neuromodulation is a suitable treatment option in those patients who have had prior onabotulinum toxin A treatment for refractory OAB, even in those for whom botulinum proved ineffective [20, 21]. Success rates were within the published range, and comparable to the results for sacral neuromodulation in patients with OAB without prior botulinum toxin treatment. Also there seems to be no difference in the efficacy of sacral neuromodulation in patients who were successful but are dissatisfied with the therapy or in those in whom botulinum toxin A treatment failed. Long-term follow-up studies are needed to confirm that sacral neuromodulation will continue to yield similar results in this specific category of patients with refractory OAB.

A Markov state transition decision analysis model was constructed using values for efficacy and complications from the literature for both SNM with the InterStim system and Botox injections [22]. Overall utility was compared monthly, and multiple 1-way sensitivity analyses were performed. For every month during the simulation, overall utility was higher for Botox than InterStim, but the authors conclude that until appropriately powered randomized controlled trials are available, both therapies are reasonable and effective strategies with comparable outcomes.

Onabotulinum Toxin Injection After Insufficient or Failed SNM

No controlled series are available that discuss the results of additional onabotulinum toxin injections after failed or partially successful SNM therapy for refractory OAB. Clinical experience indicates that this is a reasonable option if acceptable for the patient.

Similarly, concurrent pharmacotherapy is a reasonable option in patients with partially successful SNM [23]. This approach has the advantage that it can be used for a certain period of time as it may happen that some patients have temporary recurrent symptoms even if sacral neuromodulation therapy is effective. OAB symptoms may aggravate incidentally due to other factors such as UTI, psychological issues, or trouble optimizing the neuromodulatory effect.

Last Resort Solutions

In view of the successes achieved in patients with refractory OAB with the actual therapeutic modalities, there is only a limited number of patients that will need last resort solutions. In clinical practice, last resort surgical procedures have been significantly reduced, and the number of good potential candidates is small. Additional procedures that may be considered are augmentation cystoplasty, bladder replacement surgery, and urinary diversion (continent or incontinent). For these procedures, different techniques are available and specific segments of the intestine can be used. For augmentation cystoplasty, in general, a ileal patch will be utilized and acceptable results can be achieved. However, elevated residual urine prompting the need for intermittent catheterization may pose a problem and will often be associated with urinary infections and stone formation. For bladder replacement, many techniques exist and different portions of the intestinal tract can be used. Most techniques, however, use small intestine (ileum). This type of neobladder surgery can result in "urethral hypercontinence" (= urinary retention) and can cause metabolic problems that must be monitored and medically addressed.

Similarly, continent urinary diversion requires large lengths of intestine and may be prone to technical complications with stomal incontinence or stenosis, the latter of which can result in difficulty with catheterization. These types of procedures require excellent surgical skills and experience. Reinterventions at long term follow-up are common and can be challenging. Finally, an incontinent urinary diversion (Bricker procedure) may be an acceptable and reasonable last resort intervention. Even if long-term complications occur and deterioration of kidney function becomes evident, overall quality of life in patients with refractory OAB and severe symptoms may be acceptable after this type of diversion.

The advent of specific protective and absorbent materials has contributed to a decreased demand for last resort interventions and has contributed favorably to quality of life for patients with (refractory) OAB. Proper selection of the material for a given individual is essential in order to guarantee a reasonable quality of life for women with refractory OAB who cannot or do not wish to be treated in a curative fashion.

Summary

Refractory OAB remains a challenging problem for physicians and patients alike. Proper diagnostics are essential in order to choose the most appropriate treatment modality and prevent refractory problems or limit them to the minimum. Many conservative treatment modalities eventually in combination are available for OAB and should be tried maximally. If optimal conservative approaches fail, additional strategies exist. Actual algorithms fail sufficient evidence to advise a strict algorithm, but the combination of existing evidence and data from clinical and individual practice together with close consultation with the patient regarding reasonable expectations and goals can facilitate appropriate selection and sequence of treatment. Sacral neuromodulation techniques also allow for a permanent solution with excellent results. Injection with onabotulinum toxin A is a reasonable alternative solution that is well tolerated and efficacious. If these treatments fail, several last resort solutions exist, though in some patients, a conservative protective approach may be an acceptable alternative for therapy-resistant refractory OAB.

Commentary

David E. Rapp

This chapter details the challenges that practitioners often face when treating patients with refractory overactive bladder (OAB). As this chapter highlights, this begins with defining success. Although there are numerous validated questionnaires that can be used to assess patient outcomes, there is no gold-standard questionnaire and great variation exists across providers with respect to questionnaire of choice [24]. Further, outside of patient-reported measures used to assess symptom improvement, it also commonly suggested that ultimately, it is patient satisfaction that may be most important [25].

Accordingly, Dr. Van Kerrebroeck highlights the importance that patient expectation can have on outcomes and patient satisfaction. For this reason, it is not only important to define the degree of improvement that a patient considers sufficient for satisfaction, but also the symptom of primary concern to each patient. Furthermore, it is best to do this in a formal fashion *prior to* surgery. For example, once defined, this shared outcome goal can be included both in the clinic note and written on educational materials given to patients so as to serve as a reference when discussing outcomes postoperatively.

Optimizing patient satisfaction is critical as we transition into the era of quality care and reimbursement models (value-based purchasing). Indeed, urinary incontinence assessment and treatment planning are both priority measures under the Merit-based Incentive Payment Program (MIPS) in the United States [26]. Further, patient satisfaction and experience surveys (e.g., HCAHPS, Hospital Consumer Assessment of Healthcare Providers and Systems) are increasingly being used as a metric of care quality and to shape reimbursement. Although such surveys reflect numerous aspects of the overall patient experience, patient satisfaction with treatment outcome no doubt plays a significant role in survey score. Such initiatives highlight the previously discussed importance of defining patient expectations when treating OAB in order to help promote satisfaction.

A second important consideration in this era of health care is cost. This chapter provides a comprehensive discussion of advanced therapies for refractory OAB. Indeed, the introduction of treatments such as botulinum toxin and neuromodulation has allowed urologists to transform the lives of many patients in a minimally invasive fashion. While these advances should be celebrated, we also must learn to utilize these treatments in a cost-effective manner. However, we presently lack detailed evidence-based algorithms to help guide clinical strategy. As Dr. Van Kerrebroeck details, debate exists with respect to choice of initial advanced therapy and also approaches to use if botulinum toxin or neuromodulation fails. Importantly, we need quality studies to help guide these algorithms with focus not only on clinical success but also cost-effectiveness. Although there is emerging evidence to help promote a cost-effective approach [27], much more is needed.

Finally, it is important to stress another critical treatment for refractory OAB – conservative therapy. Certainly, conservative therapies (dietary modification, behavioral therapy, pelvic floor physical therapy) should be exhausted prior to considering advanced therapies. However, they must also serve as important adjunctive approaches to advanced therapies. Far too often, patients consider advanced therapies as rationale to reinstitute behaviors unfavorable to successful bladder management. For this reason, long-term follow-up after advanced therapies can be helpful as an opportunity to not only assess symptom control but also to provide re-education regarding conservative approaches.

References

1. Abrams P, Cardozo L, Fall M, Griffiths D, Rosier P, Ulmsten U, Van Kerrebroeck P, Victor A, Wein A. The standardisation of terminology of lower urinary tract function: report from the Standardisation Sub-committee of the International Continence Society. NeurourolUrodyn. 2002;21(2):167–78.
2. Van Kerrebroeck P, Abrams P, Chaikin D, Donovan J, Fonda D, Jackson S, Jennum P, Johnson T, Lose G, Mattiasson A, Robertson G, Weiss J. The standardisation of terminology in nocturia: report from the Standardisation Sub-committee of the International Continence Society. NeurourolUrodyn. 2002;21(2):179–83.
3. Bosch JL, Kelleher C, Van Kerrebroeck PE, Schurch B. What treatment should we use if drugs fail for OAB; and, what really works after drugs? NeurourolUrodyn. 2010;29(4):658–61. https://doi.org/10.1002/nau.20906.
4. Chen A, McIntyre B, De EJB. Management of postoperative lower urinary tract symptoms (LUTS) after pelvic organ prolapse (POP) repair. Curr Urol Rep. 2018;19(9):74. https://doi.org/10.1007/s11934-018-0825-9.
5. Cardozo L, Amarenco G, Pushkar D, Mikulas J, Drogendijk T, Wright M, Compion G. Severity of overactive bladder symptoms and response to dose escalation in a randomized, double-blind trial of solifenacin (SUNRISE). BJU Int. 2013;111(5):804–10. https://doi.org/10.1111/j.1464-410X.2012.11654.x. Epub 2013 Jan 7.
6. Chapple C, Khullar V, Nitti VW, Frankel J, Herschorn S, Kaper M, Blauwet MB, Siddiqui E. Efficacy of the β3-adrenoceptor agonist mirabegron for the treatment of overactive bladder by severity of incontinence at baseline: a post hoc analysis of pooled data from three randomised phase 3 trials. Eur Urol. 2015;67(1):11–4. https://doi.org/10.1016/j.eururo.2014.06.052. Epub 2014 Aug 2.
7. Andersson KE, Choudbury N, Cornu J, Huang M, Korstanje C, Siddiqui E, Van Kerrebroeck P. The efficacy of mirabegron in the treatment of urgency and the potential utility of combination therapy. Ther Adv Urol. 2018;10(8):243–56.
8. Wang AC, Wang YY, Chen MC. Single-blind, randomized trial of pelvic floor muscle training, biofeedback-assisted pelvic floor muscle training, and electrical stimulation in the management of overactive bladder. Urology. 2004;63(1):61–6.

9. O'Reilly BA, Fynes M, Achtari C, Hiscock R, Thomas E, Murray C, Dwyer PL. A prospective randomised double-blind controlled trial evaluating the effect of trans-sacral magnetic stimulation in women with overactive bladder. Int Urogynecol J Pelvic Floor Dysfunct. 2008;19(4):497–502. Epub 2007 Oct 12.
10. Peters KM, Carrico DJ, Wooldridge LS, Miller CJ, MacDiarmid SA. Percutaneous tibial nerve stimulation for the long-term treatment of overactive bladder: 3-year results of the STEP study. J Urol. 2013;189(6):2194–201. https://doi.org/10.1016/j.juro.2012.11.175. Epub 2012 Dec 3.
11. Heesakkers JPFA, Digesu GA, van Breda J, Van Kerrebroeck P, Elneil S. A novel leadless, miniature implantable tibial nerve neuromodulation system for the management of overactive bladder complaints. NeurourolUrodyn. 2018;37(3):1060–7. https://doi.org/10.1002/nau.23401. Epub 2017 Sep 1.
12. Schmidt RA, Jonas U, Oleson KA, Janknegt RA, Hassouna MM, Siegel SW, Van Kerrebroeck PE. Sacral nerve stimulation for treatment of refractory urinary urge incontinence. J Urol. 1999;162(2):352–7.
13. Hassouna MM, Siegel SW, Nÿeholt AA, Elhilali MM, Van Kerrebroeck PE, Das AK, Gajewski JB, Janknegt RA, Rivas DA, Dijkema H, Milam DF, Oleson KA, Schmidt RA. Sacral neuromodulation in the treatment of urgency-frequency symptoms: a multicenter study on efficacy and safety. J Urol. 2000;163(6):1849–54.
14. Van Kerrebroeck PE, van Voskuilen AC, Heesakkers JP, Lycklama á Nijholt AA, Siegel S, Jonas U, Fowler CJ, Fall M, Gajewski JB, Hassouna MM, Cappellano F, Elhilali MM, Milam DF, Das AK, Dijkema HE, van den Hombergh U. Results of sacral neuromodulation therapy for urinary voiding dysfunction: outcomes of a prospective, worldwide clinical study. J Urol. 2007;178(5):2029–34. Epub 2007 Sep 1.
15. Leong RK, De Wachter SG, Nieman FH, de Bie RA, van Kerrebroeck PE. PNE versus 1st stage tined lead procedure: a direct comparison to select the most sensitive test method to identify patients suitable for sacral neuromodulation therapy. NeurourolUrodyn. 2011;30(7):1249–52. https://doi.org/10.1002/nau.20979. Epub 2011 Mar 14.
16. Siegel S, Noblett K, Mangel J, Bennett J, Griebling TL, Sutherland SE, Bird ET, Comiter C, Culkin D, Zylstra S, Kan F, Berg KC. Five-year follow-up results of a prospective, multicenter study of patients with overactive bladder treated with sacral neuromodulation. J Urol. 2018;199(1):229–36. https://doi.org/10.1016/j.juro.2017.07.010. Epub 2017 Jul 11.
17. Blok B, Van Kerrebroeck P, de Wachter S, Ruffion A, Van der Aa F, Jairam R, Perrouin-Verbe MA, Elneil S. A prospective, multicenter study of a novel, miniaturized rechargeable sacral neuromodulation system: 12-month results from the RELAX-OAB study. Neurourol Urodyn. 2018. https://doi.org/10.1002/nau.23892.
18. Nitti VW, Ginsberg D, Sievert KD, Sussman D, Radomski S, Sand P, De Ridder D, Jenkins B, Magyar A, Chapple C. Durable efficacy and safety of long-term onabotulinumtoxinA treatment in patients with overactive bladder syndrome: final results of a 3.5-year study. J Urol. 2016;196(3):791–800. https://doi.org/10.1016/j.juro.2016.03.146. Epub 2016 Mar 30.
19. Amundsen CL, Komesu YM, Chermansky C, Gregory WT, Myers DL, Honeycutt EF, Vasavada SP, Nguyen JN, Wilson TS, Harvie HS, Wallace D. Two-year outcomes of sacral neuromodulation versus onabotulinumtoxinA for refractory urgency urinary incontinence: a randomized trial. Eur Urol. 2018;74(1):66–73. https://doi.org/10.1016/j.eururo.2018.02.011. Epub 2018 Feb 24.
20. Smits MAC, Oerlemans D, Marcelissen TAT, Van Kerrebroeck PEV, De Wachter SGG. Sacral neuromodulation in patients with idiopathic overactive bladder after initial botulinum toxin therapy. J Urol. 2013;190:2148–52.
21. Hoag N, Plagakis S, Pillay S, Edwards AW, Gani J. Sacral neuromodulation for refractory overactive bladder after prior intravesical onabotulinumtoxinA treatment. NeurourolUrodyn. 2017;36:1377–81.
22. Shepherd JP, Lowder JL, Leng WW, Smith KJ. InterStim sacral neuromodulation and botox botulinum-A toxin intradetrusor injections for refractory urge urinary incontinence: a decision analysis comparing outcomes including efficacy and complications. Female Pelvic Med Reconstr Surg. 2011;17(4):199–203. https://doi.org/10.1097/SPV.0b013e318224e0d7.
23. Zahner PM, Giusto LL, Goldman HB. What is the role of additional pharmacotherapy and neuromodulation in patients with marginal benefit from botulinum toxin injection? Curr Urol Rep. 2018;19(11):91. https://doi.org/10.1007/s11934-018-0842-8.
24. Malik R, Hess D, Christie A, Carmel M, Zimmern P. Domain comparison between 6 validated questionnaires administered to women with urinary incontinence. Urology. 2019;132:75–80.
25. Rapp DE, Kobashi KC. Outcomes following sling surgery: importance of the definition of success. J Urol. 2008;180(3):998–1002.
26. https://www.auanet.org/practice-resources/patient-safety-and-quality-of-care/2019-mips-toolkit. Accessed 3 Jan 2020.
27. Harvie H, Amundsen C, Neuwahi S, Honeycutt A, Lukacz E, Sung V, et al. Cost effectiveness of sacral neuromodulation versus onabotulinum toxin A for refactory urgency urinary incontinence: results of the ROSETTA randomized trial. J Urol. [Epub ahead of print].

Part III

Treatment: Fecal Incontinence

11 Treatment for Fecal Incontinence: Nonsurgical Approaches

Victoria Valinluck Lao and Dana R. Sands

Case Scenario

A 68-year-old woman presents to the office with complaints of urgency and inability to hold her bowel movements. She reports that she has soiled undergarments intermittently during the past 2 months, prior to which time, she had no bowel control problems. She notes that her stools have been more irregular and less formed. She has had two vaginal deliveries in her early 30s and no previous anorectal surgeries. She denies urinary incontinence or inability to control flatus.

Introduction

Fecal incontinence (FI) is the uncontrolled passage of feces or gas in an individual age ≥4 years old who has previously attained control, lasting for greater than 1 month [1]. The reported rates of fecal incontinence vary, depending upon the population that is examined. In the general population, the rates of fecal incontinence range between 1.4% and 18%, with the rates being higher in the elderly and in institutionalized populations. In the elderly, the prevalence is approximately 15%, whereas incontinence may affect up to 50% of institutionalized patients [2–7]. In addition, fecal incontinence is more prevalent among individuals with inflammatory bowel disease, celiac disease, irritable bowel syndrome, or diabetes than people without these disorders [7]. The largest household survey revealed that 18% of adult women had experienced at least one episode of fecal incontinence during the year prior to the survey [8].

Fecal continence is a complex condition. It requires coordinated interplay among rectal capacity, sensation, and neuromuscular function. Alterations in factors such as stool consistency, stool volume, rectal distensibility, colonic transit, anorectal sensation, anal sphincter function, and anorectal reflexes can all contribute to the development of fecal incontinence [9]. Because of this complexity, when evaluating a patient for fecal incontinence, risk factors for fecal incontinence should be elucidated. Risk factors include pregnancy, chronic diarrhea, diabetes, smoking, previous anorectal surgery, obesity, urinary incontinence, neurologic disease [2, 10]. Obstetric history is important to determine if there has been injury to the sphincters, which is overtly identified in 10% of vaginal deliveries. Up to 35% of vaginal deliveries will have occult

Commentary by Tracy L. Hull, Cleveland Clinic, Department of Colon and Rectal Surgery, Cleveland, OH, USA

V. V. Lao
Memorial Hospital West, Division of Colon and Rectal Surgery, Pembroke Pines, FL, USA

D. R. Sands (✉)
Cleveland Clinic Florida, Department of Colorectal Surgery, Weston, FL, USA
e-mail: sandsd@ccf.org

K. C. Kobashi, S. D. Wexner (eds.), *Female Pelvic Medicine*,
https://doi.org/10.1007/978-3-030-54839-1_11

injuries to the anal sphincters. Often times, there will be a long delay between onset of symptoms and the injury due to compensatory mechanisms [1, 11].

Classification of Fecal Incontinence

Many scoring systems have been developed to describe and measure the type, amount, frequency, and impact the incontinence has on a patient. The use of these scoring systems or grading scales is to help to quantify the severity of the incontinence and to select patients for treatment as well as to measure response to treatment. The authors utilize the validated Cleveland Clinic Florida Fecal Incontinence Score (CCF-FIS) [12]. The CCF-FIS factors in frequency as well as type of incontinence (liquid, sold, or gas), the impact on the patient's lifestyle, and whether the patient wears a pad (Table 11.1). It has been validated in multiple languages and is the most widely cited FI score in the world's literature. In addition, there is statistically significant correlation between the CCF-FIS and quality of life [13, 14].

In addition to scoring systems, fecal incontinence can be stratified based upon etiology of the disease in order to better understand and treat the fecal incontinence. These two groups are as follows: (1) fecal incontinence with normal pelvic floor, and (2) fecal incontinence with abnormal pelvic floor (Table 11.2) [9].

Patients with fecal incontinence who have a normal pelvic floor include elderly patients. The mechanism of incontinence is usually a chronic history of straining with subsequent injury to the pudendal nerve. Neurogenic cause of fecal incontinence is due to disturbance of motor and sensory nerve innervation of the sphincters and rectum, in the case of CNS or spinal cord disorders resulting from congenital, traumatic, or infectious causes. In patients with idiopathic incontinence, who have no structural abnormalities, it is also thought that neurologic damage results in abnormal sensation in the anal canal and rectum, causing incontinence [15, 16]. Patients with gastrointestinal diseases such as chronic diarrhea, inflammatory bowel disease, infectious colitis, and laxative abuse general also have a normal pelvic floor. Incontinence develops due to interference from these diseases in the sphincter function as well as loss of reservoir function of the rectum. History of pelvic radiation may also result in proctitis and reduced reservoir function of the rectum, leading to fecal incontinence. Patients with overflow incontinence due to fecal impaction and seepage of liquid stool around the impacted stool also fall under this category of normal pelvic floor.

Patients with fecal incontinence who have an abnormal pelvic floor tend to have a structural abnormality, whether it is congenital, due to trauma, due to prolapse or previous anorectal surgery. For example, patients with imperforate anus and subsequent surgical repair can develop fecal incontinence. Patients with previous anorectal surgeries such as lateral internal sphincterotomy, hemorrhoidectomy, or fistula surgery may have sphincter damage, resulting in incontinence. Trauma from childbirth or other source can disrupt the sphincter mechanism, leading to incontinence. Full-thickness rectal prolapse can also cause internal and external sphincter damage due to chronic dilation, as well as pudendal nerve injury.

Table 11.1 Cleveland Clinic Florida FecalIncontinence Score (CCF-FIS)

Type of incontinence	Never	Rarely	Sometimes	Usually	Always
Solid	0	1	2	3	4
Liquid	0	1	2	3	4
Gas	0	1	2	3	4
Wears pad	0	1	2	3	4
Lifestyle modification	0	1	2	3	4

Never, 0; Rarely, < 1/mo; Sometimes, < 1/d, ≥ 1/mo; Usually, <1/d, ≥ 1/wk; Always. > 1/d

Table 11.2 Stratification of fecal incontinence patients

Fecal incontinence	
With normal pelvic floor	With abnormal pelvic floor
Aging	Anorectal surgery
Gastrointestinal pathologies	Childbirth
Irradiation	Trauma
Neurogenic causes	Congenital abnormalities
Overflow incontinence and soiling	Procidentia
Idiopathic incontinence	

Approaches to Fecal Incontinence

Nonoperative Management

Medical Management

A large component of nonoperative management is medical management geared at efforts to improve stool frequency and consistency, provide skin protection, strengthen the pelvic floor and the sphincters as well as improving sensation. Appropriate medical management can improve symptoms in many patients, potentially avoiding surgical intervention.

Fecal seepage and soilage can be detrimental to the perianal skin. Wearing pads with polymers can provide skin protection by wicking moisture away from the skin as well as protection for clothing [17]. Skin irritation from fecal soilage can also be tempered with barrier creams such as zinc-oxide containing agents such as calmoseptine [18].

Fecal incontinence may be directly related to stool consistency, such as in patients with chronic diarrhea. The treatment in this case is to treat the underlying cause (in the case of inflammatory bowel disease or infectious causes) and modify the stool consistency (when other causes have been ruled out). Patients should be instructed to use a diary in order to identify and eventually avoid triggers and aggravating factors for their fecal incontinence. This detailed log and systematic changes can impact their bowel function and thereby fecal control. Example of dietary components that are often culprits with regard to diarrhea include caffeine, lactose, and sugar substitutes [19]. Fiber supplementation such as psyllium can be used as a bulking agent for the stool, in addition to antidiarrheal agents once other causes have been ruled out. Loperamide is often preferred as the first-line antidiarrheal treatment, because it does not have an effect on the central nervous system [20–22]. Diphenoxylate and codeine can also be added as stronger antidiarrheal agents but have central nervous system effects. These treatments decrease intestinal fluid secretion and slow down the colonic transit time, allowing for increased water absorption [23, 24]. In the case of patients with irritable bowel syndrome that causes diarrhea, bile acid sequestrants such as colestipol or colesevelam may be helpful. This is based upon observations that a subset of these patients has bile acid malabsorption [25]. Tricyclic antidepressants are also known to inhibit intestinal motility as well as inhibit sphincter relaxation [26]. More recently, clonidine has been used in fecal incontinence as it is thought to reduce rectal sensation and urgency [27, 28].

In patients with overflow incontinence associated with fecal impaction, management is with disimpaction and colonic cleansing. Subsequently, a consistent bowel regimen needs to be implemented to prevent recurrence. The patient needs scheduled defecation with the addition of fiber supplementation, regular sufficient water intake as well as stool softeners and laxatives, such as docusate, polyethylene glycol, and bisacodyl.

Behavioral modification is another cornerstone of medical management. Manometric or electromyography (EMG) – assisted biofeedback – is a specialized technique geared at strengthening the external anal sphincter muscle as well as the puborectalis, much like Kegels exercises, but in addition to muscle strengthening, the patient works toward enhancing rectal sensation so that progressively smaller volumes of distension will trigger the threshold of rectal sensation and shorten the response time between perception of rectal distension and voluntary contraction of the external anal sphincter [18]. Data from a randomized controlled trial suggests that manometric biofeedback is superior to Kegels exercises alone [29].

Many patients with fecal incontinence do respond well to medical management with pharmacologics, lifestyle modification, and biofeedback therapy. However, further evaluation is needed with the more invasive interventions outlined below for patients who do not respond to these conservative approaches,

Augmentation

Methods for augmentation are described in Chap. 14.

Inserts

Insertable devices have been developed to aid in the treatment of fecal incontinence. The vaginal bowel control device is a vaginal inflatable balloon and pump system that is fitted to each woman. The vaginal insert is a dynamic, low-risk, reversible, patient-controlled device that is deflated to allow for bowel movements and inflated to prevent stool leakage. A small multicenter prospective study of 61 patients showed a 50% reduction in episodes and no adverse events, with 41% of patients achieving complete continence [30–33]. Currently, there is an ongoing multicenter trial to evaluate the durability and long-term safety of the device.

Anal insert devices have also been used to aid in the treatment of fecal incontinence. Their use is limited as it is often difficult to tolerate [34]. A multicenter prospective study with a single arm cohort showed a 50% improvement in continence, with minor adverse side effects including sensation of urge 26%, displacement up into rectum 24%, irritation 13%, pain 7%, and soreness 6% [35]. Long-term efficacy data and comparative data to other modalities of treatment are still needed.

Overview of Surgical Interventions for Fecal Incontinence

Neuromodulation

Percutaneous Tibial Nerve Stimulation (PTNS) and Transcutaneous Tibial Nerve Stimulation (TTNS)

Given the success of SNS in the treatment of FI with modulation of the S3 nerve root, peripheral tibial nerve stimulation (PTNS and TTNS) has been investigated for treatment of fecal incontinence. The tibial nerve has afferent and efferent fibers originating from L4-S3 nerve roots. Therefore, it is thought that tibial nerve modulation may lead to alterations in anorectal neuromuscular function, much like SNS. TNS is nonsurgical and thereby less invasive than SNS. There are two main methods of delivering outpatient TNS treatments: percutaneous and transcutaneous. With PTNS, a needle is placed superior to the medial malleolus near the tibial nerve in the ankle and electrical stimulation is given via the needle. TTNS involves two pad electrodes placed above the medial malleolus over the tibial nerve. Outpatient treatment protocols for both PTNS and TTNS can vary in frequency and duration. Studies have shown that although TTNS resulted in improvements in some outcome measures for fecal incontinence, it is not superior to sham simulation in a large adequately powered randomized control trial [36]. With regard to PTNS efficacy, results of studies are equivocal with only one study showing statistically significant improvement in incontinence at 6 months, whereas other trials show no difference between the sham and PTNS groups when treated for shorter periods of time [3–39]. Data from the Control of Fecal Incontinence using Distal Neuromodulation Trial demonstrated no significant clinical benefit of percutaneous tibial nerve stimulation (PTNS) compared to sham stimulation in patients with fecal incontinence (FI) much like TTNS. However, reanalysis of the primary outcome excluding patients with obstructive defecation symptoms resulted in a significant clinical effect of PTNS compared to sham (48.9% vs. 18.2% response, $P = 0.002$; multivariable OR, 4.71; 95% CI, 1.71–12.93; $P = 0.003$) [40]. These data suggest that patient selection may be a key factor in the successful implementation of tibial nerve stimulation for fecal incontinence.

Fecal Diversion

In patients who have failed alternative therapies for fecal incontinence, fecal diversion with a well-created stoma at an optimal site is a surgical option. Studies show that the majority of patients who underwent stoma creation for fecal diversion for fecal incontinence had a significant improvement in their quality of life [41, 42].

Injectables

Bulking agents in the form of biomaterial injectables may be a viable option for the above patient with minor FI in order to augment passive outlet resistance. The method of injection is dependent on the agent of choice; final sites of implantation may include submucosal, intersphincteric, or intrasphincteric and the route of injection may be transmucosal, transsphincteric, or intersphincteric. Local anesthetic and/or endorectal ultrasound may be used to assist in the injection of the agent.

The use of injectable polytetrafluoroethylene was initially described in the 1990s when traditional bulking agents such as carbon, collagen, and fat demonstrated poor long-term results. Newer agents such as NASHA Dx, PTQ™ (a biocompatible silicone implant), and Durasphere™ (carbon-coated beads) are the most common injectables used worldwide; however, only NASHA Dx or Solesta® is FDA approved for use in FI in the USA [32]. NASHA Dx or nonanimal stabilized hyaluronic acid/dextranomer has been used for years as a bulking agent for urological procedures. The injection is typically performed in the office, with the patient either in left lateral or prone position. The anal canal is divided into four quadrants and using an anoscope, 1 mL of the bulking agent is injected into the deep submucosa of each of the quadrants. After injection, the needle is retained within the submucosa space for 10 seconds in order to avoid leakage through the puncture site. The use of NASHA Dx has been shown to reduce the number of FI episodes by at least 50% in 52% of patients versus a similar reduction rate in only 31% of the placebo group [43]. NASHA Dx was used in patients with moderate FI and the 36-month follow-up demonstrated a sustained reduction with significant improvement in quality-of-life measures. The percentage of patients who experienced complete continence doubled from 6% at 6 months to 13.2% at 36 months [44]. The authors contend that these results are due to the durable composition of NASHA Dx and the lack of migration resulting from its particle size.

Complications with injectable bulking agents are generally minimal and short-lived. Pertaining to NASHA Dx injections, the most commonly reported adverse events include proctalgia, rectal bleeding, diarrhea, constipation, and fever. Rare and serious adverse events include abscess development. Though these results are encouraging and are supported by other prospective trials, it should be noted that repeat injections were necessary in most patients in order to achieve such outcomes [31, 44–47]. As such, other agents are currently being explored in order to improve long-term outcomes and include stem cells and the use of self-expandable agents.

One such self-expandable agent being investigated is the Gatekeeper™ prosthesis. It is made of the inert polymer resin polyacrylonitrile and was originally intended for use to bulk the lower esophageal sphincter in the setting of gastric reflux. For FI, the material is implanted in six locations circumscribing the intersphincteric space using a specially designed delivery system. The resin material reshapes to its environment by water absorption over time and thus is purported as an ideal bulking agent. One multicenter observational study performed in Europe demonstrated greater than 75% improvement in all FI parameters at 12 months, with 13% of patients reporting full continence during the same timeframe [48]. Another observational study noted that those of whom responded to the treatment initially will likely sustain a response and demonstrate greater than 50% improvement in FI scores from baseline at least at the one-year interval [49]. The primary issue with this product is prosthesis migration with reported rates ranging from 5% to more than 50%. One small study demonstrated by endorectal ultrasound at 3 months after injection that more than half of the implanted material had migrated, though they noted no significant clinical change in their patients' FI [50]. Other risks associated with this product include pain, infection that may require removal, and dislodgement that may require extraction and/or replacement. Unfortunately, the Gatekeeper™ is currently not an available option in the USA.

Radio-frequency Tissue Remodeling

Radio-frequency tissue remodeling is a therapeutic option for mild-to-moderate FI with intact or limited sphincter defect (less than 30°) who failed conservative management and are seeking less invasive treatments. Using the SECCA® anoscope containing nickel-titanium needles, radio-frequency energy is delivered into the internal anal sphincter to approximately 85 °F in order to induce higher passive outlet resistance through remodeling in collagen deposition and thickening of the muscularis propria. Needle insertion is repeated at several levels within the upper anal canal. The specialized anoscope can detect impedance and self-thermoregulates so that it does not induce burning. This is a minimally invasive outpatient procedure that can be performed either in the operating room or in the endoscopy suite. Complications may include pain, bleeding/hematoma, infection, diarrhea, and mucosal ulceration. Though extremely rare, it also has the potential to cause rectovaginal fistula due to anterior penetration of the thermo-needle in females, especially in the presence of rectocele. Patients who have undergone biomaterial injections are excluded from radio-frequency tissue remodeling. The mechanisms of action have been elegantly delineated.

Efron et al. published the initial prospective multicenter study in the US of 50 patients (43 women) with long-standing FI who underwent radio-frequency tissue remodeling [51]. At 6 months, the mean CCF-FIS significantly improved from 14.5 to 11.1. Whereas the FI of 11.1 is considered moderate in severity, patients experienced significant improvement in quality of life. While the above study remains the largest study to date, there were other smaller sample studies on the use of radio-frequency tissue remodeling in the late 2000s through early 2010s [52–55]. Most report significant improvement in FI scores at 6-month or 12-month follow-up with the exception of one study [54]. Three of the four studies assessed for whether improvement in incontinence affected quality of life and were split in terms of whether it actually did or not [53–55]. Interestingly, one study reported that while there was a significant improvement in FI, there was no significant change in the anal manometry and rectal compliance of these patients at 3 months [52]. They suggested that there may be a tendency toward increased rectal sensitivity related to urge and the maximal tolerated volume, as a potential contributor to improvements in reported scores. Reported long-term results were variable, in terms of duration of the improvement in FI. Despite an initial response of 78% to treatment, Abbas et al. reported that over 50% of the patients required or were waiting for additional intervention at a mean follow-up time of 40 months. Another study noted that only 6% of their patients maintained their results in the same time interval [56, 57]. The longest follow-up to date was at 5 years by Takahashi-Monroy et al. and they noted significant clinical improvement in FI scores that persisted to 5 years, as well as improvements in quality-of-life measures especially in the social functioning and mental components [58]. More recently, a small study comparing radio-frequency tissue remodeling versus sham control showed no difference in quality-of-life scores and anorectal function at 6 months [59]. Table 11.3 depicts the results of different studies. Despite these varying outcomes, radio-frequency tissue remodeling may still be a worthwhile procedure for those who have failed other options, given its low rate of serious complications.

Case Discussion (Fig. 11.1)

The first step in evaluation of our patient is a detailed history of her incontinence episodes, diet, medications, comorbidities, obstetric history, and bowel habits. A digital rectal exam is performed, taking note of whether there is fecal impaction, and her resting sphincter tone and ability to squeeze. If there is no anorectal pathology on examination, such as rectal prolapse, anal

Table 11.3 Outcomes for SECCA

Author	*n*	Follow-up (months)	Fecal incontinence	Improvement
Takahashi [60]	10	12	CCF: – 13.5–5	80%
Takahashi [61]	10	24	CCF: 13.8–7.8	70%
Efron [51]	50	6	CCF: 14.6–11.1	60%
Felt-Bersma, [52]	11	12	Vaizey 18.8–11.5	55%
Takahashi, [58]	19	60	CCF: 14.3–8.26	84%
Lefebure [53]	15	12	14–12.3	13%
Kim [54]	8	6	CCF: 13.6–9.9	–
Walega [62]	20	6	CCF: 12.1–9.3	68%
Ruiz [55]	16	12	CCF: 15.6–12.9	37.5%
Abbas [56]	27	40	CCF: 16–11	22%

CCF Cleveland Clinic Incontinence score

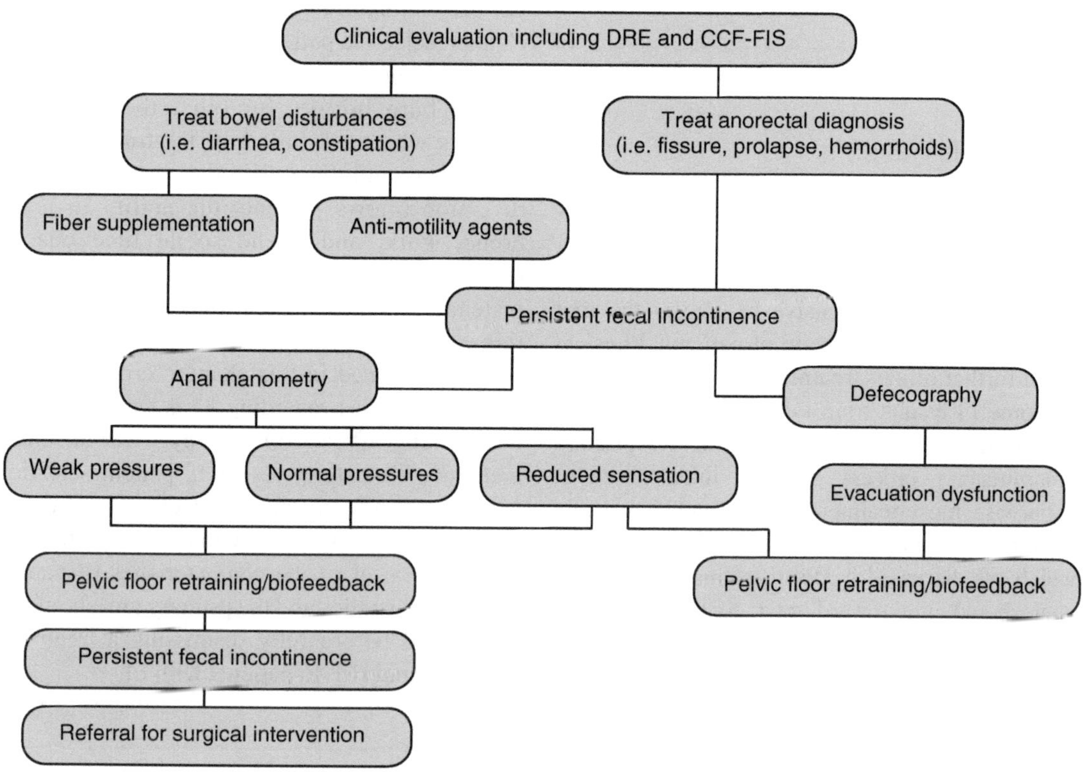

Fig. 11.1 Flow chart for nonoperative management of fecal incontinence

fissure, or significant hemorrhoids, the next step would be to treat her bowel disturbance, which is loose stools. If she has not under gone a recent colonoscopy with biopsies, she should undergo a colonoscopy with biopsies as part of her work-up to rule out microscopic colitis. Stool studies should be sent to exclude infectious diarrhea.

She can proceed with the addition of fiber supplementation such as psyllium and ensure adequate water intake daily. She should also start a diary to chart any aggravating factors to her loose stools, paying close attention to caffeine intake, lactose, and sugar alternatives.

If the diary does not identify any modifiable factors, and the fiber supplementation does not improve her continence, the next step would be to add pharmacologic modulators for her loose stools, as long as her stools studies are negative for an infectious cause and the biopsies from her colonoscopy do not reveal a gastrointestinal disease process such as inflammatory bowel disease. She can start with loperamide to slow down her bowel transit and secretions, prior to escalating to more robust agents such diphenoxylate and codeine. If IBS-D is suspected, she can also be treated with bile acid binders, tricyclic antidepressants as well as clonidine.

If after treatment with pharmacologic therapy, she has persistent fecal incontinence, she should then be referred for biofeedback pelvic floor retraining therapy.

Commentary

Tracy L. Hull

Fecal incontinence (FI) as outlined in this chapter is not uncommon. The etiology is multifactorial, and treatment is individualized for each patient. Therefore, a comprehensive history is the first step in caring for this group of patients. Physical exam further refines treatment possibilities [63].

Some FI results from inflammatory conditions like ulcerative colitis. Treatment of the primary inflammatory process is the initial therapy. Otherwise, most treatment recommendations begin with a combination of nonsurgical approaches, which are discussed in detail in this chapter. The goal should aim toward total continence. Many studies determine successful results as 50% reduction in incontinent episodes. While a 50% reduction may be an improvement, any accidental episodes of FI can be humiliating and demoralizing.

Loose stools are a factor for many patients with FI, and strategies to minimize diarrhea are part of most recommendations. As mentioned, anal skin care with protective barrier creams is sometimes a forgotten component of treatment [64]. Physical therapy utilizing auditory and/or visual feedback emphasizes retraining for improved anal strength, pelvic coordination, and optimization of rectal sensitivity. This therapy can be operator dependent and time intensive to produce an acceptable outcome. Enemas or rectal washout is also a treatment strategy that may be successfully utilized for selected patients who are motivated to use this therapy [65, 66]. As outlined in the chapter, a combination of these treatments is part of the individual approach.

To further optimize quality of life, other nonsurgical approaches may be considered. While insertion of devices into the vagina in women or anal inserts seem like attractive options to prevent stool from being expelled at unwanted times, both success and tolerance have been suboptimal [66].

With the success of sacral nerve modulation, percutaneous tibial nerve stimulation seems like an attractive less invasive treatment that should stimulate similar nerve pathways. Results have not been straightforward, but as discussed in the chapter, selective patients may benefit [67].

Nonsurgical therapies are overall safe and do not burn bridges for other therapies. For patients who have failed all treatment options or are not candidates for other therapies, fecal diversion allows patients the ability to leave home, work, and attend social functions. A stoma should not be viewed as a failure, but instead as a means to improve quality of life in this group of patients [66].

As mentioned in this chapter, critical examination of studies regarding FI is essential when determining efficacy of therapy. As with many areas of pelvic floor research, patient selection for studies may not appropriately compare like patients, especially those with FI. FI is difficult to treat. Appraisal of the characteristics of patient included in studies and the primary aim should be scrutinized before fully dismissing a treatment with minimal risk to patients with FI.

References

1. Paquette IM, Varma MG, Kaiser AM, Steele SR, Rafferty JF. The American Society of Colon and Rectal Surgeons' clinical practice guideline for the treatment of fecal incontinence. Dis Colon Rectum. 2015;58(7):623–36.
2. Ditah I, Devaki P, Luma HN, et al. Prevalence, trends, and risk factors for fecal incontinence in United States adults, 2005-2010. Clin Gastroenterol Hepatol. 2014;12(4):636–43.
3. Goode PS, Burgio KL, Halli AD, et al. Prevalence and correlates of fecal incontinence in community-dwelling older adults. J Am Geriatr Soc. 2005;53(4):629–35.

4. Markland AD, Goode PS, Burgio KL, et al. Incidence and risk factors for fecal incontinence in black and white older adults: a population-based study. J Am Geriatr Soc. 2010;58(7):1341–6.
5. Whitehead WE, Borrud L, Goode PS, et al. Fecal incontinence in US adults: epidemiology and risk factors. Gastroenterology. 2009;137(2):512–7, 517.e1–2.
6. Nelson RL. Epidemiology of fecal incontinence. Gastroenterology. 2004;126(1 Suppl 1):S3–7.
7. Menees SB, Almario CV, Spiegel BMR, Chey WD. Prevalence of and factors associated with fecal incontinence: results from a population-based survey. Gastroenterology. 2018;154(6):1672–1681.e3.
8. Brown HW, Wexner SD, Segall MM, Brezoczky KL, Lukacz ES. Accidental bowel leakage in the mature women's health study: prevalence and predictors. Int J Clin Pract. 2012;66(11):1101–8.
9. Pinto RA, Sands DR. Surgery and sacral nerve stimulation for constipation and fecal incontinence. Gastrointest Endosc Clin N Am. 2009;19(1):83–116, vi–vii.
10. Townsend MK, Matthews CA, Whitehead WE, Grodstein F. Risk factors for fecal incontinence in older women. Am J Gastroenterol. 2013;108(1):113–9.
11. Bharucha AE, Fletcher JG, Melton LJ 3rd, Zinsmeister AR. Obstetric trauma, pelvic floor injury and fecal incontinence: a population-based case-control study. Am J Gastroenterol. 2012;107(6):902–11.
12. Jorge JM, Wexner SD. Etiology and management of fecal incontinence. Dis Colon Rectum. 1993;36(1):77–97.
13. Brown HW, Wexner SD, Lukacz ES. Factors associated with care seeking among women with accidental bowel leakge. Female Pelvic Med Reconstr Surg. 2013;19(2):66–71.
14. Brown HW, Wexner SD, Segall MM, Brezoczky KL, Lukacz ES. Quality of life impact in women with accidental bowel leakage. Int J Clin Pract. 2012;66(11):1109–16.
15. Perry S, Shaw C, McGrother C, et al. Prevalence of faecal incontinence in adults aged 40 years or more living in the community. Gut. 2002;50(4):480–4.
16. Roberts RO, Jacobsen SJ, Reilly WT, Pemberton JH, Lieber MM, Talley NJ. Prevalence of combined fecal and urinary incontinence: a community-based study. J Am Geriatr Soc. 1999;47(7):837–41.
17. Shirran E, Brazzelli M. Absorbent products for the containment of urinary and/or faecal incontinence in adults. Cochrane Database Syst Rev. 2000;(2):CD001406.
18. Wald A. Diagnosis and management of fecal incontinence. Curr Gastroenterol Rep. 2018;20(3):9.
19. Rosier PF, Gajewski JB, Sand PK, et al. Executive summary: The International Consultation on Incontinence 2008--Committee on: "Dynamic Testing"; for urinary incontinence and for fecal incontinence. Part 1: Innovations in urodynamic techniques and urodynamic testing for signs and symptoms of urinary incontinence in female patients. Neurourol Urodyn. 2010;29(1):140–5.
20. Palmer KR, Corbett CL, Holdsworth CD. Double-blind cross-over study comparing loperamide, codeine and diphenoxylate in the treatment of chronic diarrhea. Gastroenterology. 1980;79(6):1272–5.
21. Read MG, Krejs GJ, Hendler RS, Davis G, Fordtran JS. A report of five patients with large-volume secretory diarrhea but no evidence of endocrine tumor or laxative abuse. Dig Dis Sci. 1982;27(3):193–201.
22. Sun WM, Read NW, Verlinden M. Effects of loperamide oxide on gastrointestinal transit time and anorectal function in patients with chronic diarrhoea and faecal incontinence. Scand J Gastroenterol. 1997;32(1):34–8.
23. Cheetham M, Brazzelli M, Norton C, Glazener CM. Drug treatment for faecal incontinence in adults. Cochrane Database Syst Rev. 2003;(3):CD002116.
24. Remes-Troche JM, Ozturk R, Philips C, Stessman M, Rao SS. Cholestyramine – a useful adjunct for the treatment of patients with fecal incontinence. Int J Color Dis. 2008;23(2):189–94.
25. Wedlake L, A'Hern R, Russell D, Thomas K, Walters JR, Andreyev HJ. Systematic review: the prevalence of idiopathic bile acid malabsorption as diagnosed by SeHCAT scanning in patients with diarrhoea-predominant irritable bowel syndrome. Aliment Pharmacol Ther. 2009;30(7):707–17.
26. Santoro GA, Eitan BZ, Pryde A, Bartolo DC. Open study of low-dose amitriptyline in the treatment of patients with idiopathic fecal incontinence. Dis Colon Rectum. 2000;43(12):1676–81.
27. Bharucha AE, Fletcher JG, Camilleri M, Edge J, Carlson P, Zinsmeister AR. Effects of clonidine in women with fecal incontinence. Clin Gastroenterol Hepatol. 2014;12(5):843–851.e2.
28. Bharucha AE, Seide BM, Zinsmeister AR. The effects of clonidine on symptoms and anorectal sensorimotor function in women with faecal incontinence. Aliment Pharmacol Ther. 2010;32(5):681–8.
29. Heymen S, Scarlett Y, Jones K, Ringel Y, Drossman D, Whitehead WE. Randomized controlled trial shows biofeedback to be superior to pelvic floor exercises for fecal incontinence. Dis Colon Rectum. 2009;52(10):1730–7.
30. Maeda Y, Laurberg S, Norton C. Perianal injectable bulking agents as treatment for faecal incontinence in adults. Cochrane Database Sys Rev. 2010;(5):CD007959.
31. Danielson J, Karlbom U, Wester T, Graf W. Efficacy and quality of life 2 years after treatment for faecal incontinence with injectable bulking agents. Tech Coloproctol. 2013;17(4):389–95.
32. Maeda Y, Laurberg S, Norton C. Perianal injectable bulking agents as treatment for faecal incontinence in adults. Cochrane Database Syst Rev. 2013;(2):CD007959.
33. Richter HE, Matthews CA, Muir T, et al. A vaginal bowel-control system for the treatment of fecal incontinence. Obstet Gynecol. 2015;125(3):540–7.

34. Deutekom M, Dobben AC. Plugs for containing faecal incontinence. Cochrane Database Syst Rev. 2015;(7):CD005086.
35. Lukacz ES, Segall MM, Wexner SD. Evaluation of an anal insert device for the conservative management of fecal incontinence. Dis Colon Rectum. 2015;58(9):892–8.
36. Leroi AM, Siproudhis L, Damon EH, et al. Transcutaneous electrical tibial stimuliation in the treatment of fecal incontinence: a randomized trial (CONSORT 1a). Am J Gastroenterol. 2012;107(12):1888–96.
37. Horrocks EJ, Bremner SA, Stevens N, et al. Double-blind randomised controlled trial of percutaneous tibial nerve stimulation versus sham electrical stimulation in the treatment of faecal incontinence: CONtrol of Faecal Incontinence using Distal NeuromodulaTion (the CONFIDeNT trial). Health Technol Assess. 2015;19(77):1–164.
38. Horrocks EJ, Chadi SA, Stevens NJ, Wexner SD, Knowles CH. Factors associated with efficacy of percutaneous tibial nerve stimulation for fecal incontinence, based on post-hoc analysis of data from a randomized trial. Clin Gastroenterol Hepatol. 2017;15(12):1915–1921.e2.
39. Thin NN, Horrocks EJ, Hotouras A, et al. Systematic review of the clinical effectiveness of neuromodulation in the treatment of faecal incontinence. Br J Surg. 2013;100(11):1430–47.
40. Horrocks EJ, Thin N, Thaha MA, Taylor SJ, Norton C, Knowles CH. Systematic review of tibial nerve stimulation to treat faecal incontinence. Br J Surg. 2014;101(5):457–68.
41. Colquhoun P, Kaiser R, Weiss EG, et al. Correlating the Fecal Incontinence Quality-of-Life Score and the SF-36 to a proposed Ostomy Function Index in patients with a stoma. Ostomy Wound Manage. 2006;52(12):68–74.
42. Norton C, Burch J, Kamm MA. Patients' views of a colostomy for fecal incontinence. Dis Colon Rectum. 2005;48(5):1062–9.
43. Graf W, Mellgren A, Matzel KE, Hull T, Johansson C, Bernstein M, et al. Efficacy of dextranomer in stabilised hyaluronic acid for treatment of faecal incontinence: a randomised, sham-controlled trial. Lancet. 2011;377(9770):997–1003. PubMed PMID: 21420555.
44. Mellgren A, Matzel KE, Pollack J, Hull T, Bernstein M, Graf W, et al. Long-term efficacy of NASHA Dx injection therapy for treatment of fecal incontinence. Neurogastroenterol Motil. 2014;26(8):1087–94. PubMed PMID: 24837493. Pubmed Central PMCID: 4371654.
45. Danielson J, Karlbom U, Sonesson AC, Wester T, Graf W. Submucosal injection of stabilized nonanimal hyaluronic acid with dextranomer: a new treatment option for fecal incontinence. Dis Colon Rectum. 2009;52(6):1101–6. PubMed PMID: 19581853.
46. Dodi G, Jongen J, de la Portilla F, Raval M, Altomare DF, Lehur PA. An open-label, noncomparative, multicenter study to evaluate efficacy and safety of NASHA/Dx gel as a bulking agent for the treatment of fecal incontinence. Gastroenterol Res Pract. 2010;2010:467136. PubMed PMID: 21234379. Pubmed Central PMCID: 3017894.
47. Schwandner O, Brunner M, Dietl O. Quality of life and functional results of submucosal injection therapy using dextranomer hyaluronic acid for fecal incontinence. Surg Innov. 2011;18(2):130–5. PubMed PMID: 21245071.
48. Ratto C, Buntzen S, Aigner F, Altomare DF, Heydari A, Donisi L, et al. Multicentre observational study of the Gatekeeper for faecal incontinence. Br J Surg. 2016;103(3):290–9. PubMed PMID: 26621029. Pubmed Central PMCID: 5063193.
49. Trenti L, Biondo S, Noguerales F, Nomdedeu J, Coret A, Scherer R, et al. Outcomes of Gatekeeper(TM) prosthesis implantation for the treatment of fecal incontinence: a multicenter observational study. Tech Coloproctol. 2017;21(12):963–70.
50. de la Portilla F, Reyes-Diaz ML, Maestre MV, Jimenez-Rodriguez RM, Garcia-Cabrera AM, Vazquez-Monchul JM, et al. Ultrasonographic evidence of Gatekeeper prosthesis migration in patients treated for faecal incontinence: a case series. Int J Color Dis. 2017;32(3):437–40. PubMed PMID: 28054134.
51. Efron JE, Corman ML, Fleshman J, Barnett J, Nagle D, Birnbaum E, et al. Safety and effectiveness of temperature-controlled radio-frequency energy delivery to the anal canal (Secca procedure) for the treatment of fecal incontinence. Dis Colon Rectum. 2003;46(12):1606–16; discussion 16–8. PubMed PMID: 14668584.
52. Felt-Bersma RJ, Szojda MM, Mulder CJ. Temperature-controlled radiofrequency energy (SECCA) to the anal canal for the treatment of faecal incontinence offers moderate improvement. Eur J Gastroenterol Hepatol. 2007;19(7):575–80. PubMed PMID: 17556904.
53. Lefebure B, Tuech JJ, Bridoux V, Gallas S, Leroi AM, Denis P, et al. Temperature-controlled radio frequency energy delivery (Secca procedure) for the treatment of fecal incontinence: results of a prospective study. Int J Color Dis. 2008;23(10):993–7.
54. Kim DW, Yoon HM, Park JS, Kim YH, Kang SB. Radiofrequency energy delivery to the anal canal: is it a promising new approach to the treatment of fecal incontinence? Am J Surg. 2009;197(1):14–8.
55. Ruiz D, Pinto RA, Hull TL, Efron JE, Wexner SD. Does the radiofrequency procedure for fecal incontinence improve quality of life and incontinence at 1-year follow-up? Dis Colon Rectum. 2010;53(7):1041–6. PubMed PMID: 20551757.
56. Abbas MA, Tam MS, Chun LJ. Radiofrequency treatment for fecal incontinence: is it effective long-term? Dis Colon Rectum. 2012;55(5):605–10. PubMed PMID: 22513440.
57. Lam TJ, Visscher AP, Meurs-Szojda MM, Felt-Bersma RJ. Clinical response and sustainability of

treatment with temperature-controlled radiofrequency energy (Secca) in patients with faecal incontinence: 3 years follow-up. Int J Color Dis. 2014;29(6):755–61. PubMed PMID: 24805249.

58. Takahashi-Monroy T, Morales M, Garcia-Osogobio S, Valdovinos MA, Belmonte C, Barreto C, et al. SECCA procedure for the treatment of fecal incontinence: results of five-year follow-up. Dis Colon Rectum. 2008;51(3):355–9. PubMed PMID: 18204954.
59. Visscher AP, Lam TJ, Meurs-Szojda MM, Felt-Bersma RJF. Temperature-controlled delivery of radiofrequency energy in fecal incontinence: a randomized sham-controlled clinical trial. Dis Colon Rectum. 2017;60(8):860–5. PubMed PMID: 28682972.
60. Takahashi T, Garcia-Osogobio S, Valdovinos MA, Belmonte C, Barreto C, Velasco L. Extended two-year results of radio-frequency energy delivery for the treatment of fecal incontinence (The Secca Procedure). Dis Colon Rectum. 2003;46(6):711–5.
61. Takahashi T, Garcia-Osogobio S, Valdovinos MA, Mass W, Jimenez R, Jauregui LA, Bobadilla J, Belmonte C, Edelstein PS, Utley DS. Radiofrequency energy delivery to the anal canal for the treatment of fecal incontinence. Dis Colon Rectum. 2002;45(7):915–22.
62. Walega P, Romaniszyn M, Siarkiewicz B, Zelazny D. Dynamic versus adynamic graciloplasty in treatment of end-stage fecal incontinence: is the implantation of the pacemaker really necessary? 12-month follow-up in a clinical, physiological, and functional study. Gastroenterol Res Pract. 2015;2015:698516.
63. Alavi K, Chan S, Wise P, Kaiser AM, Sudan R, Bordeianou L. Fecal incontinence: etiology, diagnosis, and management. J Gastrointest Surg. 2015;19(10):1910–21. PubMed PMID: 26268955.
64. Freeman A, Menees S. Fecal incontinence and pelvic floor dysfunction in women: a review. Gastroenterol Clin North Am. 2016;45(2):217–37.
65. Murad-Regadas SM, Regadas FSP, Regadas Filho FSP, Mendonça Filho JJ, Andrade Filho RS, Vilarinho ADS. Predictors of unsuccessful treatment for fecal incontinence biofeedback in females. Arq Gastroenterol. 2019;56(1):61–5.
66. Wald A. Diagnosis and management of fecal incontinence. Curr Gastroenterol Rep. 2018;20(3):9.
67. Sanagapalli S, Harrington S, Zarate-Lopez N, Emmanuel A. Posterior tibial nerve stimulation for the treatment of fecal incontinence following obstetric anal sphincter injury. Neuromodulation. 2018;21(7):688–93.

Treatment for Fecal Incontinence: Sphincteroplasty and Postanal Repair

12

Megan C. Turner and Karen L. Sherman

Case Scenario

A 45-year-old woman with a prior history of three vaginal deliveries with prior third-degree lacerations presents with fecal incontinence. She has failed conservative management including bulking agents, loperamide, and biofeedback therapy and is interested in surgical options.

Introduction

Fecal incontinence is commonly attributed to obstetrical trauma with injury to the anterior external anal sphincter. While these symptoms are underreported by patients, several surgical options are available for those who fail conservative management adjuncts such as dietary modification, medication, biofeedback, and radio-frequency therapies [1]. Sphincteroplasty, plication to repair a defect of the external sphincter muscles, has been standard therapy for fecal incontinence since its development in 1923 with several variations of technique described [2–4]. Primary approximation, separate external and internal anal sphincter approximation, and en masse repairs both anteriorly and posteriorly have been described with high success rates in short-term follow-up [5–7] but poor success in long-term follow-up (Fig. 12.1) [8]. Success, measured by improvement in fecal incontinence scores [9], is described in Chap. 4. Due to high long-term failure rates, poor efficacy, need for reoperation, and a multimodal approach, more recently, sphincteroplasty is being replaced by sacral neuromodulation [10, 11]. Despite increasing rates of fecal incontinence, sphincteroplasty rates have decreased as sacral neuromodulation has increased (Fig. 12.1). Predictors of successful outcomes have been established through institutional series, and as with all surgical disease, patient counseling is paramount (Fig. 12.2).

Patient Selection

Sphincteroplasty is a surgical option for symptomatic patients with an external anal sphincter defect identified on endoanal ultrasound. Pudendal neuropathy associated with a defect portends a poor outcome [3]. Identification of a sphincter defect alone, in the absence of fecal incontinence, is not an indication for sphincteroplasty. Many

Commentary by Massarat Zutshi, Cleveland Clinic, Department of Colorectal Surgery, Digestive Disease and Surgery Institute, Cleveland, OH, USA

M. C. Turner (✉)
Department of Surgery, Duke University Medical Center, Durham, NC, USA
e-mail: Megan.Turner@dm.duke.edu

K. L. Sherman
Duke University Hospital, Department of Surgery, Raleigh, NC, USA

K. C. Kobashi, S. D. Wexner (eds.), *Female Pelvic Medicine*,
https://doi.org/10.1007/978-3-030-54839-1_12

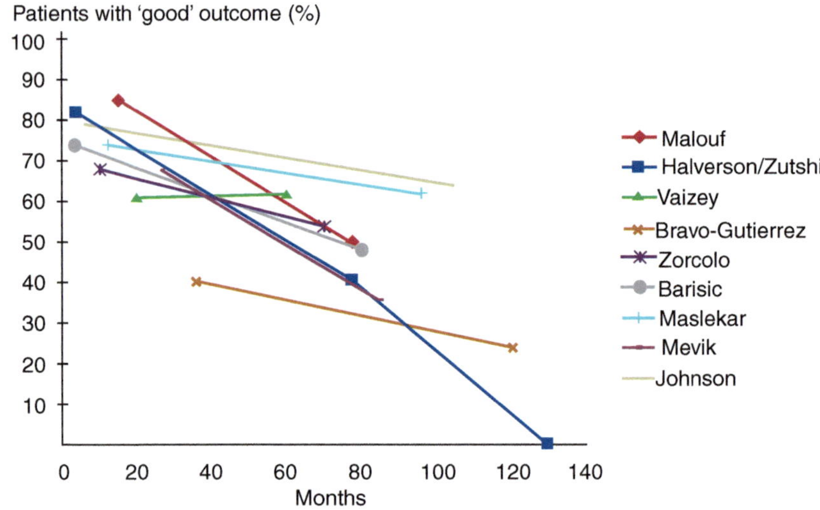

Fig. 12.1 "Good outcome" of overlapping sphincteroplasty over time. Percent "good outcome" as indicated by authors of each article including less incontinence, improved scores, and less impact on their life. Percent "good outcome" at end of study follow-up in months. (Reused with permission. Copyright Wolters Kluwer 2012 [8])

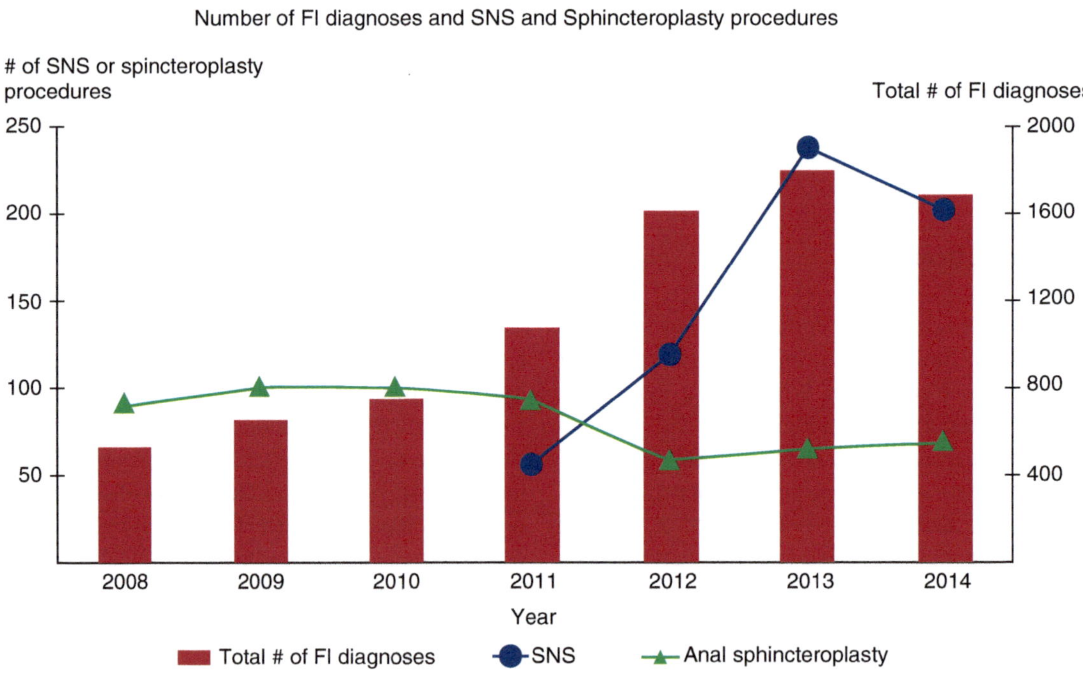

Fig. 12.2 Decreasing rates of sphincteroplasty despite increase in rate of fecal incontinence diagnoses (New York State). (Reused with permission. Copyright Wolters Kluwer 2018 [12])

patients with external anal sphincter defects, who, in the past, would have been treated with overlapping sphincteroplasty, are now being offered with sacral neuromodulation as a first-line surgical treatment. Sphincteroplasty should be considered as an alternative when sacral neuromodulation is contraindicated or has failed. In selected cases, sphincteroplasty can be utilized in conjunction with sacral neuromodulation to further improve response.

Primary Repair

Primary reapproximation of a visually disrupted external anal sphincter, specifically grade III-IV tears, can be performed immediately at the time of obstetric injury. This classic appositional repair technique involves mobilizing and diving the external anal sphincter, excising of scar tissue, and end-to-end reapproximation of the sphincter muscle [3]. Success of this intervention has attempted to be quantified objectively and subjectively with various fecal incontinence scoring systems and quality-of-life measures [8]. The best literature in aggregate suggests up to 67% success of repair in the short-term follow-up [13–15], but as low as 48% success of the repair in long-term follow-up [4, 6, 16, 17]. Once symptoms are recognized by providers, many of these patients seek further intervention with either overlapping sphincteroplasty or sacral nerve stimulation [18].

Historically, Parks postanal repair was performed by plicating the external anal sphincter posteriorly, thereby restoring the anorectal angle. This technique was performed for idiopathic and neurogenic incontinence as well as following repair of rectal prolapse [4]. While initial results were encouraging, restoration of function was poor, and may have led to progression of neurogenic damage to the pelvic floor [4, 19, 20] and this technique has been largely abandoned.

Overlapping Sphincteroplasty

Overlapping repair is conducted by division of the anterior external sphincter scar, overlap of the muscle, and layered closure with absorbable sutures; fecal diversion is not routinely required [8]. Contemporary cohort studies show a 50–86% success in short-term outcomes, 50% success in the long term. Preoperative evaluation includes physical exam, colonoscopy, endoanal ultrasound, and electromyography for persistent anterior sphincter defect and adequate functioning of the remainder sphincter complex, and pudendal nerve motor latency testing [14]. Timing to repair can be immediate in the setting of grade 3b or 4 obstetric tears, or delayed until failure of conservative management, imaging studies identify a sphincter defect, and anal manometry demonstrates decreased external anal sphincter tone.

The operative technique has been described in several ways, but an established technique includes placing the patient in lithotomy (or prone jackknife) following a standard mechanical bowel preparation and preoperative administration of intravenous antibiotics (Fig. 12.3) [3, 21]. The buttocks are taped widely apart. A curvilinear incision is made anterior to the anus and a retractor can be used to facilitate exposure. The internal and external anal sphincter muscles are identified, and the external anal sphincter is isolated (Fig. 12.4). The external sphincter scar is transected at the site of the defect and then mobilized for length; after this, 2–0 absorbable monofilament mattress sutures are used to secure the overlap. The wound is then closed with 2–0 or 3–0 sutures, either leaving an opening or placing a passive drain [19, 22]. Leaving scar tissue in situ maintains bulk for the repair, decreasing the opportunity for suture disruption [3]. Fecal diversion is not required [3]. Bowel confinement with loperamide, codeine, and clear liquid diet for 3 days postoperatively is associated with delayed bowel movement but increased pain with first bowel movement, and longer hospital stay and is not recommended [23, 24] Postoperative antibiotics, such as ciprofloxacin and metronidazole three times daily, are commonly utilized for 7–10 days [25].

Redo Procedures

Several surgical options exist for patients with persistent fecal incontinence following anterior overlapping repair including repeat overlapping anterior anal sphincter repair, sphincter augmentation, dynamic graciloplasty, artificial sphincters, nerve stimulation, and diversion [14]. Sphincter augmentation, graciloplasty, artificial sphincters, and diversion are described elsewhere in this book. The following discussion will focus on redo and nerve stimulation in the setting of failed sphincteroplasty.

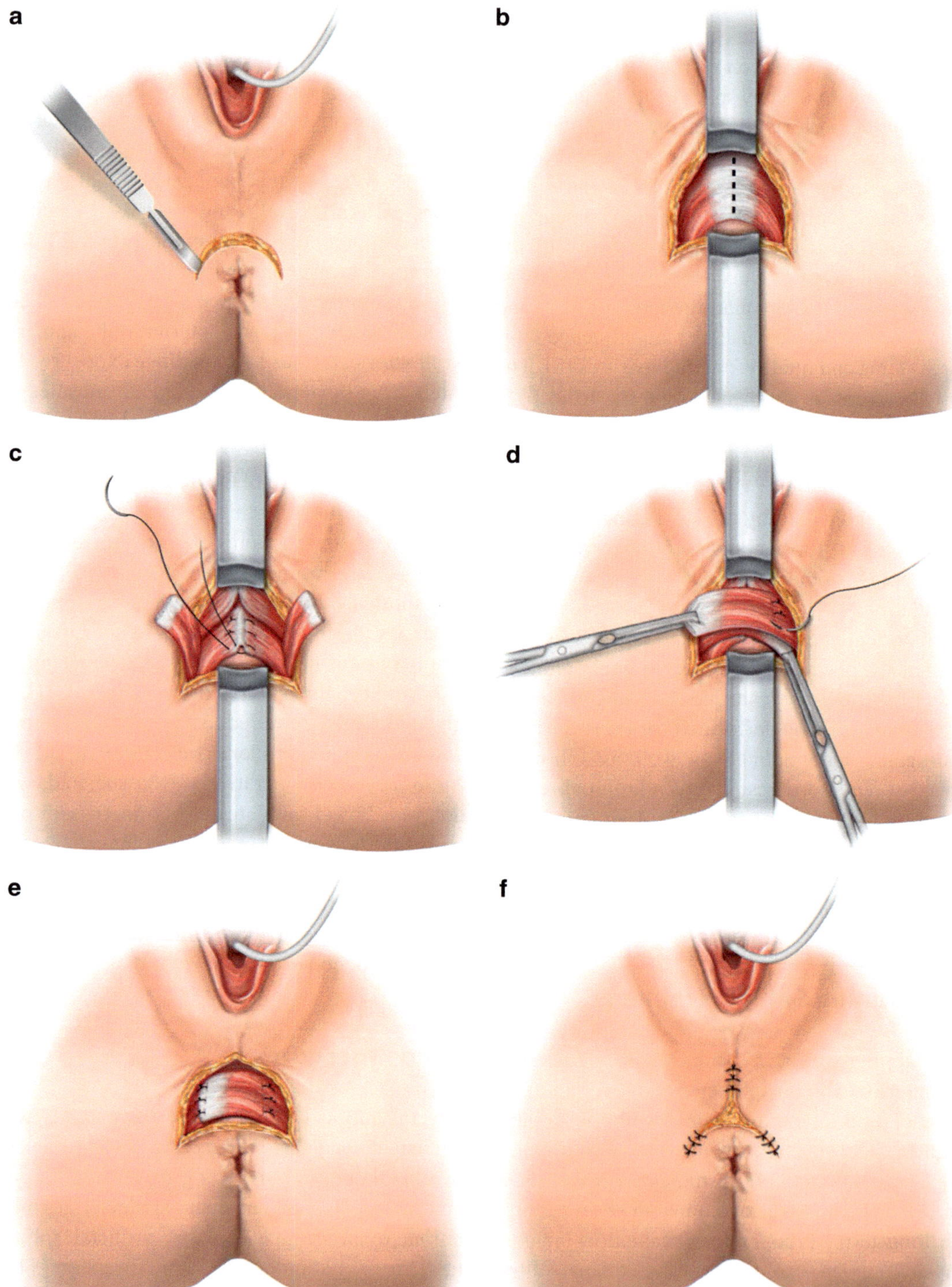

Fig. 12.3 Technique of overlapping sphincteroplasty. (**a**) Curvilinear incision made along the perineal body. (**b**) Sphincter scar divided but not excised. (**c**) Overlapping repair of the anal sphincter with mattress sutures. (**d**) Internal anal sphincter imbricated when a layered repair is performed. (**e**) External anal sphincter overlapped. (**f**) Edges of the wound approximated in a V-shape or longitudinally with interrupted 3–0 absorbable mattress sutures. The center of the wound is left open for drainage. The perineal body is bulkier than it was preoperatively. (Reused with permission. Copyright Wolters Kluwer 2018 [21])

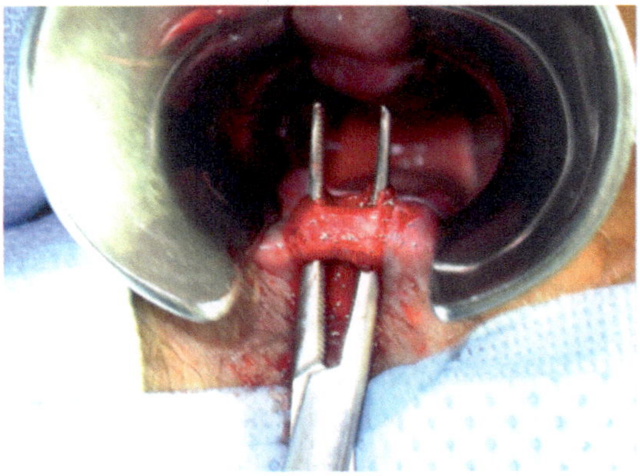

Fig. 12.4 Identification of the external anal sphincter

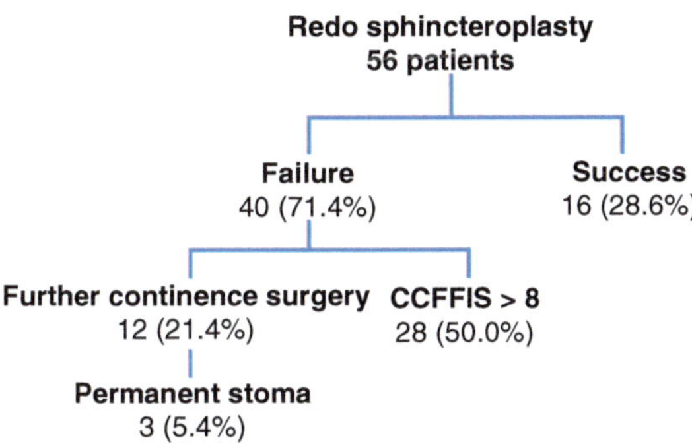

Fig. 12.5 Diagram of outcomes for patients with redo sphincteroplasty [26]

Redo repairs have been described up to seven additional times following the index procedure. Redo procedures are associated with poor long-term functional outcome, with a greater than 70% failure rate (Fig. 12.5), with an association with worse outcome at >2 repairs compared to </=2 repairs [14, 26]. The preoperative evaluation and technique remains the same as index procedures for these patients.

Prior guidelines have suggested redo sphincteroplasty for recalcitrant symptoms; however, in light of poor long-term outcomes, other approaches may be more appropriate [26]. For amenable patients, sacral neuromodulation can be combined with sphincteroplasty for those with inadequate response. Neuromodulation is further detailed in Chap. 13.

Predictors of Successful Outcomes

Despite mediocre overall outcomes, there are predictors associated with inferior continence that have been described in individual studies and meta-analyses [8]. Identified preoperative anterior defects and resolution of anterior defect are associated with superior continence [15, 27, 28]. Improved squeeze pressure postoperatively [22] and short-term improvements in incontinence scores are associated with good long-term outcomes [9]. Poor short- and long-term outcomes are associated with low preoperative fecal incontinence scores [29], obesity [26], residual defect [28], and pudendal neuropathy [3, 6, 13, 30]. Increasing age is associated with decreased anal canal pressures, decreased rectal compliance, increased sclerosis of the internal anal sphincter, and atrophy of the external anal sphincter, but disagreement exists whether age itself is a risk of poor outcome [3, 4, 8]. No correlation with postoperative outcomes has been determined with number of vaginal deliveries, episiotomy, preoperative pudendal nerve terminal motor latency (PNTML) [14]. While redo procedures initially do not affect success rates, greater than two repairs are associated with poor continence at each subsequent repair [14]. While resolution of sphincter defects on endoanal ultrasound does not portend improved prediction of continence, this technique remains essential to diagnostics [8].

Patient Counseling

Expectations are an important component of management of fecal incontinence. Patients should be aware that surgery is rarely curative, and often requires a multimodal approach, but that improvements in symptom severity and quality of life can be made in selected patients. Redo operations into the future may only improve but not resolve their symptoms. For women who intend to have subsequent pregnancies, vaginal deliveries are safe but incur a 4–8% risk of recurrent sphincter injury [31]. Despite decreasing continence scores overtime, and need for adjunctive procedures, most patients are satisfied with their decision to undergo sphincteroplasty [8].

Summary

Sphincteroplasty may no longer be the standard of care for surgical management of fecal incontinence with an anterior external anal sphincter defect, but it has a persistent role. Sphincteroplasty should be considered for selected patients in which sacral neuromodulation is contraindicated or has failed, used in combination with sacral neuromodulation, or less often, can be repeated in the setting of recurrent symptoms. Continued training in this operation is essential as it represents one of several management options for management of fecal incontinence.

Commentary

Massarat Zutshi

The chapter on sphincteroplasty is well written with a focus on why it is no longer a gold standard in the treatment of fecal incontinence. In the era of neuromodulation and the success associated with this treatment, sphincteroplasty does fade from the algorithm of procedures to treat fecal incontinence. With poor long-term outcomes, which may be a result of poor tissues, advancing age, and muscle atrophy, the authors make a valid point about its efficacy. There are very few single surgeon reports that show a good long-term outcome. That it is no longer considered a primary procedure is without doubt. In young patients after an obstetric injury or as part of a recto-vaginal fistula repair, it does still have a place and if done well can achieve good results. However, there are places in the world where neuromodulation may not be available or cost-effective, or it may be that certain patients do not want or cannot have a device, or have an allergy to the metal used; hence, knowledge of the procedure should be part of the curriculum.

The authors describe the operative procedure very well. It should however be noted that often, there may not be scar tissue in the midline that needs to be divided. Often the external sphincter is retracted and has to be identified and dissected. Most often, the sphincter complex is dissected en mass as it is difficult to dissect. Care should be taken to avoid overdissection of the muscle belly to prevent neurological damage, leading to further atrophy. During approximation, the sutures are placed without tension to prevent ischemic necrosis. As end-to-end repairs have been shown to be equally efficient to overlapping tension should be avoided at all costs. If the muscle tissue is insufficient to begin with, augmenting the sphincter with a biologic mesh may be considered [32–40].

Redo repairs require expertise as often the anatomy is distorted. Redo sphincteroplasty should be undertaken if the patient has had a previous good outcome and the muscle tissue appears sufficient on an endoanal ultrasound. Redo repair on muscle that looks poor or if the previous repair is still holding is bound to be unsuccessful.

A successful sphincteroplasty should always be followed by biofeedback with electrical stimulation to increase muscle tissue. Good bowel management also contributes to a good outcome.

References

1. Van Koughnett JA, Wexner SD. Current management of fecal incontinence: choosing amongst treatment options to optimize outcomes. World J Gastroenterol. 2013;19(48):9216–30.
2. Lockhart-Mummery JP. Diseases of the rectum and colon and their surgical treatment: W. Wood and company; London, England 1934.
3. Jorge JM, Wexner SD. Etiology and management of fecal incontinence. Dis Colon Rectum. 1993;36(1):77–97.
4. Baig MK, Wexner SD. Factors predictive of outcome after surgery for faecal incontinence. Br J Surg. 2000;87(10):1316–30.
5. Österberg A, Eeg-Olofsson KE, Graf W. Results of surgical treatment for faecal incontinence. Br J Surg. 2000;87(11):1546–52.

6. Nikiteas N, Korsgen S, Kumar D, Keighley MR. Audit of sphincter repair. Factors associated with poor outcome. Dis Colon Rectum. 1996;39(10):1164–70.
7. Young CJ, Mathur MN, Eyers AA, Solomon MJ. Successful overlapping anal sphincter repair. Dis Colon Rectum. 1998;41(3):344–9.
8. Glasgow SC, Lowry AC. Long-term outcomes of anal sphincter repair for fecal incontinence: a systematic review. Dis Colon Rectum. 2012;55(4):482–90.
9. Oliveira L, Pfeifer J, Wexner S. Physiological and clinical outcome of anterior sphincteroplasty. Br J Surg. 1996;83(4):502–5.
10. Altomare DF, De Fazio M, Giuliani RT, Catalano G, Cuccia F. Sphincteroplasty for fecal incontinence in the era of sacral nerve modulation. World J Gastroenterol. 2010;16(42):5267–71.
11. Brouwer R, Duthie G. Sacral nerve neuromodulation is effective treatment for fecal incontinence in the presence of a sphincter defect, pudendal neuropathy, or previous sphincter repair. Dis Colon Rectum. 2010;53(3):273–8.
12. Xu Z, Fleming FJ, Justiniano CF, Becerra AZ, Boodry CI, Aquina CT, et al. Trends in surgeon-level utilization of sacral nerve stimulator implantation for fecal incontinence in New York state. Dis Colon Rectum. 2018;61(1):107–14.
13. Gilliland R, Altomare DF, Moreira H Jr, Oliveira L, Gilliland JE, Wexner SD. Pudendal neuropathy is predictive of failure following anterior overlapping sphincteroplasty. Dis Colon Rectum. 1998;41(12):1516–22.
14. Giordano P, Renzi A, Efron J, Gervaz P, Weiss EG, Nogueras JJ, et al. Previous sphincter repair does not affect the outcome of repeat repair. Dis Colon Rectum. 2002;45(5):635–40.
15. Goetz LH, Lowry AC. Overlapping sphincteroplasty: is it the standard of care? Clin Colon Rectal Surg. 2005;18(1):22–31.
16. Lamblin G, Bouvier P, Damon H, Chabert P, Moret S, Chene G, et al. Long-term outcome after overlapping anterior anal sphincter repair for fecal incontinence. Int J Color Dis. 2014;29(11):1377–83.
17. Halverson AL, Hull TL. Long-term outcome of overlapping anal sphincter repair. Dis Colon Rectum. 2002;45(3):345–8.
18. Fitzpatrick M, O'Herlihy C. Short-term and long-term effects of obstetric anal sphincter injury and their management. Curr Opin Obstet Gynecol. 2005;17(6):605–10.
19. Wexner SD, Marchetti F, Jagelman DG. The role of sphincteroplasty for fecal incontinence reevaluated: a prospective physiologic and functional review. Dis Colon Rectum. 1991;34(1):22–30.
20. Browning GG, Parks AG. Postanal repair for neuropathic faecal incontinence: correlation of clinical result and anal canal pressures. Br J Surg. 1983;70(2):101–4.
21. Wexner SD, Fleshman JW, editors. Colon and rectal surgery: anorectal operations. 2nd ed. Philadelphia: Wolters Kluwer; 2019.
22. Gearhart S, Hull T, Floruta C, Schroeder T, Hammel J. Anal manometric parameters: predictors of outcome following anal sphincter repair? J Gastrointest Surg. 2005;9(1):115–20.
23. Nessim A, Wexner SD, Agachan F, Alabaz O, Weiss EG, Nogueras JJ, et al. Is bowel confinement necessary after anorectal reconstructive surgery? A prospective, randomized, surgeon-blinded trial. Dis Colon Rectum. 1999;42(1):16–23.
24. Mahoney R, Behan M, O'Herlihy C. Randomized, clinical trial of bowel confinement vs laxative use after primary repair of a third-degree obstetrics anal sphincter tear. Dis Colon Rectum. 2004;47:12–7.
25. Maldonado PA, Mcintire D, Corton MM. Long-term outcomes after overlapping sphincteroplasty for cloacal-like deformities. Female Pelvic Med Reconstr Surg. 2019;25(4):271–8.
26. Hong K, Dasilva G, Dollerschell JT, Maron D, Wexner SD. Redo sphincteroplasty: are the results sustainable? Gastroenterol Rep. 2016;4(1):39–42.
27. Saldana Ruiz N, Kaiser AM. Fecal incontinence - challenges and solutions. World J Gastroenterol. 2017;23(1):11–24.
28. Engel A, Kamm M, Sultan A, Bartram C, Nicholls R. Anterior anal sphincter repair in patients with obstetric trauma. BJS. 1994;81(8):1231–4.
29. McManus BP, Allison S, Hernanchez-Sanchez J. Anterior sphincteroplasty for fecal incontinence: predicting incontinence relapse. Int J Color Dis. 2015;30(4):513–20.
30. Sangwan YP, Coller JA, Barrett RC, Roberts PL, Murray JJ, Rusin L, et al. Unilateral pudendal neuropathy. Impact on outcome of anal sphincter repair. Dis Colon Rectum. 1996;39(6):686–9.
31. Harvey MA, Pierce M, Alter JE, Chou Q, Diamond P, Epp A, et al. Obstetrical Anal Sphincter Injuries (OASIS): prevention, recognition, and repair. J Obstet Gynaecol Can JOGC = Journal d'obstetrique et gynecologie du Canada: JOGC. 2015;37(12):1131–48.
32. Oom DM, Steensma AB, Zimmerman DD, Schouten WR. Anterior sphincteroplasty for fecal incontinence: is the outcome compromised in patients with associated pelvic floor injury? Dis Colon Rectum. 2010;53:150–5.
33. Parks A, McPartlin J. Late repair of injuries of the anal sphincters. Proc R Soc Med. 1971;64:1187–89.
34. Engel AF, Kamm MA, Sultan AH, Bartram CI, et al. Anterior anal sphincter repair in patients with obstetric trauma. Br J Surg. 1994;81:1231–4.
35. Simmang C, Birnbaum EH, Kodner IJ, Fry RD, et al. Anal sphincter reconstruction in the elderly: does advancing age affect outcome? Dis Colon Rectum. 1994;37:1065–9.
36. Nikiteas N, Korsgen S, Kumar D, Keighley MR. Audit of sphincter repair. Factors associated with poor outcome. Dis Colon Rectum. 1996;39:1164–70.
37. Giordano P, Renzi A, Efron J, Gervaz P, et al. Previous sphincter repair does not affect the outcome of repeat repair. Dis Colon Rectum. 2002;45:635–40.

38. Maslekar S, Gardiner AB, Duthie GS. Anterior anal sphincter repair for fecal incontinence: good long-term results are possible. J Am Coll Surg. 2007;204:40–6.
39. Zutshi M, Ferreira P, Hull T, Gurland B. Biological implants in sphincter augmentation offer a good short-term outcome after a sphincter repair. Colorectal Dis. 2012;14:866–71.
40. Zutshi M, Hull T, Gurland B. Anal encirclement with sphincter repair (AESR procedure) using a biological graft for anal sphincter damage involving the entire circumference. Colorectal Dis. 2012;14:592–5.

Treatment for Fecal Incontinence: Muscle Transposition, Artificial Bowel Sphincter, Magnetic Sphincter, and Stem Cell Regeneration

13

Lucia Camara Castro Oliveira

Introduction

Fecal incontinence (FI) is a distressing condition associated with a negative impact on quality of life [1]. Although the incidence in the literature indicates that approximately 7% of patients suffer from FI episodes, the true incidence is likely worse, with up to 20% of patients living with this silent affliction [2, 3]. The largest internet-based survey among healthy adult females demonstrated that the incidence of FI in this population is 18% [4]. Many of these women have never discussed incontinence episodes with their doctors. The difficulty and embarrassment that these patients experience is usually an impeding factor in our understanding of the true incidence, and many patients remain incontinent with no effective treatment.

The magnitude of the problem can have an economic impact due to the cost of devices and hospital admissions, specifically in the elderly population. Conservative and clinical treatment is initiated for all patients, but based on the etiology and severity of the case, several surgical and minimally invasive options are also available (Table 13.1) [5]. Overlapping sphincteroplasty is one of the most commonly performed procedures, with a maximum 76% short-term success rate, which decreases to as low as 15% during subsequent years [6–8]. Although this procedure is "simple" for the experienced colorectal surgeon, it is not a durable operation with deterioration of the results after 5 years [9, 10]. Other minimally invasive procedures, such as injection of bulking agents and radiofrequency tissue remodeling, will be discussed in other chapters. Management can be divided into repair, augmentation, replacement, stimulation, and bypass (diversion) (Table 13.1) [11].

Difficult and complex cases refractory to initial treatment options may require neuromodulation, sphincter replacement, or encirclement procedures. A recent algorithm of treatment has been proposed, with neuromodulation being the most promising available option (Fig. 13.1). In this chapter, we will discuss the more complex surgical procedures.

Commentary by Donato F. Altomare, Azienda Ospedaliero Universitaria Policlinico Bari, Department of Emergency and Organ Transplantation, University Aldo Moro of Bari, Bari, Italy

L. C. C. Oliveira (✉)
Anorectal Physiology Department, CEPEMED,
Rio de Janeiro, Brazil

K. C. Kobashi, S. D. Wexner (eds.), *Female Pelvic Medicine*,
https://doi.org/10.1007/978-3-030-54839-1_13

Table 13.1 Treatment options for fecal incontinence [12]

Repair	Sphincteroplasty
	Postanal repair
Augmentation	Injectables
	Radiofrequency remodeling
Replacement	Adynamic muscle transfers (gracilis or gluteus)
	Dynamic graciloplasty
	Artificial bowel sphincter
	Magnetic anal sphincter
Stimulation	Sacral nerve stimulation
	Posterior tibial nerve stimulation (percutaneous or transcutaneous)
Diversion	Standard stoma
	Antegrade stoma procedure

Case Scenario

A 56-year-old female patient who is married and a schoolteacher presents with complaints of FI for the last 5 years. She reports weekly episodes of incontinence to gas and stool, and daily use of pads, which has significantly impacted her social and professional life. She reports monthly episodes of liquid diarrhea and bloating, requiring Imodium and gas relief medications.

She had two pregnancies and had two vaginal births (weighing 3.6 and 4 kg), both of which were accompanied by episiotomies. She underwent an anterior sphincteroplasty 10 years ago for FI, an anal fistulectomy at the age of 50 with

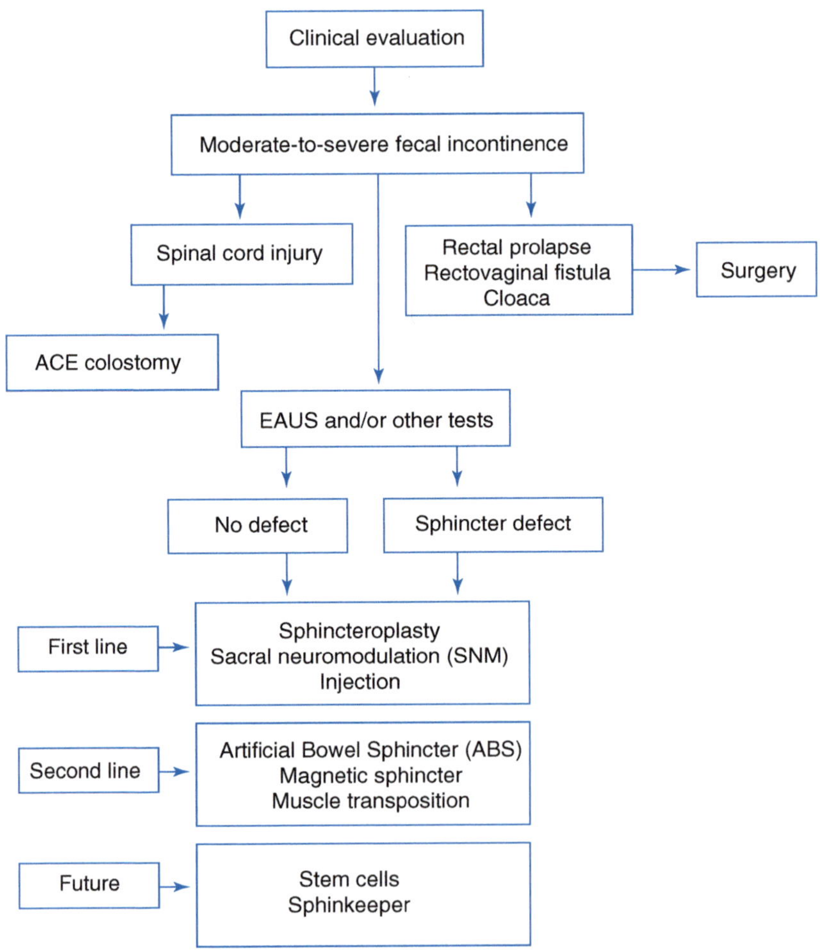

Fig. 13.1 Treatment algorithm

difficult and prolonged recovery, and a cholecystectomy 2 years ago. Her BMI was 28 kg/m^2, and her abdominal evaluation was unremarkable. Proctologic examination revealed a depressed scar in the perineal body region and another wound in the left lateral quadrant. The anus was patulous, and voluntary contraction was very poor (Fig. 13.2). Digital examination confirmed a hypotonic sphincter and asymmetry of the anal canal. The rectosigmoidoscopy was normal, without any tumors or polyps. She underwent colonoscopy at age 50 that revealed rare diverticulum in the left colon. At this point of the clinical evaluation, in order to assess severity and quality of life, the patient was given the Cleveland Clinic Florida-Fecal Incontinence Score (CCF-FIS) and the Fecal Incontinence Severity Index (FISI) for quality-of-life assessment [12, 13]. Her CCF-FIS score was 16, translating into a significant negative impact on her quality of life. The most important factor that helps to maintain anal continence is the sphincter mechanism, represented by the external anal sphincter (EAS) and the internal anal sphincter (IAS), the puborectalis, and the intact respective innervation. Therefore, any traumatic, congenital, or iatrogenic injury to the sphincters can produce FI. In this case, the patient has important traumatic and postsurgical events in her history. She also has important adjunct factors such as a previous cholecystectomy and being overweight.

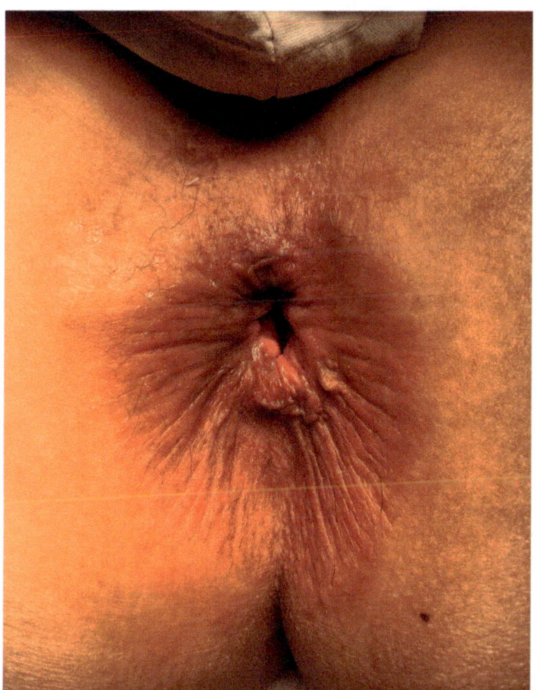

Fig. 13.2 Patulous anus

Obstetrical trauma and prior surgical procedures are the most common causes of disruption of the anal sphincter mechanism, leading to FI. Disruption of the anal canal musculature produces incontinence due to the loss of the anal canal high-pressure zone, alterations in normal sampling mechanisms, or both. Isolated sphincter dysfunction needs to be differentiated from metabolic or neurologic disorders that may clinically manifest as FI. In most patients with sphincter injury, clinical evaluation by an experienced surgeon is all that is required for preoperative evaluation and planning. Direct inspection of the perineum with adequate illumination is essential. Spreading the buttocks may reveal the presence of dermatitis, a patulous anus, loss of the perineal body, and muscular deficit in the anorectal ring. The presence of perineal soiling, scars from previous surgery or trauma, mucosal ectropion, prolapsing hemorrhoids, or complete rectal prolapse should be noted. A single glance at the perianal skin and undergarments may help to assess the degree and type of incontinence. Sensory alterations in the perianal area can be examined by gentle touch and pinprick. The patient should be asked to strain in order to evaluate the presence of perineal descent, rectocele, or cystocele. In female patients, vaginal digital examination is important to assess the perineal body and the anterior sphincter bulk. Digital examination during resting and squeezing should be performed. The external anal sphincter and the more proximal puborectalis muscle should also each be examined. Digital rectal examination may also exclude fecal impaction. Anoscopy and proctosigmoidoscopy may reveal the presence of inflammatory or neoplastic conditions, or other disorders such as solitary rectal ulcer syndrome, colitis, cystica profunda, or rectoanal intussusception.

In this case, a defect of the IAS in the left lateral quadrant was suspected, in addition to a disrupted perineal body. Digital examination revealed a hypotonic and asymmetric sphincter. The patient also had perineal descent on straining, without any other prolapsed organ or associated urinary incontinence.

Because of her history of previous sphincteroplasty and a visible weak sphincter, anal manometry was performed to objectively document IAS and EAS tone, as well as to assess sphincter fatigue and asymmetry (Fig. 13.3). Anorectal manometry can help in the selection of candidates for biofeedback therapy.

At this point, with a documented weak sphincter, anal ultrasound was performed, revealing an IAS defect at the left lateral quadrant, as well as a thin perineal body with a persistent EAS defect in the anterior quadrant Fig. 13.4.

Anal ultrasonography is a painless and relatively simple method of evaluating anal sphincter morphology and has been increasingly utilized in the assessment of incontinent patients, replacing anal EMG in many cases [14].

Selection of patients who will benefit from a surgical procedure is important, especially among female patients. A 35% incidence of sphincter injury after vaginal delivery was reported in the literature and could be detected by anal ultrasonography [14]. These isolated anterior sphincter defects can be managed by overlapping sphincteroplasty, with successful outcomes of around 69–97% [15–19].

Long-term functional outcome after anterior sphincteroplasty is unsatisfactory, and many studies have documented that only 50% of patients remain continent after 5 years [10, 15]. Until recently, surgical techniques for patients with failed anterior sphincteroplasty included the implantation of an artificial anal/bowel sphincter (ABS), stimulated graciloplasty, or sacral neuromodulation (SNM) [20–25]. The first two techniques are complex surgical procedures associated with very high morbidity and have

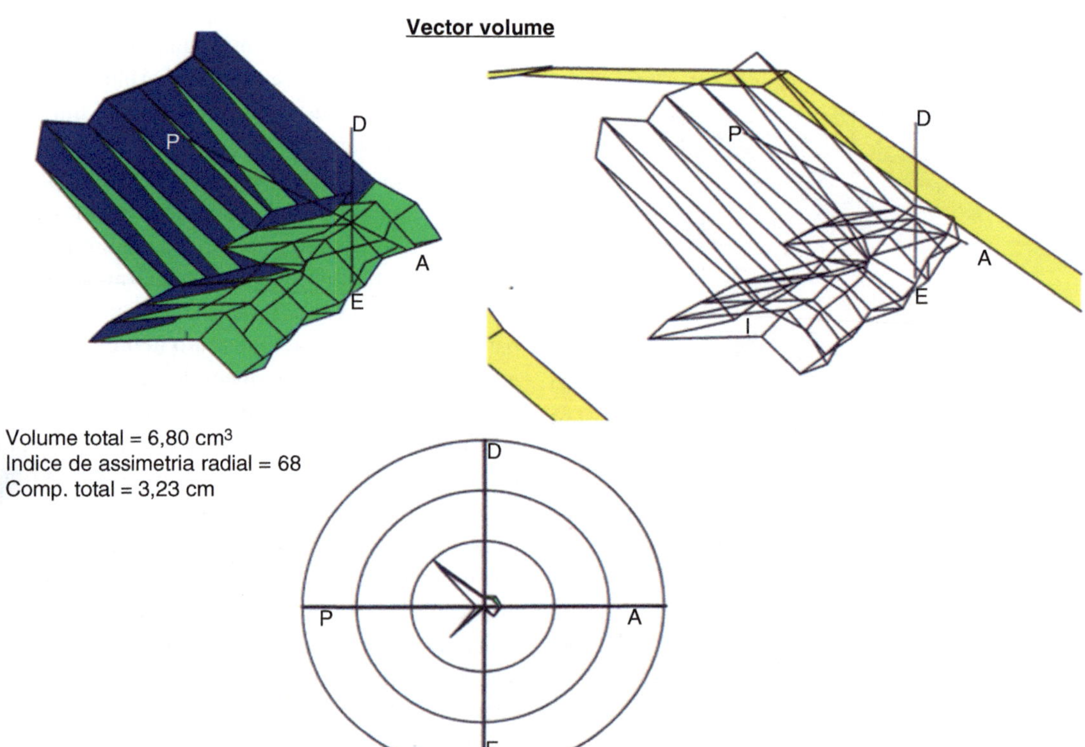

Fig. 13.3 Anal manometry to assess sphincter fatigue and asymmetry

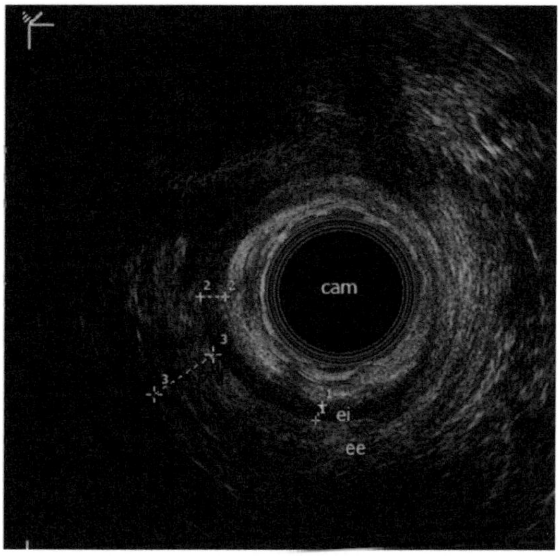

Fig. 13.4 Anal ultrasound showing an IAS defect at the left lateral quadrant, as well as a thin perineal body with a persistent EAS defect in the anterior quadrant

been employed in a very highly selective group of patients. SNM is now considered the gold standard for the treatment of FI and will be discussed in another chapter [23]. In fact, as already mentioned, a new algorithm proposed for FI has been changing the treatment of these patients (Fig. 13.1). Due to the complications associated with ABS and stimulated graciloplasty, new surgical procedures have been proposed such as the implantation of a magnetic anal sphincter and other encirclement procedures. However, one of the important caveats in the surgical treatment of FI is to establish when direct sphincter repair is not possible, because it is absent or failed. Such severe cases can be associated with congenital anal atresia, severe traumatic destruction, or when the sphincter is anatomically intact but functionally inactive and does not respond to electrostimulation techniques (sacral or the posterior tibial nerve). In addition, sacral nerve or tibial stimulation may not be available or affordable.

The current patient already had a sphincteroplasty, and the fistulectomy may have further damaged her already weak sphincter. In cases of severe FI with significant impairment of quality of life, it is necessary to recreate a neosphincter either with an autologous muscle or by implantation of a device. Severe damage to the anal sphincter muscles, with multiple defects in different quadrants of the anal circumference, is usually not amenable to direct repair. In these situations, a number of neosphincter operations are available. These are complex operations with very high morbidity rates related mainly to infection, problems with the device, and rupture of the wraps, among others [24, 25]. Despite this high morbidity, dynamic graciloplasty is still regarded as having a role in selected cases of end-stage FI when undertaken by an experienced team, as demonstrated by multicenter trials [22, 26, 27]. Regardless of the technique employed, the encirclement should be dynamic rather than static.

Free Muscle Transplantation

Free transplantation of a portion of the sartorius muscle or the palmaris longus was popularized by Hakelius and Olsen [28] mainly for the treatment of severe FI resulting from congenital absence or traumatic injury to the puborectalis muscle. Successful transplantation depends on reinnervation of the transplanted muscle following transplantation into the functional position of the puborectalis muscle. After reinnervation has taken place, the muscle becomes part of the reflex mechanism.

Gluteus Maximus Transposition

Transposition of the gluteus maximus was described by Chetwood [29] in 1902 and became the most common example of muscle transposition in the first half of this century. The transposition of this muscle is facilitated because anatomically it is localized very close to the anal canal and because it has a proximal single innervation. Compared to the gracilis muscle, there are some advantages of using the gluteus maximus muscle: it is a large and strong muscle and the proximity to the perianal area eliminates the need for thigh incisions. Therefore, anal encirclement with this muscle allows voluntary contraction and provides good functional outcomes.

Indications are usually neurogenic incontinence, multiple failed previous repairs, and severe sphincter defects. However, selection of patients is very important, as the most common complication is wound infection. Despite the potential risk of failure of the procedure, in general, those cases can be managed without the need for fecal diversion. Overall success rates of restoration of complete and partial continence are 60% and 36%, respectively [30–42]. One series wherein patients had a longer history of FI reported 11 patients who underwent augmented unilateral gluteoplasty and were followed for 6–18 months [42]. Improvement was demonstrated in almost 73% of patients with low morbidity. A randomized trial comparing total pelvic floor repair and gluteus maximus transposition demonstrated that both procedures significantly improved continence in 24 women with neuropathic incontinence [43]. However, when compared with graciloplasty, the results of a multicenter prospective trial demonstrated that the results of gluteoplasty were less successful and should be limited to investigational purposes. The gluteus maximus is a physically active muscle that contains at least 52% type I fibers (resistant to fatigue); less than the external sphincter (78%), but more than the sartorius (50%), rectus abdominis (46%), and gracilis (43%). Its anatomical and physiological characteristics, its natural synergism in the mechanism of continence, and the technical possibility to carry out its transposition make it an appropriate muscle for the construction of a neosphincter [44].

The largest series was reported by Devesa and colleagues [42] in 1997. Their results in 20 incontinent patients were not as remarkable as those described by Pearl et al. [39], and failures were related to suture disruption, poor muscular contraction, and intractable constipation. With the current information, it is not possible to establish the true value of gluteoplasty for severe FI, but according to the published series, approximately two-thirds of patients significantly improve their status. However, only a very low percentage may reach optimal levels of continence. In addition, it cannot be established which is the best of the techniques described.

Gracilis Muscle Transposition

Gracilis muscle transposition was initially described by Pickerel in 1952 for the treatment of incontinent children with neurological and congenital anomalies. The rationale of the operation was to encircle the anal canal with the muscle to produce a dynamic sling and to create a natural barrier to the passage of stool similar to the Thiersch repair [45]. However, the advantage is that anal encirclement is performed with autologous viable tissue, rather than foreign material. Since the first description, this operation has been used for the treatment of FI secondary to trauma, neurologic causes, or patients with anorectal agenesis.

The gracilis muscle is wrapped around the anus and fixed to the contralateral or ipsilateral ischial tuberosity (Fig. 13.5). Both legs are prepared and draped free to allow repositioning during the operative procedure. The superficial medial location of the gracilis muscle in the thigh and the muscle's proximal blood supply allow division of the distal insertion site and proximal mobilization of the muscle without compromising viability. The position of the muscle is first traced on the surface of the thigh from the pubic arch to the upper medial tubercle of the tibia. Two 3–5-cm long incisions are made – one in the

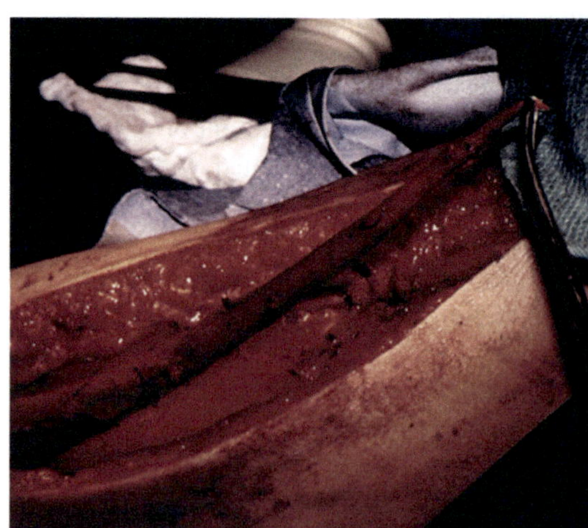

Fig. 13.5 The gracilis muscle is wrapped around the anus and fixed to the contralateral or ipsilateral ischial tuberosity

upper medial thigh overlying the gracilis neurovascular pedicle and one in the distal medial thigh overlying the gracilis tendon. Care should be taken not to cross the knee joint with the distal incision. The tendon of the gracilis muscle is identified distally and severed from its insertion on the tibia. The muscle is carefully mobilized until the neurovascular bundle is encountered in the proximal third of the muscle. The neurovascular bundle is carefully preserved and defines the cephalad limit of the gracilis muscle dissection. For the proximal transfer of the distal tendon, the perforating vessels are controlled with an energy device; there are usually between 1 and 3 of these vessels.

Two incisions approximately 1.5–2 cm from the anal verge are made on the right and left sites. A tunnel is fashioned between the two perianal incisions and the proximal dissection of the gracilis muscle. The distal tendinous portion of the gracilis is then passed through this tunnel and under the anterior and posterior raphe to encircle the anus in the ischioanal space. The leg is then fully adducted to minimize tension on the gracilis, and the tendinous end of the muscle is anchored to the contralateral tibial tuberosity with strong nonabsorbable suture. When complete, the anal canal should allow one finger to pass snugly. Incisions are closed primarily without the use of drains. Immediate postoperative care consists of bed rest for 48 hours, followed by gradual ambulation. Although considered a "living Thiersch" procedure, the gracilis muscle can sometimes be relaxed purposely at the time of defecation by assuming the squatting position and avoiding abduction of the thigh. Suppositories or enemas can be used to help establish a regular pattern of defecation and to promote complete evacuation of the rectum. Functional results are not as good as expected as most patients can only control solid stool. Selected patients may benefit from gracilis transposition when other means have failed, or inadequate sphincter muscle is available for a classic sphincter repair. Unfortunately, stimulated graciloplasty is no longer an option.

Artificial Bowel Sphincter

The initial experience with artificial sphincter for FI was undertaken by using an inflatable prosthesis in animal models [46]. Subsequent clinical studies led to the development of a subcutaneous cuff to be placed around the anal canal [21, 47]. The indications were usually related to neurogenic incontinence or severe traumatic injuries of the anal sphincter. This prosthesis is an implantable, fluid-filled, solid silicone elastomer device, consisting of three components: a cuff, a control-pump, and a pressure-regulating balloon, attached together by kink-resistant tubing (Fig. 13.6). This device simulates normal sphincter function by opening and closing the anal canal according to patient control.

The operation is relatively simple, beginning by the implantation of the occlusive cuff around the anal canal; a variety of cuff sizes are available. Next, the pressure-regulating balloon is implanted in the prevesical space, controlling the amount of pressure exerted by the occlusive cuff. Finally, the control pump is implanted in the soft tissue of the scrotum or vaginal greater labium. The upper part of the control pump contains the resistor and valves needed to transfer fluid to and from the cuff. It also contains the deactivation button. The patient squeezes and releases the bulb at the bottom half of the control pump to transfer fluid within the device. A septum at the bottom of the control pump is designed to allow the insertion of small amount of fluid if needed in the postoperative period.

Although continence was improved in the majority of patients, morbidity was high, especially infectious complications, mechanical malfunctions of device, and evacuatory problems. Although there was no associated mortality and the percentage of successes maintained in the long term was higher than with myoplasties, the Acticon AMS artificial sphincter is no longer available and only the A.M.I. Soft Anal Band® remains for clinical use, in very selected cases.

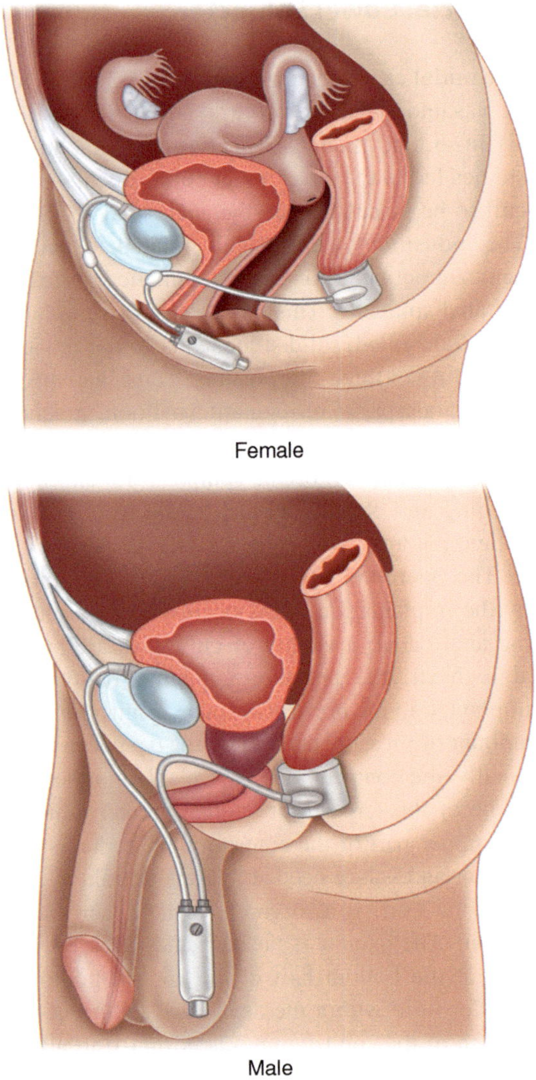

Fig. 13.6 Artificial bowel sphincter in females *(top)* and males *(bottom)*. The cuff is placed to encircle the anus, while the balloon is located in the space of Retzius. The button is placed in the labia in females and in the scrotum in males. (Reused with permission. Copyright Springer Nature)

Synthetic Encirclement Procedures

Several investigators have attempted to correct damaged nonfunctioning sphincter musculature by encirclement procedures, using synthetic material.

Synthetic encirclement of the anus was originally described by Thiersch [48] in 1891, for the treatment of rectal prolapse associated with anal incontinence.

This author imagined that circumanal wiring would give support to the anus and contain the prolapse while the reaction to the foreign material by the tissues would create a fibrosis that would provide additional support to the wire. However, due to the high incidence of wire breaking, different types of materials were proposed to overcome this complication such as steel wire, nylon, and dacron-impregnated silastic. Clearly, synthetic material cannot be expected to function as normal muscle and, to date, the results have been suboptimal. Improvement in continence with this procedure appears to rely on narrowing of the anal canal as a result of postoperative scarring. Although a silastic sling is not free of infection and erosion risk, it appears to be the most reasonable material as the static properties of wire can be overcome by the elasticity of this material, allowing defecation. The operative procedure involves incision over both ischioanal fossae and the creation of a tunnel deep enough to accommodate a 2-cm strip of silastic material, which is encircled around the anus. The dacron sheet is tightened around the tip of an index finger and secured with staples. The wounds are closed in layers, and the patient is discharged home after the first bowel movement. There is a high incidence of infection and extrusion of the implant. Thus, this operation has little to offer the patient and should be abandoned or performed only in very selected circumstances.

Although sophisticated techniques such as the artificial anal sphincter or the magnetic anal sphincter have been associated with successful results, these devices are no longer available in the market. Experienced surgeons have been utilizing newer materials, such as a simple silicone drain or the Jackson Pratt drain [49].

Magnetic Sphincter

Since muscle transposition techniques and artificial sphincters have been associated with high morbidity, with complications resulting in the necessity for explantations and revisions, newer and simpler encirclement procedures have been developed in the last few years. One of the new and promising devices was the magnetic anal sphincter (Fig. 13.7) [50–52]. Compared to the other implantable devices, the magnetic sphincter procedure is more less complicated and with an acceptable safety profile. According to investigators, the magnetic anal sphincter device was designed to augment the native anal sphincter. The device consists of a series of titanium beads with magnetic cores linked together with independent titanium wires. In order to defecate, the force generated by straining separates the beads to open up the anal canal. The technique of

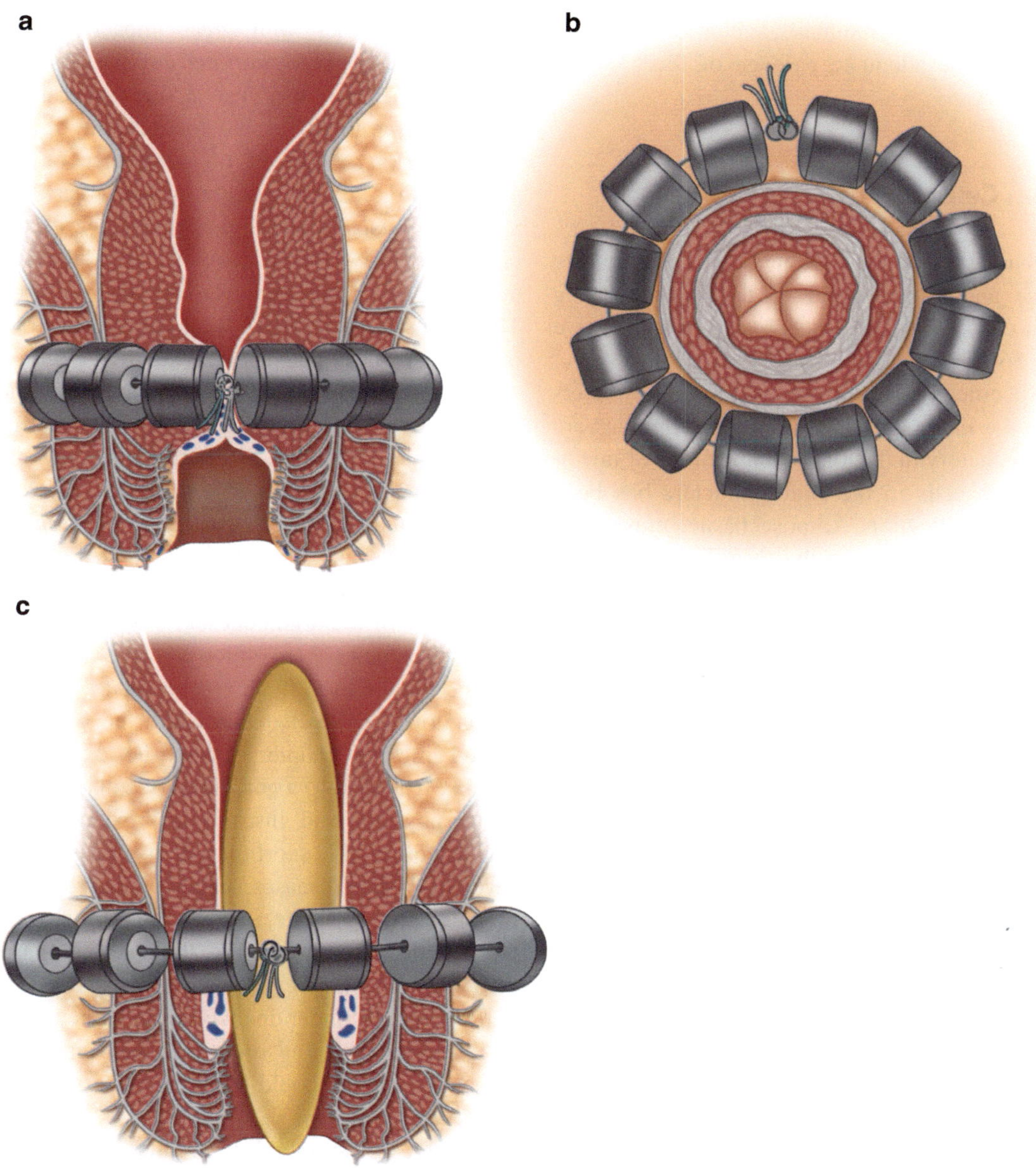

Fig. 13.7 Magnetic anal sphincter. Magnetic anal sphincter. (**a**) In the resting state, the magnets keep the anal canal closed. (**b**) Axial view to demonstrate placement of the magnetic sphincter outside the sphincter complex. (**c**) With bowel movements and Valsalva, the magnets expand to allow passage of stool. (Reused with permission. Copyright Springer Nature [59])

implantation is simple with no need for adjustments. Although it is a promising new option for patients with severe impairment of sphincter function, such in the case presented here, it has not been approved for clinical use in the United States by the Food and Drug Administration (FDA). Nevertheless, it has been associated with successful results in initial series and in the first feasibility study, as it is an expandable device that can help to maintain a closed anus, but allowing the adequate passage of feces, when necessary.

Stem Cells

Regeneration of the lost anal sphincter muscle tissue and improvement of its function using stem cells has been considered as an alternative [53–56].

Specifically, because repairing the sphincters with the many available surgical techniques are unsatisfactory in the long term, the idea of injecting stem cells in the anal sphincters has been under investigation. Adipose tissue, muscle, or mesenchymal stem cells (MSCs) have been shown to improve functioning of the heart and the urinary sphincter in animal models, leading researchers to test their effects in regenerating the anal sphincter.

Summary

In summary, despite the etiology, once the sphincter mechanism is damaged, the perfect restoration of continence is a challenge to the colorectal surgeon. In order to offer the best option to each individual patient, clinical evaluation is an important initial step. Plication of a weak and denervated sphincter will probably be insufficient to maintain reasonable continence. Although neuromodulation and recovery of bowel control have been considered the best options for most severe cases, other options such as the magnetic anal sphincter and regeneration of the anal sphincter using stem cells may play an increasingly important role.

Commentary

Donato F. Altomare

Fecal incontinence is one of the most distressing functional diseases with great impact on the patients' quality of life, working ability, and social and sexual life. Nevertheless, the interest of researchers on this topic has focused only in the last 30 years because of the reluctance of the patients to discuss their disability with their doctors, and because of the poor knowledge of the pathophysiology of fecal incontinence and the lack of reliable treatments, particularly in the long term. These considerations make fecal incontinence one of the most challenging condition to treat.

This excellent chapter is written by one of the most renowned experts in this field and focuses on the management of a difficult case of fecal incontinence in a mid-age woman. The case is analyzed and described with great experience and any possible diagnostic and therapeutic option is critically discussed showing profound knowledge of the argument and a wise proposal of the possible surgical options.

The author uses this case report to demonstrate how a difficult patient like the one presented in this chapter should be examined, starting from taking a good history and performing a physical and instrumental examination. The use of reliable scoring systems to assess the severity of the diseases, and its effect on the patient's quality of life, is crucial not only to follow up the effectiveness of the treatment, but also to choose the best surgical option for each patient. A fecal incontinence of moderate severity but with profound impact on the quality of life, for example, could justify the use of some invasive procedures.

In the case reported by Dr. Oliveira, the possible surgical options are gone through, explaining the pros and cons of each surgical technique, including some old and obsolete treatments like the gluteoplasty or the unstimulated graciloplasty. The addition of continuous low-frequency electrostimulation of this muscle in the early 1990s by Cor Baeten and by Norman Williams represented a significant step forward in the treatment of difficult cases like the one presented in this chapter; however, the high percentage of complications and the insufficient long-term results have limited the diffusion of this technique to very few specialized centers, making the production of the electrostimulator device from Medtronic® economically inconvenient. For that reasons, the company recently stopped its production and distribution.

Similarly, the attempts of mimicking the anal sphincter function by an implantable dynamic artificial bowel sphincter resulted in poor long-term outcome and unacceptable percentage of complications [57].

Therefore, several researchers came back to the old idea of the anal encirclement but using new elastic materials or a magnetic beads ring as described in this chapter. But any foreign material placed in that region of the body is destined to fail. Another more conservative option includes the injection of bulking agents or, more recently, the perianal injection of expandable prosthesis. This minimally invasive technique has been reported to achieve good functional result [58] although the correct indication is still questioned.

The proposal of using autologous myoblast stem cells to regenerate the anal sphincter is pretty new and very intriguing. However, the procedure to expand and inject human stem cells is still experimental and very expensive, even if the few researcher experts in this field have reported excellent results [59].

Finally, this chapter does not discuss the use of sacral nerve stimulation for fecal incontinence because it is reported in a separate chapter. However, this surgical option could have been considered in a patient like this, after failure of a sphincteroplasty [19]. The complex and poorly known mechanism of action of this electrostimulation could help patient with different types of incontinence, even if the long-term outcome, like all the techniques described, is disappointing [60].

References

1. Oliveira L. Quality of life issues. In: Wexner SD, Zbar A, Pescatori M, editors. Complex Ano-rectal disorders. London: Springer; 2005. p. 595–605.
2. Johanson JF, Lafferty J. Epidemiology of fecal incontinence: the silent affliction. Am J Gastroenterol. 1996;91(1):33–6.
3. Kang HW, Jung HK, Kwon KJ, Song EM, et al. Prevalence and predictive factors of fecal incontinence. J Neurogastroenterol Motil. 2012;18(1): 86–93.
4. Brown HW, Wexner SD, Segall MM, Brezoczky KL, Lukacz ES. Accidental bowel leakage in the mature women's health study: prevalence and predictors. Int J Clin Pract. 2012;66(11):1101–8.
5. Paquette IM, MaVarma MG, Kaiser AM, Steel SR, Rafferty JF. The American Society of Colon and Rectal Surgeons'clinical practice guideline for the treatment of fecal incontinence. Dis Colon Rectum. 2015;58:623–36.
6. Oliveira L, Pfeifer J, Wexner SD. Physiological and clinical outcome of anterior sphincteroplasty. Br J Surg. 1996;83:1244–51.
7. Londono-Schimmer EE, Garcia-Duperly R, Nicholls RJ, Thomson JPS, Hawley PR. Overlapping anal sphincter repair for faecal incontinence due to sphincter trauma: five year follow-up of functional results. Int J Color Dis. 1994;9:110–3.
8. Oom DM, Gosselink MP, Schouten WR. Anterior sphincteroplasty for fecal incontinence: a single center experience in the era of sacral neuromodulation. Dis Colon Rectum. 2009;52(10):1681–7.
9. Halverson AL, Hull TL. Long-term outcome of overlapping anal sphincter repair. Dis Colon Rectum. 2002;45(3):345–8.
10. Bravo Gutierrez A, Madoff RD, Lowry AC, Parker SC, Buie WD, Baxter NN. Long-term results of anterior sphincteroplasty. Dis Colon Rectum. 2004;47(5):727–31.
11. Wexner SD. Percutaneous tibial nerve stimulation in faecal incontinence. Lancet. 2015;386(10004):1605–6.
12. Jorge JMN, Wexner SD. Etiology and management of fecal incontinence. Dis Colon Rectum. 1993;36:77–97.
13. Rockwood TH, Church J, Fleshman JW, Kane RL, Mavrantonis C, Thorson AG, Wexner SD, Bliss D, Lowry AC. Fecal incontinence quality of life scale. Quality of life instrument for patients with fecal incontinence. Dis Colon Rectum. 2000;43:9–17.
14. Enck P, von Giesen HJ, Schäfer A, Heyer T, Gantke B, Flesch S, et al. Comparison of anal sonography with conventional needle electromyography in the evaluation of anal sphincter defects. Am J Gastroenterol. 1996;91(12):2539–43.
15. Sultan AH, Kamm MA, Hudson CN, et al. Anal-sphincter disruption during vaginal delivery. N Engl J Med. 1993;329(26):1905–11.

16. Glasgow SC, Lowry AC. Long-term outcomes of anal sphincter repair for fecal incontinence: a systematic review. Dis Colon Rectum. 2012;55(4):482–90.
17. Fleshman JW, Peters WR, Shemesh EI, et al. Anal sphincter reconstruction: anterior overlapping muscle repair. Dis Colon Rectum. 1991;34:739–43.
18. Engel AF, Kamm AM, Sultan AH, Bartram CI, Nicholls RJ. Anterior sphincter repair in patients with obstetric trauma. Br J Surg. 1994;81:1231–4.
19. Hong K, Dasilva G, Dollerschell JT, Maron D, Wexner SD. Redo sphincteroplasty: are the results sustainable? Gastroenterol Rep (Oxf). 2016;4(1):39–42.
20. Pescatori LC, Pescatori M. Sphincteroplasty for anal incontinence. Gastroenterol Rep (Oxf). 2014;2(2):92–7.
21. Wong WD, Jensen LL, Bartolo DCC, Rothenberger DA. Artificial anal sphincter. Dis Colon Rectum. 1996;39:1352–5.
22. Rongen MJ, Uludag O, El Naggar K, Geerdes BP, Konsten J, Baeten CG. Long-term follow-up of dynamic graciloplasty for fecal incontinence. Dis Colon Rectum. 2003;46:716–21.
23. Matzel KE, Stadelmaier U, Hohenfellner M, Gall FP. Electrical stimulation of sacral spinel nerves for treatment of fecal incontinence. Lancet. 1995;346:1124–7.
24. Maeda Y, O'Connell PR, Lehur PA, Matzel KE, Laurberg S, European SNS Bowel Study Group. Sacral nerve stimulation for faecal incontinence and constipation: a European consensus statement. Color Dis. 2015;17(4):O74–87.
25. Devesa JM, Rey A, Hervas PL, Halawa KS, Larranaga I, Svidler L, Abraira V, Muriel A. Artificial anal sphincter complications and functional results of a large personal series. Dis Colon Rectum. 2002;45:1154–63.
26. Altomare DF, Dodi G, La Torre F, et al. Multicenter retrospective analysis of the outcome of artificial anal sphincter implantation for severe faecal incontinence. Br J Surg. 2001;88:1481–6.
27. Wexner SD, Baeten C, Bailey R, et al. Long-term efficacy of dynamic graciloplasty for fecal incontinence. Dis Colon Rectum. 2002;45:809–18.
28. Hakelius L, Olsen L. Free autogenous muscle transplantation in children. Long-term results. Eur J Pediatr Surg. 1991 Dec;1(6):353–7.
29. Chetwood CH. Plastic operation of the sphincter ani: report of a case. Med Rec. 1902;61:529.
30. Schoemaker J. Un nouveau procede operatoire pour la reconstituition du sphincter anal. Semin Med. 1909;29:160.
31. Bistrom O. Plastichesarzatz des M. sphincter ani. Acta Chir Scand. 1944;90:431–8.
32. Bruining HA, Bos KE, Colthoff EG, et al. Creation of an anal sphincter mechanism by bilateral proximaly based gluteal muscle transposition. Plast Reconstr Surg. 1981;67:70–3.
33. Prochiantz A, Gross P. Gluteal myoplasty for sphincter replacement: principles, results and prospects. J Pediatr Surg. 1982;17:25–30.
34. Hentz VR. Construction of rectal sphincter using the origin of the gluteus maximus muscle. Plast Reconstr Surg. 1982;70:82–5.
35. Skef Z, Radhakrishnan J, Reyes HM. Anorectal continence following sphincter reconstruction utilizing the gluteus maximus muscle: a case report. J Pediatr Surg. 1983;18:779–81.
36. Iwai N, Kaneda H, Tsuto T, Yanagihara J, Takahashi T. Objective assessment of anorectal function after sphincter reconstruction using the gluteus maximus muscle. Report of a case. Dis Colon Rectum. 1985;28:973–7.
37. Chen YL, Zhang XH. Reconstruction of rectal sphincter by transposition of gluteus muscle for fecal incontinence. J Pediatr Surg. 1987;22:62–4.
38. Onishi K, Maruyama Y, Shiba T. A wrap-around procedure using gluteus maximus muscle for the functional reconstruction of the sphincter in a case of anal incontinence. Acta Chir Plast. 1989;31:56–63.
39. Pearl RK, Prasad ML, Nelson RL, Orsay CP, Abcarian H. Bilateral gluteus maximus transposition for anal incontinence. Dis Colon Rectum. 1991;34:478–81.
40. Christiansen J, Hansen CR, Rassmussen O. Bilateral gluteus maximus transposition for anal incontinence. Br J Surg. 1995;82:903–5.
41. Devesa JM, Vicente E, Enriquez JM, Nuno J, Bucheli P, de Blass G, et al. Total fecal incontinence-new method of gluteus maximus transposition: preliminary results and report of previous experience with similar procedures. Dis Colon Rectum. 1992;35:339–49.
42. Devesa JM, Madrid JM, Gallego BR, Vicente E, Nuno J, Enriquez JM. Bilateral gluteoplasty for fecal incontinence. Dis Colon Rectum. 1997;40:883–8.
43. Maddof RD, Rosen HR, Baeten CG, La Fontaine LJ, Cavina E, Devesa M, Rouanet P, Christiansen J, et al. Safety and efficacy of dynamic muscle plasty for anal incontinence: lessons from a prospective multicenter trial. Gastroenterology. 1999;116:549–56.
44. Yoshioka K, Ogunbiyi OA, Keighley MR. A pilot study of total pelvic floor repair or gluteus maximus transposition for postobstetric neuropathic fecal incontinence. Dis Colon Rectum. 1999;42(2):252–7.
45. Pickrell KL, Broadbent TR, Masters FW, Metzger JT. Construction of a rectal sphincter and restoration of anal continence by transplanting the gracilis muscle. Report of four cases in children. Ann Surg. 1952;135:853–62.
46. Christiansen J, Lorentzen M. Implantation of artificial sphincter for anal incontinence. Lancet. 1987;1:244–5.
47. Lehur PA, Michot F, Denis P, et al. Results of artificial sphincter in severe anal incontinence. Report of 14 consecutive implantations. Dis Colon Rectum. 1996;39:1352–5.
48. Thiersch C. Concerning prolapse of the rectum with special emphasis on the ope-ration by Thiersch. Dis Colon Rectum. 1988;31(2):154–5.

49. Devesa JM, Lopez-Hervas P, Vicente R, et al. Anal encirclement with a simple rectal sling for faecal incontinence. Tech Coloproctol. 2011;15:17–22.
50. Lehur PA, McNevin S, Buntzen S, Mellgren AF, Laurberg S, Madoff RD. Magnetic anal sphincter augmentation for the treatment of fecal incontinence: a preliminary report from a feasibility study. Dis Colon Rectum. 2010;53(12):1604–10.
51. Pakravan F, Helmes C. Magnetic anal sphincter augmentation in patients with severe fecal incontinence. Dis Colon Rectum. 2015;58(1):109–14.
52. Kim M, Lehur PA. How to size the anal canal circumference when implanting a magnetic anal sphincter for fecal incontinence. Evolution and update of a new surgical technique. Dis Colon Rectum. 2016;59(9):901–3.
53. Frudinger A, Kolle D, Schwaiger W, Pfeifer J, Paede J, Halligan S. Muscle-derived cell injection to treat anal incontinence due to obstetric trauma: pilot study with 1 year follow-up. Gut. 2010;59(1):55–61.
54. Park EJ, Kang J, Baik SH. Treatment of faecal incontinence using allogeneic-adipose-derived mesenchymal stem cells: a study protocol for a pilot randomised controlled trial. BMJ Open. 2016;6(2):e010450.
55. Sarveazad A, Newstead GL, Mirzaei R, Joghataei MT, Bakhtiari M, Babahajian A, et al. A new method for treating fecal incontinence by implanting stem cells derived from human adipose tissue: preliminary findings of a randomized double-blind clinical trial. Stem Cell Res Ther. 2017;8(1):40.
56. Paquette IM, Bordeianou L. Evaluation and treatment of FI. In: Steele SR, Hull TL, Read TE, Saclarides TJ, Senagore AJ, Whitlow CB, editors. The ASCRS textbook of colon and rectal surgery. 3rd ed. New York: Springer Nature; 2016.
57. Altomare DF, Binda GA, Dodi G, La Torre F, Romano G, Rinaldi M, Melega E. Disappointing long-term results of the artificial anal sphincter for faecal incontinence. Br J Surg. 2004;91(10):1352–3.
58. Ratto C, Buntzen S, Aigner F, Altomare DF, Heydari A, Donisi L, Lundby L, Parello A. Multicentre observational study of the Gatekeeper for faecal incontinence. Br J Surg. 2016;103(3):290–9.
59. Frudinger A, Marksteiner R, Pfeifer J, Margreiter E, Paede J, Thurner M. Skeletal muscle-derived cell implantation for the treatment of sphincter-related faecal incontinence. Stem Cell Res Ther. 2018;9(1):233.
60. Altomare DF, Giuratrabocchetta S, Knowles CH, Muñoz Duyos A, Robert-Yap J, Matzel KE; European SNS Outcome Study Group. Long-term outcomes of sacral nerve stimulation for faecal incontinence. Br J Surg. 2015;102(4):407–15.

14 Treatment for Fecal Incontinence: Neuromodulation

Vanessa W. Hui and Giovanna da Silva

Case Scenario

A 67-year-old woman with a history of three vaginal deliveries presents with symptoms of solid and liquid stool leakage requiring daily pad use. In addition, she complains of urge urinary incontinence. Anal manometry reveals low sphincter pressures and ultrasound does not demonstrate sphincter defect.

Origins, Trends, and Epidemiology

Sacral neuromodulation (SNM) is currently the surgical treatment of choice for patients with fecal incontinence (FI) without an anal sphincter defect or a defect less than or equal to 120°. It is reserved for patients who are not candidates for biofeedback therapy, injectable bulking agents, or sphincteroplasty, or in whom these modalities have failed. Originally developed by urologists in 1979, SNM was originally approved by the Food and Drug Administration (FDA) in 1999 for urinary incontinence [1, 2]. When this "bladder pacemaker" was repositioned to the sacral area from the perineum in an attempt to reduce inflammatory complications, patients with concurrent FI noted improvements in control and function of both the bladder and the anus [3]. When it was approved by the FDA for treatment of FI more than a decade after its approval for urinary incontinence, there was a notable practice shift toward SNM implantation with an accompanying decline in the use of sphincteroplasty. As of 2010, there have been approximately 85,000 SNM devices implanted worldwide [4–8]. Some studies have subsequently shown, a trend towards lower Cleveland Clinic Florida Fecal Incontinence Scores (CCF-FIS) in patients who undergo SNM as compared to sphincteroplasty for idiopathic FI [9].

Mechanism of Action

Although SNM has been in use for over a decade for FI, its mechanism of action is not clearly understood. There are three postulated mechanisms: stimulation of the somato-visceral reflex, direct effect on the anal sphincter complex, and afferent neuromodulation (Fig. 14.1).

The effects of SNM include changes in muscle type from fast to slow twitch, reducing muscle fatigue. It causes sensory changes in rectal

Commentary by Tracy L. Hull, Cleveland Clinic, Department of Colon and Rectal Surgery, Cleveland, OH, USA

V. W. Hui
University of Miami, Department of General Surgery, Division of Colorectal Surgery, Miami, FL, USA

G. da Silva (✉)
Department of Colorectal Surgery, Cleveland Clinic Florida, Weston, FL, USA
e-mail: dasilvg@ccf.org

K. C. Kobashi, S. D. Wexner (eds.), *Female Pelvic Medicine*, https://doi.org/10.1007/978-3-030-54839-1_14

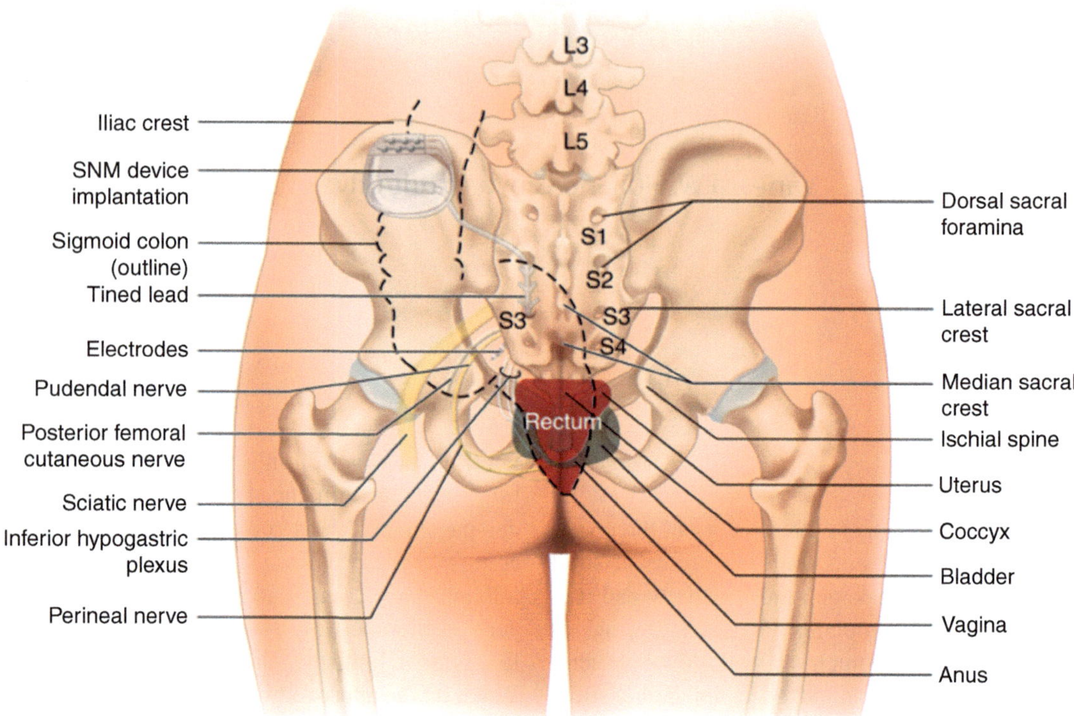

Fig. 14.1 Sacral nerve modulation: the lead is ideally placed through the S3 foramen and the implantable pulse generator is placed below the iliac crest and lateral to the sacrum. (Reused with permission. Copyright Springer Nature [52])

filling so that patients experience the urge to defecate at higher rectal volumes. SNM also induces retrograde colonic propagating sequences and slows colonic transit [10].

Basic scientists propose that there is a significant amount of central nervous system modulation from SNM. Several studies suggest that continuous low-flow stimulation of somatic afferent fibers that induce anal sphincter contraction may permanently modify the ascending supraspinal control of defecation [11]. This is supported by increased locoregional cerebral flood flow activity noted on PET during active nerve stimulation with continued increased PET activity after two weeks of continuous activity. These changes in cerebral activity are consistent with its effects on afferent projections of the vagus nerve. Initial activity in the frontal cortex may reflect focused attention, whereas subsequent activation of the caudate nucleus may reflect recruitment mechanisms involving learning and reward processing [12]. These alterations may contribute to improved continence over time [13]. All this modulation translates to increasing stimulatory threshold for the anal canal and decreased anal sensitivity, leading to significantly improved FI scores [12, 14].

The lasting effects of SNM in neuromodulation have been demonstrated in mouse models in which continuous stimulation has been shown to augment anal representation in the sensory cortex and restore afferent pathways following injury [15]. Some postulate that with long periods of stimulation, the cerebral neuroplasticity may be remolded to restore the neural circuitry to its pre-incontinent state. However, studies on this remain inconclusive [16, 17].

Procedure

Implantation of the InterStim™ system is performed in two stages – test and implantation phases – by most surgeons. Percutaneous nerve evaluation (PNE) can be done as an outpatient procedure to reduce the number of necessary operations for a patient and seems to have a lower infection rate compared to a two-stage approach [18]. The two-stage procedure in the operating room offers several advantages. First, an operative test phase has been shown to reduce the number of false negatives by reducing the incidence of temporary wire migrations. Second, the duration of the test phase could be extended because tined leads do not carry an increased risk of infection. Third, these electrode leads are permanent and do not require replacement in the second stage [19].

The test phase is performed under light sedation with local anesthesia. The tined lead is placed into the S3 foramen in the operating room via fluoroscopic and patient-directed guidance. Electrostimulation is commonly demonstrated by sphincter bellowing with plantar flexion of the hallux. A temporary device is implanted for two weeks in order to assess response. Fast responders may potentially undergo permanent pulse generator implantation as early as 1 week, but it is not clear whether this rapid response is predictive of long-term sustained outcome [20]. Thus, most surgeons wait two weeks to assess true persistent response prior to returning to the operating room for permanent implantation.

The second stage essentially requires the exchange of the temporary to the permanent pulse generator device. Caution must be exercised when electrocautery is used during the procedure as inadvertent damage to the lead, its extension, the implant, or nerve roots may occur with the conducted current. The settings of the permanent pulse generator may be reset with the electric current; thus, the company recommendation is to avoid use of electrocautery within 15 cm of the device. It should be noted that a meaningful clinical response does not necessitate a complete intraoperative motor response of all four active electrode poles. However, it has been shown that when all electrode poles are active during permanent implantation, the threshold needed for continued stimulation is diminished, which reduces the cost of SNM by prolonging the battery life [21]. SNM programming can be adjusted as an outpatient. It may be turned on and off, and its amplitude can be changed. Patients may also choose from preset programs of the device, depending on their symptomatology. The average battery life is approximately six years, accounting for both cyclical and subsensory stimulation.

Efficacy

Compared to non-invasive medical therapies such as pelvic floor exercises, bulking agents, and dietary changes, SNM has been able to improve symptoms in patients with FI. A randomized clinical trial of 120 patients in Australia compared patients with severe FI treated with SNM versus optimal combined medical therapies of pelvic floor exercises, bulking agents, and dietary modification. Patients who underwent SNM had significant reductions in the number of incontinent episodes per week from a mean of 9.5 to 3.1 ($p < 0.0001$) and in the mean number of incontinent days per week from 3.3 to 1 ($p < 0.0001$), with improvement in overall FI quality-of-life scores at 12 months. Patients demonstrated significant improvement within all four FI quality-of-life index domains, which include lifestyle, coping/behavior, depression/self-perception, and embarrassment, as early as 3 months after SNM implantation. These improvements persisted at the 6- and 12-month follow-up. By contrast, there was no significant improvement in frequency of incontinence or quality-of-life scores in patients who did not undergo SNM. Furthermore, 47.2% of the SNM patients were noted to have achieved full continence at the 12-month follow-up [6].

An early short-term prospective study of 50 patients showed at least a 50% reduction in symptoms in more than half of the patients who underwent permanent SNM implantation. Furthermore, 26% of this group was able to achieve full the continence at the 17-month follow-up. These patients noted a reduction in median FI episodes per fortnight from 14 to 2 ($p < 0.0001$), with significantly greater ability to control and defer defecation ($p < 0.0001$). Unfortunately, more than a quarter of the overall cohort did not respond or were dissatisfied after the initial test stage [22]. However, the SNM Study Group was able to demonstrate a 90% success rate after the initial test stage and was able to evaluate the long-term efficacy of SNM for FI via a prospective study of 120 patients from 14 centers in North America and Australia. Therapeutic success was defined as at least a 50% reduction in incontinent episodes per week compared to baseline. At 12 months, therapeutic success was noted in 83% of patients, with 41% achieving complete continence. These results persisted at 24 months with a therapeutic success rate of 85%. Therapeutic success rates of 86% and 89% were also noted over the long-term follow-up periods of three and five years, respectively. In addition, 36% of SNM patients maintained complete continence at five years, illustrating the potential durable effects of SNM [23–25].

In terms of other measures of success, the study was notable for demonstrating a reduction in the number of FI episodes per week from a mean from 9.4 per week at baseline to a mean of 1.9 per week post-SNM at the initial 12-month follow-up. These results were sustained at five years, with a significant decrease from a mean of 9.1 at baseline to a mean 1.7 episodes per week [23–25]. These findings were corroborated in a Finnish multicenter trial of 317 patients who underwent, SNM in which 59.3% of patients who underwent the permanent implantation stage reported significant alleviation of their FI symptoms at a mean follow-up of 2.4 years (range 8 days to 13.3 years) [26].

The European Outcome Study Group for SNM has established the durable effects of SNM via a 10-year prospective follow-up from 10 participating centers with sustained therapeutic success in 71.3% of the 407 patients, in which 50% of the patients achieved full continence. The number of FI episodes per week was significantly reduced from a median of 7 to 0.25 per week, with the median CCF-FIS decreasing from 16 to 7 and the St. Mark's score also decreasing significantly from 19 to 6 (all $p < 0.001$) [27].

Similarly, several studies published from St. Mark's Hospital have also noted a test stage success rate of 82–92%, which led to permanent SNM implantation. Over 90% of patients had at least a 50% reduction in incontinent episodes per week at 1 year after permanent implant. Eighty-three percent of patients had persistent therapeutic success at the 10-year follow-up, with a reported 48–61% of patients achieving full continence [28, 29]. These studies prove that patients who achieve significant improvement during the test stage may achieve long-lasting impactful outcomes after permanent implantation.

Predictors

Some studies were not able to identify predictors of success after implantation of SNM [27, 30], while others have not been able to corroborate these predictors. Studies have shown that a low threshold intensity to obtain motor response during the test stage may be associated with improved implantation stage outcomes [31–33]. Pudendal nerve terminal latency has been shown to be a predictor for long-term patient satisfaction after SNM implantation [34]. Patients who have loose stool consistency may have more favorable outcomes with SNM [32]. Pre-SNM anal manometry demonstrates lower resting and squeeze pressures in patients with FI, but these findings do necessarily predict success/failure of SNM [26]. Notable short-term improvement in FI scores at 6 months from baseline has been shown to be a significant positive predictor of success [odds ratio (OR): 6.29; 95% confidence interval (CI): 1.33–34.3; $p = 0.025$], particularly improvement of FI scores from three to six months (OR: 41.5; 95% CI: 3.51–811; $p = 0.007$). In addition, improvement in urge incontinence during the test phase has also been shown to be a potential positive predictor for reduction in FI (OR: 10.8; 95% CI: 1.72–132; $p = 0.036$) [33].

Potential predictors of failure may include patients who require repeated test stage procedures and those with minimal improvement during the test stage. While some studies note that evidence of significant anal sphincter trauma is a negative predictor, other studies contend there is no difference in clinical outcomes in patients with or without sphincter defects [31]. Increasing age has also been demonstrated as a negative predictive factor in at least one study, where for every 1-year increase in age, the odds of successful outcomes at five years decrease by 4.3% (OR: 0.96; 95% CI: 0.92–0.99; $p = 0.016$) [27, 31, 33]. However, the safety profile of SNM is such that it should be at least attempted in patients who are candidates for the procedure.

Complications

Comorbidities associated with permanent SNM implantation are low. Surgeons commonly field complaints of pain at the implantation site, postoperative hematoma, and wound infection, among others. Of the reportable events from various studies, the most common event was loss of efficacy at 37%, lack of efficacy or suboptimal efficacy at 12.1–27.1%, and pain/discomfort ranging from 13–21.7% [33, 35]. Early infection rates were reportedly as high as 10.8%, [36] but other studies suggest that infection rates after permanent implantation may range as low as 1.6–3.9% [22, 35, 37].

Additional procedures may be an unexpected complication related to SNM. Patients may require revision, replacement, and/or removal of their device. The most common cause for surgical revision is device migration. Replacement of the device is most commonly related to battery depletion, as the average battery life lasts for six years. The most common reason for device explantation is lack of efficacy [21, 25].

Lead migration, erosion, and loss of efficacy can occur in both stages. However, meaningful outcomes can still be achieved after lead reimplantation with significant decrease in CCF-FIS, although these changes may not be as in substantial as in those patients who did not require additional procedures. Furthermore, patients who require lead reimplantation before the implantation stage tend to have worse functional outcomes than those who require reimplantation after the implantation stage [38].

Adverse stimulation is also a rare event. This may be confused with pain at the implant site and can be differentiated by turning off the device and may require a change in the stimulation programming. Electrical shock may occur if insulation breaks at the connection of the lead and extension. High pulse widths and high-frequency stimulations may lead to irreversible nerve damage. Poor result or leg pain early in the postoperative course may lead to more unfavorable long-term outcomes [39]. If patients have initially good results but then lose efficacy, it is necessary to evaluate for potential lead or battery dislocation, damage, trauma, or the stimulation programming for possible readjustment.

Comparison to Other Nerve Stimulation

A recent systematic review and meta-analysis comparing SNM to percutaneous tibial nerve stimulation (PTNS) for the treatment of idiopathic FI demonstrated that both modalities provided symptomatic improvement, without any difference in efficacy. However, SNM was shown to have a greater reduction in the number of weekly FI episodes, greater CCF-FIS improvement, and better FI quality of life scores, especially in the coping and depression domains [40]. Patients who fail PTNS and subsequently undergo SNM may still experience significant therapeutic benefit with improvement in FI scores [41]. A randomized controlled trial of PTNS versus sham noted a mild advantage with PTNS in terms of CCF-FIS improvement, but not necessarily in the mean number of incontinent episodes per week [42]. PTNS is not currently FDA approved for use in the United States, and its effectiveness remains to be seen.

Cost and Quality of Life

Even if there is no significant difference in physical scores or significant changes in FI symptoms, SNM patients tend to demonstrate higher mental health scores including vitality, social function, lifestyle, and depression domains [29, 43, 44]. Some patients explain that they were able to have a more active social life after SNM therapy, though their functional outcomes did not drastically change based on various bowel diaries/ scores. Patient perspectives of their overall bowel health improve dramatically with improvement in FI episodes and FI scores [45]. In addition, there have been demonstrable positive effects on sexual function with substantial improvements in arousal, satisfaction, and pain, with a trend toward increased desire in women with pelvic floor disorders after SNM treatment [46]. In addition to the improvements in quality of life, SNM is actually cost-effective for patients plagued with long-term FI. In a cost analysis study performed in France, the average cost of SNM for the treatment of FI was €6581 more (95% confidence interval €2077–11,084; $p = 0.006$) for the first two years compared to alternative treatments. However, in those patients in whom there is greater than 50% improvement in their incontinence severity scores, the incremental cost-effectiveness ratio was €185,160 at 24 months [47]. The enhancements in quality of life and significant long-term cost-effectiveness justify the early costs for patients impaired with moderate-to-severe FI.

SNM for Other Etiologies

Several small-volume studies were performed in patients undergoing SNM for FI after pelvic surgery. Overall, patients who did not require a proctectomy demonstrated a greater improvement in CCF-FIS after SNM implantation. In those who underwent a proctectomy, patients with nonmalignant disease fared better than those in whom the resection was performed for cancer. All studies showed that SNM did improve functional and quality-of-life scores, but not necessarily improve anal manometry scores. The effects of radiation in response to SNM are unclear, as most of these studies were performed on a heterogeneous population undergoing pelvic surgery for various etiologies [48–50]. SNM implantation has been reported in patients with inflammatory bowel disease-associated FI with some demonstrable success, but long-term outcomes remain to be seen [51].

Summary

SNM has had a tremendous impact on the treatment of FI since its inception. For the patient in our case with moderate-to-severe FI, it may be highly effective and also benefit her urinary incontinence. SNM may be life-changing in patients crippled both physically and mentally by FI, as demonstrated in various long-term follow-up studies. Although the device may require additional procedures and adjustments, its risks are relatively low. In patients who demonstrate a greater than 50% improvement in their symptoms, this modality is cost-effective with highly replicable results.

Commentary

Tracy L. Hull

Fecal incontinence (FI), although not life threatening, can be a devastating condition. The anguish unleashed from the fear of FI can lead to social isolation and emotional desolation. The etiology of FI is multifactorial, and treatment must be individualized and based on a careful history, physical exam, and selected testing [53]. Many factors influence the ability to control stool and gas. These include diet, stool consistency, other bowel surgery, injury, and other unknown factors. Most treatment starts with diet manipulation, reducing diarrhea, and physical therapy training (biofeedback) [53]. However, while these treatments can improve FI, in many instances, it does not result in sufficient reduction to alleviate the anguish of FI. Innovations to improve the quality of life of those with FI have evolved over the years. Repair of an injured sphincter muscle is still included in the treatment armamentarium. Surgeons can repair a sphincter defect, but long-term results are disappointing [54]. The artificial bowel sphincter, stimulated gracilis wrap, and magnetic sphincter have all had variable success in treating FI, but are no longer available treatments in the United States [55].

Stimulation of the sacral nerves (typically S3) was an accepted treatment of urinary incontinence [56]. The observation that bowel function was improved with this therapy led to trials utilizing sacral neuromodulation (SNM) for FI. Initially, the speculation was that direct stimulation of the muscle occurred with SNM (like a pacemaker for the anal sphincter). While the exact mechanism of action is unknown, direct afferent stimulation to the brain with resultant brain stimulation is felt to be mechanism of action. The beauty of this therapy is that it is done in two stages and allows a trial of stimulation and, if improvement is recorded, the permanent device can be implanted. Additionally, SNM is approved for patients with a sphincter defect of up to 60°, but even patients with a defect up to 120° have reportedly had successful results [57]. Lastly, 35% of SNM patients assessed at 5-year follow-up achieved complete continence, an outcome not matched with other current therapies [25].

SNM has minimal morbidity. Problems with lead erosion or displacement along with the need to replace the battery about every 5 years remain long-term factors that require continuous contact with these patients [38, 58]. New rechargeable batteries are now available. Numerous published studies from many countries have corroborated the optimistic results with SNM since the mid 1990s. SNM is currently the therapy of choice for most patients with FI who fail nonsurgical therapy.

References

1. Schmidt RA, Bruschini H, Tanagho EA. Sacral root stimulation in controlled micturition. Peripheral somatic neurotomy and stimulated voiding. Investig Urol. 1979;17(2):130–4. PubMed PMID: 468511.
2. Schmidt RA, Jonas U, Oleson KA, Janknegt RA, Hassouna MM, Siegel SW, et al. Sacral nerve stimulation for treatment of refractory urinary urge incontinence. Sacral Nerve Stimulation Study Group. J Urol. 1999;162(2):352–7. PubMed PMID: 10411037.
3. Matzel KE, Stadelmaier U, Hohenfellner M, Gall FP. Electrical stimulation of sacral spinal nerves for treatment of faecal incontinence. Lancet. 1995;346(8983):1124–7. PubMed PMID: 7475602.
4. Thaha MA, Abukar AA, Thin NN, Ramsanahie A, Knowles CH. Sacral nerve stimulation for faecal incontinence and constipation in adults. Cochrane Database Syst Rev. 2015;(8):CD004464. PubMed PMID: 26299888.
5. Thin NN, Horrocks EJ, Hotouras A, Palit S, Thaha MA, Chan CL, et al. Systematic review of the clinical effectiveness of neuromodulation in the treatment of faecal incontinence. Br J Surg. 2013;100(11):1430–47. PubMed PMID: 24037562.
6. Tjandra JJ, Chan MK, Yeh CH, Murray-Green C. Sacral nerve stimulation is more effective than optimal medical therapy for severe fecal incontinence: a randomized, controlled study. Dis Colon Rectum. 2008;51(5):494–502. PubMed PMID: 18278532.
7. Hetzer FH. Fifteen years of sacral nerve stimulation: from an open procedure to a minimally invasive technique. Colorectal Dis. 2011;13 Suppl 2:1–4. PubMed PMID: 21284794.
8. Xu Z, Fleming FJ, Justiniano CF, Becerra AZ, Boodry CI, Aquina CT, et al. Trends in surgeon-level utilization of sacral nerve stimulator implantation for fecal incontinence in New York state. Dis Colon Rectum. 2018;61(1):107–14. PubMed PMID: 29215481.
9. Rodrigues FG, Chadi SA, Cracco AJ, Sands DR, Zutshi M, Gurland B, et al. Faecal incontinence in patients with a sphincter defect: comparison of sphincteroplasty and sacral nerve stimulation. Colorectal Dis. 2017;19(5):456–61. PubMed PMID: 27620162.
10. Patton V, Wiklendt L, Arkwright JW, Lubowski DZ, Dinning PG. The effect of sacral nerve stimulation on distal colonic motility in patients with faecal incontinence. Br J Surg. 2013;100(7):959–68. PubMed PMID: 23536312.
11. Carrington EV, Evers J, Grossi U, Dinning PG, Scott SM, O'Connell PR, et al. A systematic review of sacral nerve stimulation mechanisms in the treatment of fecal incontinence and constipation. Neurogastroenterol Motil. 2014;26(9):1222–37. PubMed PMID: 25167953.
12. Langlois LD, Le Long E, Meleine M, Antor M, Atmani K, Dechelotte P, et al. Acute sacral nerve stimulation reduces visceral mechanosensitivity in a cross organ sensitization model. Neurogastroenterol Motil. 2017;29(4). PubMed PMID: 27997083.
13. Lundby L, Moller A, Buntzen S, Krogh K, Vang K, Gjedde A, et al. Relief of fecal incontinence by sacral nerve stimulation linked to focal brain activation. Dis Colon Rectum. 2011;54(3):318–23. PubMed PMID: 21304303.
14. Haas S, Brock C, Krogh K, Gram M, Lundby L, Drewes AM, et al. Does sacral nerve stimulation improve continence through enhanced sensitivity of the anal canal? A pilot study. Dis Colon Rectum. 2016;59(11):1039–46. PubMed PMID: 27749479.
15. Evers J, Devane L, Carrington EV, Scott SM, Knowles CH, O'Connell PR, et al. Reversal of sensory deficit through sacral neuromodulation in an animal model of fecal incontinence. Neurogastroenterol Motil. 2016;28(5):665–73. PubMed PMID: 26821877.
16. Altomare DF, Giannini I, Giuratrabocchetta S, Digennaro R. The effects of sacral nerve stimulation on continence are temporarily maintained after turning

the stimulator off. Colorectal Dis. 2013;15(12):e741–8. PubMed PMID: 24102954.
17. Kahlke V, Topic H, Peleikis HG, Jongen J. Sacral nerve modulation for fecal incontinence: results of a prospective single-center randomized crossover study. Dis Colon Rectum. 2015;58(2):235–40. PubMed PMID: 25585083.
18. Rice TC, Quezada Y, Rafferty JF, Paquette IM. Dynamic article: percutaneous nerve evaluation versus staged sacral nerve stimulation for fecal incontinence. Dis Colon Rectum. 2016;59(10):962–7. PubMed PMID: 27602927.
19. Everaert K, Kerckhaert W, Caluwaerts H, Audenaert M, Vereecke H, De Cuypere G, et al. A prospective randomized trial comparing the 1-stage with the 2-stage implantation of a pulse generator in patients with pelvic floor dysfunction selected for sacral nerve stimulation. Eur Urol. 2004;45(5):649–54. PubMed PMID: 15082209.
20. Lambrescak E, Wyart V, Meurette G, Faucheron JL, Thomas C, Atienza P, et al. Sacral nerve stimulation for fecal incontinence: how long should the test phase be? Dis Colon Rectum. 2017;60(12):1314–9. PubMed PMID: 29112568.
21. Duelund-Jakobsen J, Lundby L, Lehur PA, Wyart V, Laurberg S, Buntzen S. Is the efficacy of sacral nerve stimulation for faecal incontinence dependent on the number of active electrode poles achieved during permanent lead insertion? Colorectal Dis. 2016;18(11):O414–O9. PubMed PMID: 27619970.
22. Boyle DJ, Knowles CH, Lunniss PJ, Scott SM, Williams NS, Gill KA. Efficacy of sacral nerve stimulation for fecal incontinence in patients with anal sphincter defects. Dis Colon Rectum. 2009;52(7):1234–9. PubMed PMID: 19571698.
23. Wexner SD, Coller JA, Devroede G, Hull T, McCallum R, Chan M, et al. Sacral nerve stimulation for fecal incontinence: results of a 120-patient prospective multicenter study. Ann Surg. 2010;251(3):441–9. PubMed PMID: 20160636.
24. Mellgren A, Wexner SD, Coller JA, Devroede G, Lerew DR, Madoff RD, et al. Long-term efficacy and safety of sacral nerve stimulation for fecal incontinence. Dis Colon Rectum. 2011;54(9):1065–75. PubMed PMID: 21825885.
25. Hull T, Giese C, Wexner SD, Mellgren A, Devroede G, Madoff RD, et al. Long-term durability of sacral nerve stimulation therapy for chronic fecal incontinence. Dis Colon Rectum. 2013;56(2):234–45. PubMed PMID: 23303153.
26. Kirss J Jr, Pinta T, Varpe P, Rautio T, Kairaluoma M, Hyoty M, et al. Outcomes of treatment of faecal incontinence with sacral nerve stimulation - a Finnish multicentre study. Colorectal Dis. 2019;21(1):59–65. PubMed PMID: 30192431.
27. Altomare DF, Giuratrabocchetta S, Knowles CH, Munoz Duyos A, Robert-Yap J, Matzel KE, et al. Long-term outcomes of sacral nerve stimulation for faecal incontinence. Br J Surg. 2015;102(4):407–15. PubMed PMID: 25644687.
28. Hollingshead JR, Dudding TC, Vaizey CJ. Sacral nerve stimulation for faecal incontinence: results from a single centre over a 10-year period. Colorectal Dis. 2011;13(9):1030–4. PubMed PMID: 20718837.
29. George AT, Kalmar K, Panarese A, Dudding TC, Nicholls RJ, Vaizey CJ. Long-term outcomes of sacral nerve stimulation for fecal incontinence. Dis Colon Rectum. 2012;55(3):302–6. PubMed PMID: 22469797.
30. Roy AL, Gourcerol G, Menard JF, Michot F, Leroi AM, Bridoux V. Predictive factors for successful sacral nerve stimulation in the treatment of fecal incontinence: lessons from a comprehensive treatment assessment. Dis Colon Rectum. 2014;57(6):772–80. PubMed PMID: 24807603.
31. Dudding TC, Pares D, Vaizey CJ, Kamm MA. Predictive factors for successful sacral nerve stimulation in the treatment of faecal incontinence: a 10-year cohort analysis. Colorectal Dis. 2008;10(3):249–56. PubMed PMID: 17655722.
32. Gallas S, Michot F, Faucheron JL, Meurette G, Lehur PA, Barth X, et al. Predictive factors for successful sacral nerve stimulation in the treatment of faecal incontinence: results of trial stimulation in 200 patients. Colorectal Dis. 2011;13(6):689–96. PubMed PMID: 20236144.
33. Maeda Y, Lundby L, Buntzen S, Laurberg S. Outcome of sacral nerve stimulation for fecal incontinence at 5 years. Ann Surg. 2014;259(6):1126–31. PubMed PMID: 23817505.
34. Duelund-Jakobsen J, van Wunnik B, Buntzen S, Lundby L, Laurberg S, Baeten C. Baseline factors predictive of patient satisfaction with sacral neuromodulation for idiopathic fecal incontinence. Int J Color Dis. 2014;29(7):793–8. PubMed PMID: 24743849.
35. Maeda Y, Matzel K, Lundby L, Buntzen S, Laurberg S. Postoperative issues of sacral nerve stimulation for fecal incontinence and constipation: a systematic literature review and treatment guideline. Dis Colon Rectum. 2011;54(11):1443–60. PubMed PMID: 21979192.
36. Wexner SD, Hull T, Edden Y, Coller JA, Devroede G, McCallum R, et al. Infection rates in a large investigational trial of sacral nerve stimulation for fecal incontinence. J Gastrointest Surg. 2010;14(7):1081–9. PubMed PMID: 20354809.
37. Michelsen HB, Thompson-Fawcett M, Lundby L, Krogh K, Laurberg S, Buntzen S. Six years of experience with sacral nerve stimulation for fecal incontinence. Dis Colon Rectum. 2010;53(4):414–21. PubMed PMID: 20305440.
38. Cracco AJ, Chadi SA, Rodrigues FG, Zutshi M, Gurland B, Wexner SD, et al. Outcomes of sacral neurostimulation lead reimplantation for fecal incontinence: a cohort study. Dis Colon Rectum. 2016;59(1):48–53. PubMed PMID: 26651112.
39. Maeda Y, Lundby L, Buntzen S, Laurberg S. Suboptimal outcome following sacral nerve stimulation for faecal incontinence. Br J Surg. 2011;98(1):140–7. PubMed PMID: 21136568.

40. Simillis C, Lal N, Qiu S, Kontovounisios C, Rasheed S, Tan E, et al. Sacral nerve stimulation versus percutaneous tibial nerve stimulation for faecal incontinence: a systematic review and meta-analysis. Int J Color Dis. 2018;33(5):645–8. PubMed PMID: 29470730.
41. Hotouras A, Murphy J, Thin NN, Allison M, Horrocks E, Williams NS, et al. Outcome of sacral nerve stimulation for fecal incontinence in patients refractory to percutaneous tibial nerve stimulation. Dis Colon Rectum. 2013;56(7):915–20. PubMed PMID: 23739200.
42. van der Wilt AA, Giuliani G, Kubis C, van Wunnik BPW, Ferreira I, Breukink SO, et al. Randomized clinical trial of percutaneous tibial nerve stimulation versus sham electrical stimulation in patients with faecal incontinence. Br J Surg. 2017;104(9):1167–76. PubMed PMID: 28703936.
43. Lim JT, Hastie IA, Hiscock RJ, Shedda SM. Sacral nerve stimulation for fecal incontinence: long-term outcomes. Dis Colon Rectum. 2011;54(8):969–74. PubMed PMID: 21730785.
44. Duelund-Jakobsen J, van Wunnik B, Buntzen S, Lundby L, Baeten C, Laurberg S. Functional results and patient satisfaction with sacral nerve stimulation for idiopathic faecal incontinence. Colorectal Dis. 2012;14(6):753–9. PubMed PMID: 21883814.
45. Devroede G, Giese C, Wexner SD, Mellgren A, Coller JA, Madoff RD, et al. Quality of life is markedly improved in patients with fecal incontinence after sacral nerve stimulation. Female Pelvic Med Reconstr Surg. 2012;18(2):103–12. PubMed PMID: 22453321.
46. Khunda A, McCormick C, Ballard P. Sacral neuromodulation and sexual function: a systematic review and meta-analysis of the literature. Int Urogynecol J. 2019;30(3):339–52. PubMed PMID: 30535791.
47. Leroi AM, Lenne X, Dervaux B, Chartier-Kastler E, Mauroy B, Normand LL, et al. Outcome and cost analysis of sacral nerve modulation for treating urinary and/or fecal incontinence. Ann Surg. 2011;253(4):720–32. PubMed PMID: 21475012.
48. Mizrahi I, Chadi SA, Haim N, Sands DR, Gurland B, Zutshi M, et al. Sacral neuromodulation for the treatment of faecal incontinence following proctectomy. Colorectal Dis. 2017;19(5):O145–O52. PubMed PMID: 27885800.
49. Thomas GP, Bradshaw E, Vaizey CJ. A review of sacral nerve stimulation for faecal incontinence following rectal surgery and radiotherapy. Colorectal Dis. 2015;17(11):939–42. PubMed PMID: 26201673.
50. Schiano di Visconte M, Santoro GA, Cracco N, Sarzo G, Bellio G, Brunner M, et al. Effectiveness of sacral nerve stimulation in fecal incontinence after multimodal oncologic treatment for pelvic malignancies: a multicenter study with 2-year follow-up. Tech Coloproctol. 2018;22(2):97–105. PubMed PMID: 29313165.
51. Gu P, Kuenzig ME, Kaplan GG, Pimentel M, Rezaie A. Fecal incontinence in inflammatory bowel disease: a systematic review and meta-analysis. Inflamm Bowel Dis. 2018;24(6):1280–90. PubMed PMID: 29617820.
52. Paquette IM, Bordeianou L. Evaluation and treatment of FI. In: Steele SR, Hull TL, Read TE, Saclarides TJ, Senagore AJ, Whitlow CB, editors. The ASCRS textbook of colon and rectal surgery. 3rd ed. New York: Springer Nature; 2016.
53. Alavi K, Chan S, Wise P, Kaiser AM, Sudan R, Bordeianou L. Fecal incontinence: etiology, diagnosis, and management. J Gastrointest Surg. 2015;19(10):1910–21.
54. Zutshi M, Hull T, Bast J, Halverson A, Na J. Ten year outcome after anal sphincter repair for fecal incontinence. Dis Colon Rectum. 2009;52(6):1089–94.
55. Kaiser AM, Orangio GR, Zutshi M, Alva S, Hull TL, Marcello PW, Margolin DA, Rafferty JF, Buie WD, Wexner SD. Current status: new technologies for the treatment of patients with fecal incontinence. Surg Endosc. 2014;28(8):2277–301.
56. Skull A, Hull TL. Sacral nerve stimulation for fecal incontinence. Expert Rev Med Devices. 2012;9(5):477–82.
57. Chan MK, Tjandra J. Sacral nerve stimulation for fecal incontinence: external anal sphincter defect vs intact anal sphincter. Dis Colon Rectum. 2008;51(7):1015–24; discussion 1024–5.
58. Le Fouler A, Duchalais E, Loong TH, Baayen C, Wyart V, Kubis C, Meurette G, Lehur PA. Long-term outcome following implanted pulse generator change in patients treated with sacral nerve modulation for fecal incontinence. Neuromodulation. 2018;21(7):694–9.

Part IV

Treatment: Pelvic Organ Prolapse

Approach to Pelvic Organ Prolapse

15

Claire S. Burton and Jennifer T. Anger

Case Scenario

A 53-year-old woman with a history of three vaginal deliveries presents with a bothersome bulge and sensation of pelvic heaviness for 3 years. On exam she has multicompartment prolapse (POP-Q Aa+2, Ba+2, C0, Ap0, Bp0, gh5, pb2, tvl9), Stage 3. She is interested in surgical repair.

Introduction

The pelvic organs are supported by the pelvic floor muscles. The support of the vagina and uterus can be classified into three levels as described by DeLancey (Fig. 15.1). Level I support of the vaginal apex is dependent on the strength of the uterosacral and cardinal ligaments. Level II support of the midvagina is via the connection of the posterior endopelvic fascia to the lateral pelvic sidewalls. And finally, level III support is the fusion of the endopelvic fascia to the perineal body and pubic symphysis [1].

Pelvic organ prolapse (POP) refers to the progressive descent of pelvic organs into the vaginal canal, and is typically categorized into three compartments. Anterior compartment prolapse, also referred to as cystocele or cystourethrocele, refers to descent of the bladder or urethra. Posterior compartment prolapse (rectocele) refers to a descent of the rectum or small bowel, which causes the posterior vaginal wall to bulge into the vagina. And lastly, descent of the uterus or vaginal apex is referred to as uterine or vault (in the absence of a uterus) prolapse, respectively. Vault prolapse may also contain descent of small bowel, which is referred to as an enterocele.

Pelvic organ prolapse affects 30–40% of women in their lifetimes. One in nine women will undergo surgery for POP [2, 3]. Parity is a major risk factor for the development of POP. Other risk factors include vaginal delivery, obesity, chronic constipation, increasing age, and prior pelvic surgery [4]. There also may be a degree of heritability, as women with affected first-degree relatives have a two- to threefold increase of developing prolapse, and a positive family history is associated with earlier onset and more rapid progression of symptoms [5]. The *COL1A1* (collagen type I, alpha I) and *COL3A1* (collagen type 3 alpha 1) have been associated with increased POP risk [6, 7].

Commentary by Benjamin M. Brucker, Division of Female Pelvic Medicine and Reconstructive Surgery and Neurourology, New York University Langone Health, Department of Urology and Obstetrics and Gynecology, New York, NY, USA

C. S. Burton
University of California – Los Angeles, Department of Urology, Los Angeles, CA, USA

J. T. Anger (✉)
Cedars-Sinai Medical Center, Department of Surgery, Division of Urology, Los Angeles, CA, USA
e-mail: Jennifer.anger@cshs.org

K. C. Kobashi, S. D. Wexner (eds.), *Female Pelvic Medicine*,
https://doi.org/10.1007/978-3-030-54839-1_15

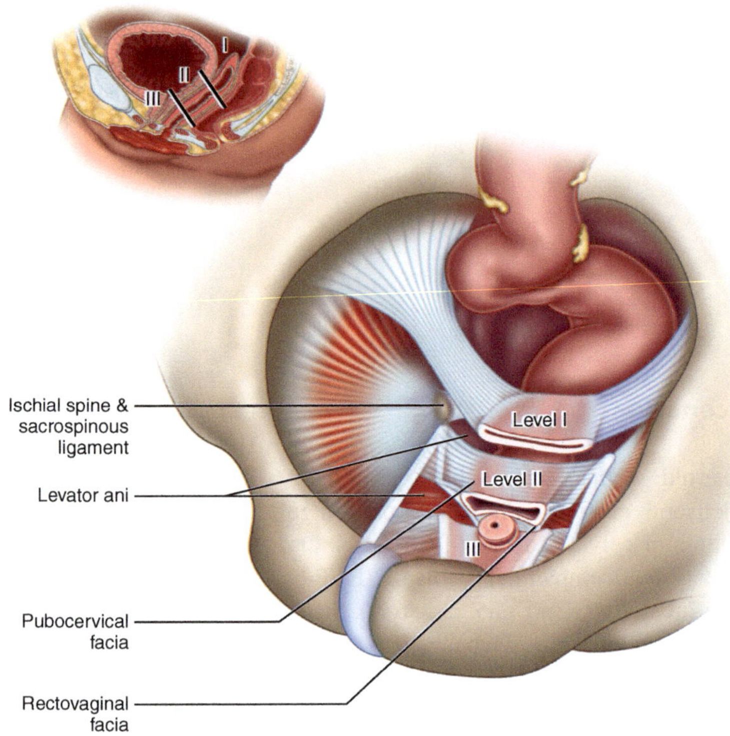

Fig. 15.1 DeLancey's three levels of pelvic support. (Reprinted with permission. Copyright 1992 with permission from Elsevier [1]. Source: Linda M. Szymanski, Jessica L. Bienstock: *The Johns Hopkins Handbook of Obstetrics and Gynecology*: www.obgyn.mhmedical.com. Copyright © McGraw-Hill Education. All rights reserved.)

There are multiple means to measure success after repair of POP, but the most commonly utilized, and probably most important, is subjective improvement by the patient. Although most diagnostic of POP is the sensation of a vaginal bulge, common patient symptoms may also include voiding difficulty, defecatory dysfunction, dyspareunia, or a feeling of pelvic heaviness, pressure, and/or pain. Many patients will continue to have a small degree of prolapse even after surgery, but improvement in symptoms and the absence of the feeling of a "bulge" is associated with patient satisfaction and improvements in quality of life [8]. Other more strict definitions of success of prolapse repair are anatomic, with some studies classifying success only if the leading edge is above or at the hymen, though most women only develop symptoms when the leading edge is more than 0.5 cm beyond the hymen [9]. Conversely, the most liberal definition of failure would be the need for repeat prolapse surgery.

The success of a surgical repair is in part dependent upon a correct assessment of the specific sector defect and degree of prolapse. The Pelvic Organ Prolapse Quantification System (POP-Q) (Fig. 15.2) is commonly utilized to define the location and degree of prolapse. There is no cutoff point for which surgical repair is recommended. Rather, it is considered a quality-of-life procedure that should be repaired based upon patient preference. Other management options include observation or pessaries.

The following chapter will highlight the surgical options for POP, and the indications and options for vaginal, abdominal, or perineal repair.

Anterior Compartment Prolapse

Vaginal Approach

Anterior vaginal prolapse or cystocele can occur because of a (1) central defect in the vaginal

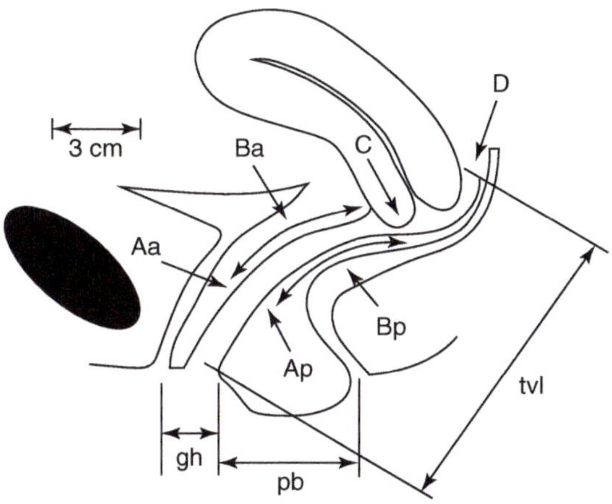

Fig. 15.2 POP–Q system examination. Aa, point A anterior, Ap, point A posterior, Ba, point B anterior; Bp, point B posterior; C, cervix or vaginal cuff; D, posterior fornix (if cervix is present); gh, genital hiatus; pb, perineal body; tvl, total vaginal length. (Copyright Carol Davila University Press [96]) [This is an open-access article distributed under the terms of the Creative Commons Attribution License, which permits unrestricted use, distribution, and reproduction in any medium, provided the original work is properly cited.]

wall, (2) a defect in the lateral attachments of the pubocervical fascia to the arcus tendineus fascia pelvis, or (3) a transverse defect in the separation between the pubocervical fascia and the cervix. Proper identification of the location of defect is crucial for selecting the appropriate repair [10, 11].

Native Tissue Repair

A transvaginal approach is ideal to address an anterior compartment central defect. First performed by Kelly in 1913, plication has been a mainstay of central cystocele repair. Although there is no truly standardized procedure, anterior colporrhaphy is generally performed by making a midline incision in the anterior vaginal wall and dissecting laterally on each side to expose the prolapsed prevesical fascia [12]. The dissection should be carried out to the arcus tendineous fascia pelvis bilaterally. Absorbable sutures (usually 2–0) are used to plicate the muscularis and adventitia of the anterior vaginal wall (Fig. 15.3).

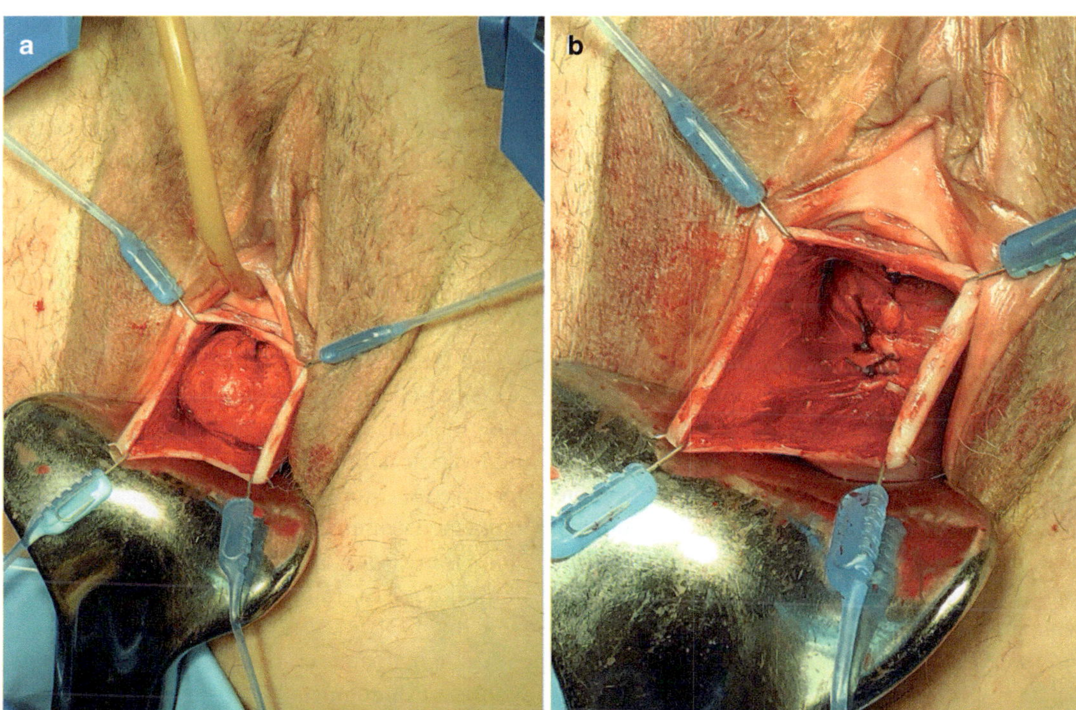

Fig. 15.3 (**a**) Cystocele with (**b**) native tissue plication of anterior vaginal wall. (Courtesy of Jennifer T. Anger MD)

A Kelly plication refers to additional sutures placed at the bladder neck and urethra to treat incontinence [13]. Anterior repair should always be accompanied by cystoscopy to ensure ureteral patency, as sutures placed too deep can cause ureteral obstruction [14]. The excess skin of the anterior vaginal wall is removed and the mucosa is reapproximated.

The majority of first time prolapse surgery is performed using the patient's own tissue, also known as native tissue repair, though high recurrence rates (20–30%) have led surgeons to augment repairs with mesh or biografts for added support [15, 16]. Historically, long-term success for first time repair of native tissue anterior colporrhaphy is lower (30%) when strict anatomic definitions (leading edge at least 2 cm above the hymen) are used. When patients were reevaluated with less strict definitions though, 95% of patients report no bulge symptoms with a standard anterior colporrhaphy [17, 18]. Techniques such as utilization of slower absorption or permanent sutures may improve outcomes [19]. Song et al. showed that the use of a purse string suture in addition to plication increased success to 98% at 4 years [20]. Additionally, the role of apical support in anterior prolapse has now been well defined. Support of the apex can improve anterior wall prolapse 63% of the time, and women with combined anterior and apical repair have lower reoperation rates than anterior repair alone (11.6% vs. 20.2%) [15, 21].

Mesh Repair

Because of the historically limited success of transvaginal anterior repair, mesh-augmented repairs gained popularity. Additionally, the inclusion of mesh in anterior repair helps to address both lateral and central defects, while plication alone really only addresses the central component. Mesh repair for anterior compartment prolapse is usually performed with the use of a kit with pre-prepared mesh and anchors. Each kit varies slightly, but most involve placing a piece of polypropylene mesh between the vaginal epithelium and underlying fascia and anchoring it in a tension-free manner to a connective tissue structure such as the sacrospinous ligament, obturator internus membrane, iliococcygeus ligament, or arcus tendineus fascia lata [22, 23]. Unfortunately, high complications rates related to polypropylene mesh such as extrusion (exposure of graft material in the vagina) and erosion (presence of graft material in the urinary tract) led to the FDA to issue two warnings in 2008 and 2011, ultimately leading to an increase in the classification of polypropylene mesh from Class II (moderate risk) to Class III (high risk) [24]. Most recently, in April of 2019, the FDA mandated an immediate recall of mesh utilized specifically for transvaginal repair of prolapse. This mandate did not include transvaginal mesh slings or abdominally placed mesh for prolapse repair [25].

In comparing surgical outcomes of native tissue and mesh repairs, mesh has better anatomic outcomes, but equivalent or decreased functional outcomes compared to native tissue repairs [26–30]. In a Cochrane Review of anterior compartment prolapse from 2016, women had increased rates of anterior prolapse recurrence (32–45% vs. 13%), prolapse awareness (18–30% vs. 13%), and need for repeat surgery within 1–3 years (2–7% vs. 2%) with native tissue repair compared to women with mesh repair [31]. Conversely, women with mesh-augmented repairs had an 11% mesh exposure rate, with a need for repeat surgery of 7.3% for mesh exposure. Similarly, in another comparison of native tissue versus mesh, the 5-year risk of need for repeat surgery was higher in the mesh group due to mesh complications (15.2% vs. 9.8%) [32].

A NSQIP analysis of 6849 women during the period 2006–2013 with either mesh or native tissue anterior repair reported increase in 30-day complications in patients receiving mesh, and on multivariate analysis mesh was associated with negative postoperative outcomes such as unplanned intubation, prolonged ventilation, blood transfusion, and overall surgical complications, though overall rates of these complications were low [33].

Though anatomic outcomes may be better with a mesh-augmented repair, the PROSPECT (PROlapse Surgery: Pragmatic Evaluation and randomized Controlled Trials) trial compared 865 women with mesh versus native tissue repair and demonstrated no improvement in patient-reported symptoms or quality of life over a 2-year period [34]. Given this, many studies have repeatedly concluded that the risks of bladder injury, repeat surgery, and mesh complications do not outweigh the benefits of improved anatomic outcome without any correlating symptom or quality-of-life improvement [31, 34, 35].

Biograft Repair

As polypropylene mesh kits have since been removed from the market, there has been increased interest in the use of absorbable mesh or biografts to achieve improved anatomic outcomes without the complications associated with mesh [36]. Unfortunately, absorbable mesh has not shown a decrease in complications and in fact has shown high rates of mesh extrusion [37, 38].

Biografts also theoretically offer an alternative to mesh in terms of increasing support beyond native tissue alone without the risk of erosion or exposure. The PROSPECT randomized trial arm comparing 673 women with standard native tissue versus Biological-graft-augmented repair found no improvement in symptom or quality-of-life scores but did in fact find an increased rate of women reporting "something coming down" in the graft arm compared to native tissue at 2 years (40 vs. 31%, $p = 0.04$). Other RCTs of cadaveric fascia lata and porcine dermis used for augmentation of anterior repair have similarly failed to show significant improvement in outcomes compared to native tissue repair [39–41].

The use of autologous fascia lata has demonstrated durable success for recurrent anterior prolapse, but the morbidity of a fascial harvest has made this option less attractive for an initial repair [42]. Thus, native tissue repair with central plication remains the mainstay of surgical treatment for the initial presentation of anterior compartment prolapse with a central defect without significant apical prolapse.

Paravaginal Repair

For lateral defects, the transabdominal paravaginal repair offers the best visualization and will be discussed later. A vaginal approach for a paravaginal repair is performed by dissecting laterally to the limits of the pubic rami and then plicating the suburethral and paravaginal connective tissue to the midline [43]. While the vaginal approach is feasible and associated with low rates of reoperation (7%), the poor visualization has been associated with an increase in complications [44–47]. In a series of 100 consecutive women undergoing vaginal paravaginal repair, 22% had recurrence within 1 year, and there were 21 major and 14 minor complications [46]. In another series of 135 women with 9 years of follow-up, anatomic recurrence was 45% and symptomatic recurrence was 26% [44]. This is likely due to the fact that paravaginal defects are associated with loss of apical support (uterine or vaginal vault prolapse), and paravaginal repair may not be sufficient to address apical support defects.

Abdominal Approach

Open abdominal paravaginal repair was popularized by Richardson in the 1970s [48, 49], and with the advent of minimally invasive surgery, laparoscopic paravaginal repair remains a valuable option for lateral anterior defects. A transperitoneal approach is utilized, and the retropubic space is dissected by opening the peritoneum between the obliterated umbilical arteries and entering the space of Retzius until the obturator internus fascia and arcus tendineus fascia pelvis (ATFP) is visualized. The assistant places a finger vaginally to palpate the ischial spine and manually elevate the lateral sulcus. Interrupted sutures are then placed through the pubocervical fascia, obturator internus fascia, and Cooper's ligament.

Bedford and colleagues reported on long-term outcomes of 223 women who underwent laparoscopic paravaginal repair at the time of uterosacral colpopexy or hysteropexy and reported 73% subjective failure at a median of 18 months; 37% required reoperation for recurrent anterior prolapse and 60% required any prolapse reoperation [50].

Posterior Compartment Prolapse

Prolapse of the posterior vaginal wall is due to a defect in the rectovaginal fascia that can be classified into low (hymen to perineal body), mid (due to weakness of the lateral attachment to the arcus tendineus), or high (due to weakening of the uterosacral and cardinal ligament complex) vaginal defects [51]. The levator muscular sling serves to pull forward the distal vagina and creates the posterior angulation of the vagina. While prolapse of the posterior vagina may include enterocele or sigmoidocele, rectocele is the most common, and is generally used to describe any posterior wall prolapse. Symptoms of rectocele include constipation, difficulty evacuating stool, and presence of a vaginal bulge. The goal of posterior prolapse surgery is to restore the vaginal axis, preserve vaginal depth, and prevent narrowing or stenosis of the vagina.

Native Tissue Repair

Transvaginal native tissue rectocele repair is the most common approach. This is performed by incising the posterior vaginal epithelium and performing a midline plication of the fascia with absorbable suture (Fig. 15.4). Care must be taken not to diminish the length or caliber of the vaginal vault. Additionally, rectal injury is possible, so it is wise to perform a rectal exam after plication has been completed. Transvaginal rectocele repair has better long-term anatomic success than cystocele repair, but the most common side effect of dyspareunia can be seen in 8–33% of patients [52, 53].

In an effort to reduce the morbidity of transvaginal rectocele repair, Richardson proposed site-specific repair, wherein interrupted sutures are placed only at the site of discrete and palpable fascial defects [51]. Unfortunately, in a retrospective study, patients with site-specific

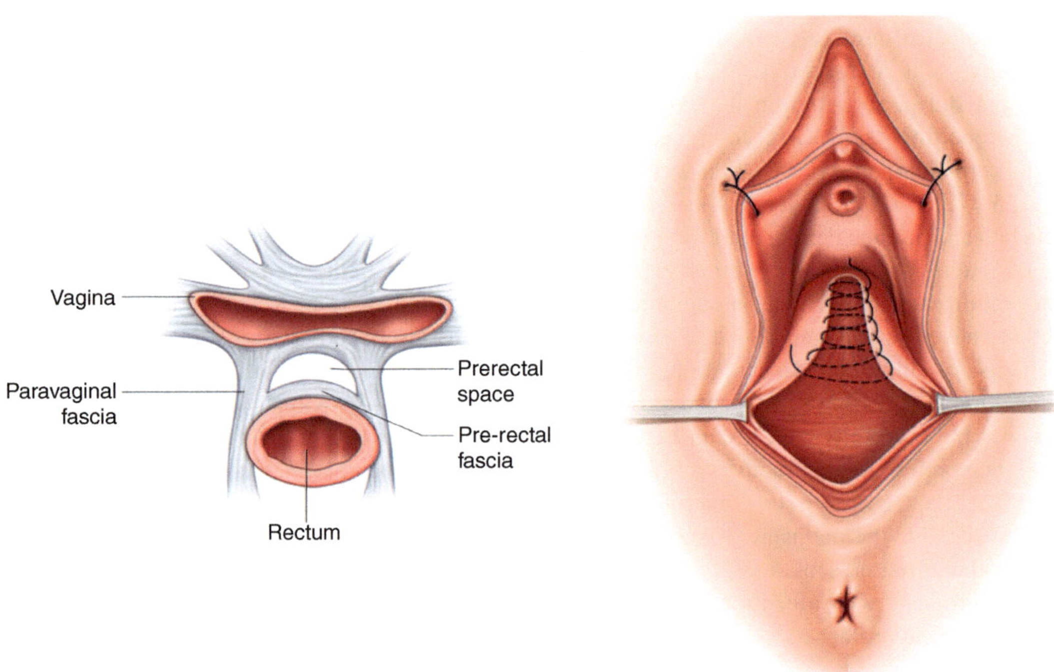

Fig. 15.4 Diagram of native tissue repair of rectocele defect by incorporating pararectal and prerectal fascia with running, locking suture. (Reused with permission. Copyright Springer Nature [56])

repair had increased recurrence rates and no improvement in complication rates or dyspareunia compared to a traditional posterior colporrhaphy [54]. Transanal repair has also been proposed as a mechanism to decrease postoperative dyspareunia, but recurrence rates are significantly higher (42% vs. 10%) and thus should be avoided [55].

Because of the high rates of postoperative dyspareunia, the risks and benefits of repair of asymptomatic posterior prolapse at the time of an anti-incontinence procedure or anterior repair should be discussed with the patient. The advantages of repair include restoration of the normal vaginal axis and creation of a more solid pelvic floor, which can reduce rates of prolapse recurrence and potentially improve outcomes of anti-incontinence surgery [56]. In women with a widened genital hiatus, posterior repair together with perineorrhaphy will also restore vaginal anatomy and improve sensation during sexual intercourse.

Mesh and Biograft Repair

As the subjective and anatomic success of native tissue repair for posterior prolapse is quite high (~90%), mesh- or biograft-augmented repairs are unlikely to provide any further benefit [55]. A 2018 Cochrane review and meta-analysis compared native tissue and mesh-augmented repairs and found no difference in recurrence, need for repeat surgery, awareness of prolapse, or dyspareunia [55, 57]. Similarly, biografts have failed to demonstrate any improvements in anatomic or subjective outcomes [58, 59]. In a randomized controlled trial of 160 women comparing standard native tissue repair to porcine graft repair, there was no difference in anatomic failure (12% vs. 9%) or vaginal bulge symptoms (3% vs. 7%) in graft versus control at 12 months [59]. Although there is no specific harm associated with biologic graft augmentation, the Choosing Wisely Campaign advises against mesh and biologic graft use in primary repair of the posterior compartment [60].

Apical/Vault Prolapse

Apical prolapse includes prolapse of the uterus or, after hysterectomy, the vaginal vault.

The cardinal-uterosacral ligament complex serves as the main support structure for the apex of the vagina. After hysterectomy, this ligament complex detaches from the vaginal cuff at the level of the ischial spine and can lead to vault prolapse. Vault prolapse (posthysterectomy apical prolapse) often includes an enterocele as well, as the endopelvic fascia is weakened after hysterectomy and allows the peritoneum to protrude through the fascial defect. The rate of apical repairs has increased as it has become more apparent that missed apical defects are a cause of surgical failures, and that the inclusion of apical repair is associated with improved outcomes compared to anterior or posterior repair alone [61]. The optimal approach for apical prolapse is undetermined as of yet, though abdominal sacral colpopexy with mesh appears to have the lowest rates of anatomic failure, symptomatic failure, and reoperation rates (Table 15.1) [9]. Both abdominal and vaginal approaches, with and without mesh, will be discussed in this section.

Vaginal Approach

Native Tissue Repair

Transvaginal apical prolapse repair is generally accomplished via uterosacral ligament suspension (USLS) or sacrospinous ligament fixation (SSLF). USLS can be performed either intra- or extraperitoneally. Sutures are placed through the uterosacral ligament, pubocervical fascia, and rectovaginal fascia bilaterally, bringing the vaginal cuff to the level of the ischial spine (Fig. 15.5). This may cause kinking of the distal ureter, so it is crucial to perform intraoperative cystoscopy to ensure ureteral integrity, as demonstrated by efflux of urine from the ureteral orifices.

SSLF is performed by placing sutures through the sacrospinous ligament, medial to the ischial

Table 15.1 Comparison of apical support approaches

Author	Type of study	*N*	Comparison	Follow-up	Anatomic recurrence (%)	Symptom recurrence (%)	Overall recurrence[a] (%)	Retreatment (%)
Lavelle [86], 2018	Retrospective review	756	Laparoscopic or robotic ASC vs. USLS	41 weeks (median)	7.4 vs. 17.1[b]			
Maher [87], 2011	RCT	108	Laparoscopic ASC vs. vaginal mesh (Prolift)	24 months	33 vs. 67[b]			5 vs. 22[b]
Maher [88], 2004	RCT	95	ASC vs. SSLF	24 months	24 vs. 31	6 vs. 9		
Coolen [89], 2017	RCT	74	Laparoscopic ASC vs. open ASC	12 months		5 vs. 11	16 vs. 11	11 vs. 27
Rondini [90], 2015	RCT	110	ASC vs. high USLS	12 months	0 vs. 17.5[b]			5.6 vs. 17[b]
Ow [91], 2018	RCT	82	ASC vs. extraperitoneal USLS with mesh	12 months		6 vs. 9	35 vs. 59[b]	12 vs. 20
Tate [92], 2011	RCT	58	Autologous fascia ASC vs. mesh ASC	60 months	38 vs. 7[b]	10 vs. 3		
Deprest [93], 2009	Prospective cohort	129	Biograft (porcine intestine or dermal collagen) ASC vs. mesh ASC	33 months (mean)	49 vs 34			12 vs. 0[b]
Culligan [78], 2005	RCT	100	Autologous fascia ASC vs. mesh ASC	12 months	32 vs. 8[b]			
To [94], 2017	Retrospective review	413	Lap ASC with mesh vs. transvaginal mesh (elevate)	12 months	3 vs. 3.4		4.5 vs. 4.8	2.6 vs. 4.1
Jelovsek [66], 2018	RCT	196	USLS vs. SSLF	60 months	47.5 vs. 61.8	37.4 vs. 41.8	61.5 vs. 70.3	11.9 vs. 8.1
Gutman [71], 2013	RCT	65[c]	Vaginal colpopexy (USLS or SSLF) vs. vaginal colpopexy with mesh (Prolift)	36 months	29 vs. 15	19 vs. 8		0 vs. 13
Halaska [72], 2012	RCT	151	SSLF vs. transvaginal mesh	12 months	39.4 vs. 16.9[b]			4 vs. 1
Svabik [73], 2014	RCT	72	SSLF vs. transvaginal mesh (Prolift) in post hysterectomy levator ani avulsion	12 months	65% vs. 3%[b]			
Detollenaere [67], 2015	RCT	208	Vaginal sacrospinous hysteropexy vs. TVH with USLS	12 months	50 vs. 44		11 vs. 17	1 vs. 4
Dietz [95], 2010	RCT	66	Vaginal sacrospinous hysteropexy vs. TVH with USLS	12 months	27 vs. 3[b]			11 vs. 7
Lo [68], 2015	Retrospective review	146	SSLF with hysterectomy vs. SSLF with hysteropexy	60 months	27.5 vs. 50[b]	32.5 vs. 50		1 vs. 0

RCT randomized controlled trial, *ASC* abdominal sacral colpopexy, *USLS* uterosacral ligament suspension, *SSLF* sacrospinous ligament fixation, *TVH* transvaginal hysterectomy

[a]Overall recurrence refers to a composite of anatomic and symptomatic recurrence

[b]Statistically significant $p < 0.05$

[c]Study terminated early due to >15% mesh exposure rate

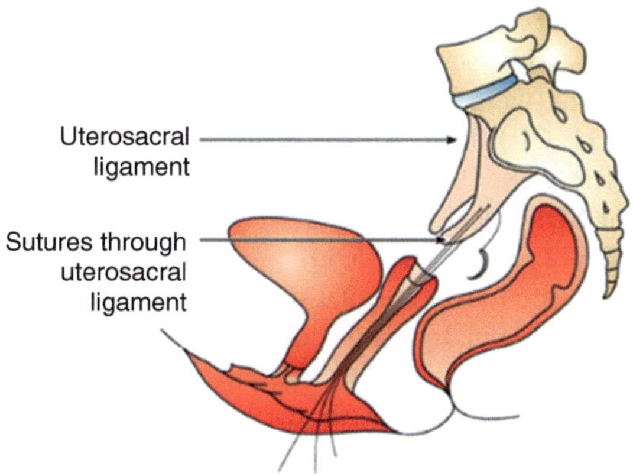

Fig. 15.5 Diagram of uterosacral ligament suspension. (Reused with permission. Copyright Springer Nature [97])

spine and the vaginal muscularis. While this fixation method was popular with the use of mesh-based kits, it is also used in native tissue repairs. Self-capture suture devices, such as the Capio ®, can assist in suture placement in the ligament. Although the classic SSLF is a unilateral procedure, this procedure can be performed unilaterally or bilaterally [62].

A third option for apical support is the iliococcygeus fascia fixation. Initially described by Sze and Karram, the vaginal apex is sutured to the iliococcygeal fascia, just below the ischial spine. The advantage of this approach is the decreased likelihood of injury to the pudendal nerve. The procedure also offers good success, with cure of up to 89% at 5 years [63]. In a review of 158 women, ileococcygeus fixation success was better if hysterectomy was performed at the same time (100% for mild prolapse, 91.2% for advanced prolapse) [64].

The OPTIMAL Trial is a multicenter randomized controlled trial that compared treatment of vault prolapse with either USLS or SSLF in 374 women. Adverse events were also equivalent, but all cases of ureteral obstruction (3.7%) occurred in the USLS arm [65]. Extended 5-year outcomes from the trial were reported in 309 women. Rates of surgical failure (defined as POP-Q point C descended more than one-third vaginal length, POP Aa/Ba/Ap/Bp beyond the hymen, bothersome bulge, or re-treatment) rose each year. At 5 years, surgical failure was 64.8% in the USLS group and 71.2% in the SSLF group ($p = 0.25$). When anatomic and bothersome bulge symptoms were evaluated separately, there was still no difference between approaches (5-year anatomic failure: 51.1% vs. 59.7%, $p = 0.11$; 5-year bothersome bulge symptoms 42.1% vs. 47.8%, $p = 0.60$). Five-year re-treatment rates were 11.9% for USLS and 8.1% for SSLF [66].

While most of these repairs are commonly done at the time of or after hysterectomy, some women prefer to retain their uterus. Vaginal sacrospinous hysteropexy is performed by incising the posterior vaginal wall deep to the rectovaginal fascia (or superficial if posterior repair is also planned) and then bluntly dissecting the right pararectal space until the ischial spine is palpated and the sacrospinous ligament can be identified. Two permanent or delayed absorbable sutures are then placed through the sacrospinous ligament (under direct vision or with a ligature carrier) and the posterior cervix, with care to make sure that the sutures are not protruding through the vaginal wall.

In a multicenter randomized controlled trial of 208 women with POP, Detollenaere and colleagues compared outcomes of sacrospinous hysteropexy and vaginal hysterectomy with USLS. At 12 months of follow-up, hysteropexy was found to be noninferior to hysterectomy in terms of bothersome bulge, need for repeat surgery, quality-of-life measurements, or complications [67]. In a retrospective review of 146 women with either sacrospinous hysteropexy versus vaginal hysterectomy with SSLF, hysteropexy was associated with a significantly lower rate of objective cure at 5-year follow-up (50% vs. 72.5%, $p = 0.03$), but subjective cure was not significantly different [68].

Mesh-Augmented Repair

As with anterior and posterior repair, the use of mesh-augmented repairs gained popularity in the early 2000s. The rationale behind transvaginal mesh kits was the combination of an apical suspension with mesh augmentation, all from an extraperitoneal and potentially safer approach. However, complications were reported at a high rate, resulting in two safety notifications in 2008 and 2011 by the FDA. This preceded media attention and massive litigation, resulting in the withdrawal of the majority of apical mesh products from the market and the ultimate FDA ban of mesh for transvaginal prolapse repair [69].

Even when transvaginal mesh was utilized more frequently, its benefit was debated, though many series showed that outcomes were superior to nonmesh approaches [26]. Zhu and colleagues evaluated their experience with transvaginal sacrospinous ligament fixation with polypropylene mesh in 60 patients, and found durable anatomic improvement as well as improvement in quality-of-life scores with low rates of postoperative pain (3.3%) and mesh exposure (3.3%) at 2 years [70]. The Vaginal Mesh for Prolapse Repair Trial compared transvaginal mesh to native tissue repair for women with multicompartment and apical prolapse and found no significant improvement in symptomatic or anatomic success [71]. Other smaller RCTs demonstrated decreased failure rates with mesh versus native tissue (3–16.9% vs. 39.4–65%), but mesh exposure rates of up to 20% [72, 73]. A 2016 Cochrane review of apical prolapse found that in 6 RCTs with 598 women comparing mesh to native tissue vaginal repair, there was no difference in prolapse awareness, repeat surgery for prolapse, or repeat surgery for SUI [9].

Transvaginal mesh was also used for hysteropexy in patients who desired uterine sparing surgery. For example, the Uphold Lite (Boston Scientific) was placed by dissecting the anterior vaginal wall and suturing the mesh to the sacrospinous ligaments, cervix, and fibromuscular layer on the bladder. In a prospective cohort study of 76 vaginal versus 74 laparoscopic mesh hysteropexies, vaginal mesh hysteropexy had 80% anatomic success, 95% symptomatic success, and 6.6% mesh exposure at 1-year follow-up [74].

Abdominal Approach

Abdominal sacral colpopexy (ASC) is arguably the most durable repair for apical prolapse, and as mentioned above, transabdominal mesh placed for prolapse repair remains a viable option. A 2016 Cochrane review of 583 women concluded that, with sacral colpopexy compared to vaginal repair, women had less prolapse awareness (RR 2.11, CI 1.06–4.21), less need for repeat surgery (RR 2.28, CI 1.20–4.32), and fewer complaints of SUI (RR 1.86, CI 1.17–2.94) or dyspareunia (RR 2.53, CI 1.17–5.50). The disadvantages of ASC are longer hospital stay and recovery times.

Abdominal sacral colpopexy can be performed: open, laparoscopically, or robotically. Regardless of approach, the key elements of the procedure include securing a graft, usually a y-shaped microporous, monofilament mesh, to the sacral promontory and vaginal apex/cervix as well as reducing any enterocele and performing a culdoplasty. Care must be taken to suture the graft without any tension (Fig. 15.6). If performed open, it is commonly done through a Pfannenstiel incision, though a low midline incision can also be used. Supracervical hysterectomy can also be performed at the time of ASC without increased complications compared to sacral colpopexy with prior hysterectomy [75]. When performing a concomitant hysterectomy, a supracervical approach (versus total) will significantly reduce mesh-related complications, from over 20% in the total hysterectomy group to 5% in the supracervical group [76].

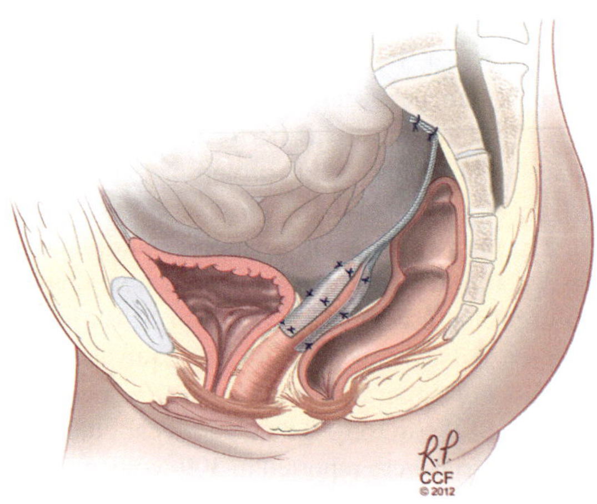

Fig. 15.6 Diagram of abdominal sacral colpopexy with Y-mesh to the vaginal cuff. (Reused with permission, Cleveland Clinic Center for Medical Art & Photography © 2018–2019. All Rights Reserved)

Native Tissue Repair

While mesh sacrocolpopexy is the gold standard, mesh litigation has led to an interest in performing ASC with autologous fascia. The advantages of autologous fascia are decreased risk of mesh infection and decreased rates of erosion, as there has been no reported case of autologous fascia erosion at the time of this publication. There has been little investigation into the long-term outcomes of autologous fascia, but a small case series demonstrated 90% cure rate [77]. In an RCT comparing synthetic mesh versus autologous fascia, ASC mesh had superior anatomic outcomes. This was also true in a comparison of cadaveric fascia lata versus synthetic mesh, with a 9% mesh failure rate compared to a 32% fascia lata anatomic failure rate [78].

Autologous fascia can be harvested from either the rectus fascia or fascia lata. Rectus fascia is advantageous if the ASC is being performed open, as a single incision can be used. Alternatively, fascia lata can be harvested from a small leg incision if ASC will be performed laparoscopically or robotically.

Mesh Sacral Colpopexy

In the Colpopexy and Urinary Reduction Efforts (CARE) trial of 223 women, mesh erosion for ASC was noted to be 10.5% at 7 years, and reoperation was noted to be 4.4%. This is compared to quoted rates of surgical failure of 40–60% and reoperation rates of 5% for transvaginal apical repair [65, 79]. In a large population-based study from Ontario, Canada, women with transvaginal mesh required reoperation more frequently than women with abdominal mesh or native tissue repair. Still, 10% of women with both vaginal and abdominal mesh required surgical revision or excision [80].

Linder and colleagues performed an NSQIP analysis of 6390 women who underwent non-mesh vaginal apical repairs or minimally invasive sacral colpopexy (MISC) during the period 2010–2016. Those undergoing MISC were more likely to be younger and undergo concomitant urethral sling placement. MISC was also associated with lower 30-day minor complications (3.9% vs. 5.6%, $P = 0.004$) and lower rates of prolonged hospitalization >2 days (5.2% vs. 7.9%, $p < 0.001$), but higher rates of progressive renal insufficiency or acute renal failure, requiring dialysis. On multivariate analysis, there was no difference among 30-day complications, prolonged hospitalization, readmission, or reoperation [81].

As with vaginal hysteropexy, laparoscopic mesh hysteropexy is an option for uterine preservation. Gutman and colleagues also evaluated the 12-month outcomes of 74 women undergoing laparoscopic sacral hysteropexy and found 77% anatomic success, 90% symptomatic success, and 2.7% mesh exposure [74].

Perineal Procedures

Perineocele

Herniation of abdominal organs through the perineum is a known complication of abdomino-perineal resection or pelvic exenteration but may also occur in the absence of prior procedures. Perineocele may present with bulging of the perineum and a widened distance between the posterior fourchette of the vagina and the anus greater than 4 cm [82]. Symptoms include perineal pressure, constipation, and need to splint and manually reduce the perineocele for defecation. Repair is performed by creating an inverted Y incision between the posterior vagina and either side of the rectum. By developing the ischiorectal fossae, the levator musculature can be exposed and the pararectal space entered. The posterior levator fascia is then sutured to the transverse perineal muscle and external anal sphincter so as to re-create the central perineal tendon. A series of 6 patients reported successful repair and resolution of symptoms with this surgical approach [82].

Colpocleisis

Women with bothersome prolapse who are not able to undergo a more invasive repair such as a sacral colpopexy and who are not interested in future penetrative intercourse or a functional vagina may be the best candidates for obliterative vaginal surgery, or colpocleisis, which can be performed under regional anesthesia. LeFort, or partial colpocleisis, is the most common approach when the uterus is present to allow cervical discharge to exit. Colpectomy can be performed if the uterus is absent. The anterior and posterior vaginal epithelia are removed and the walls are then sutured together to obliterate the vaginal cavity and reduce the prolapse. An aggressive perinorrhaphy is then performed (Fig. 15.7).

The procedure is generally well tolerated with few complications. On telephone follow-up at almost 4 years after surgery, 90% of women reported satisfaction [83]. Another series of 47 women undergoing LeFort colpocleisis reported 91.5% subjective cure at 14.8 months [84]. Another option for women who do not desire a functional vagina is to perform a constricting perineal procedure after any necessary anterior,

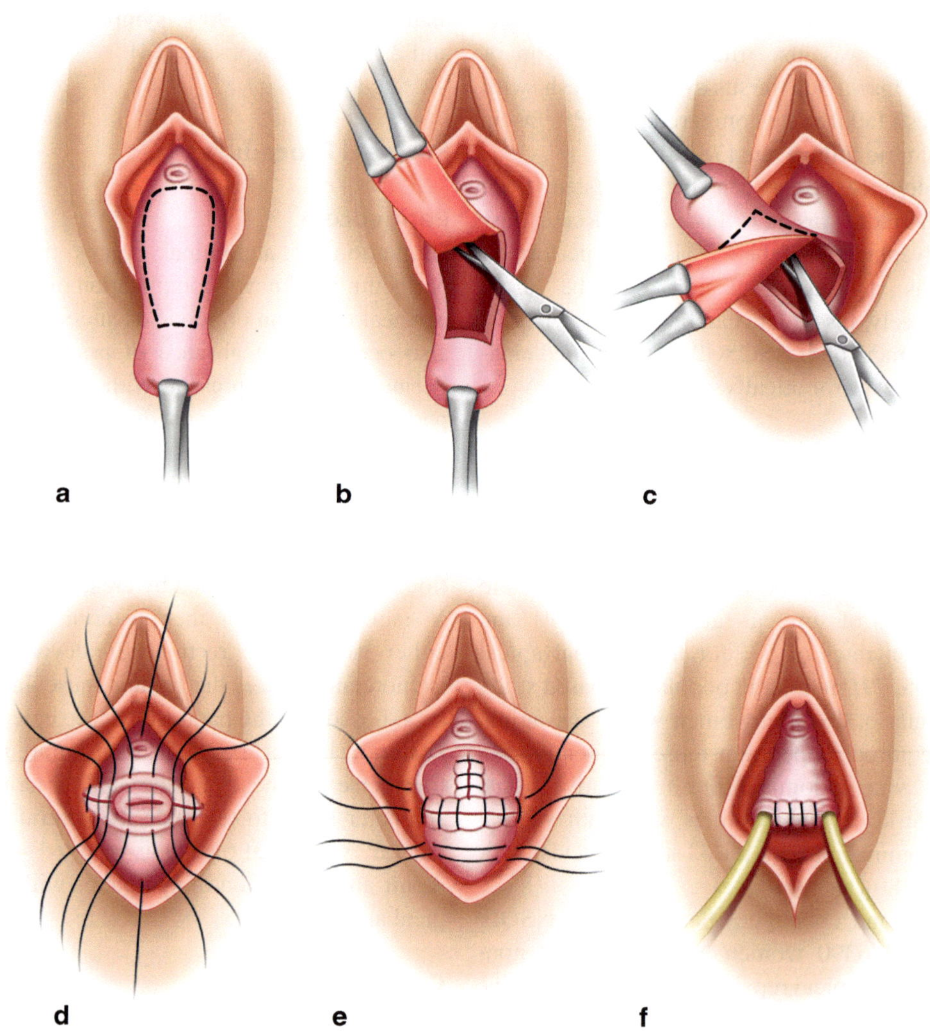

Fig. 15.7 LeFort colpocleisis: (**a**) The vagina is everted and the anterior vaginal mucosa is incised and (**b**) separated from the underlying fascia. (**c**) The same is repeated posteriorly. (**d**) The vaginal mucosal edge is then reapproximated in front of the cervix. (**e**) The anterior and posterior vaginal wall edges are reapproximated horizontally, and plication sutures are placed beneath the bladder neck. (**f**) The outer mucosal edges are closed, leaving tunnels on either side of the vagina. (Reused with permission. Copyright Wolters Kluwer Health [98])

posterior, or apical repair, in which much of the excess vaginal tissue is excised and the vaginal epithelium is reapproximated narrowly, leaving a 1-cm genital hiatus [85].

Summary

In the case of the 53-year-old woman with anterior prolapse, the patient elected for a robotic ASC and hysterectomy with mesh with concomitant posterior colporrhaphy. For all women considering surgery for POP, a shared decision-making approach outlining the advantages and disadvantages of mesh or graft-augmented repair is critical.

Commentary

Benjamin M. Brucker

Pelvic organ prolapse is a very common condition. Cross-sectional data suggest that 25% of women have significant anatomical prolapse, with the leading edge of the prolapse at the hymenal ring or below [99]. Not all women with pelvic organ prolapse will require a surgical intervention, but it is estimated that at least 10% of the female population will eventually undergo surgical correction, presumably because of bothersome symptoms or derangements of normal pelvic floor/organ functions. As the population of the United States ages, and women remain more active later in life, the importance of understanding how to manage women with pelvic organ prolapse is more pertinent than ever before [100]. The authors of this chapter do a fantastic job laying out the surgical approaches to treating women with pelvic organ prolapse. This chapter touches on the myriad approaches that surgeons use to treat pelvic organ prolapse. The data pertaining to these options are clearly summarized and presented in an easy-to-understand format (i.e., Table 15.1).

When choosing from the various approaches to surgical correction of pelvic organ prolapse, one critical question patients and clinicians ask is "how successful is this surgery?" The stage is set for analyzing the data presented when the authors explain the range of definitions of "success" that are commonly used in publications. As we read the data and compare the approaches, we must remind ourselves of the importance of considering what definition is being used in a given series. It is also important to look at studies with consideration of length of follow-up, taking into account the underlying disease process of pelvic organ prolapse. Additionally, understanding any bias each study may have, inherent to the study design and/or patient population, is critical. Finally, other factors, such as rates and severity of complications and the availability of patient-reported outcomes, add branches to our expanding decision tree. The complexity of the comparison does not end there. As members of a healthcare community, we need to consider cost of treatment choices [101]. Further, as providers sitting in front of an individual patient, we add unique patient factors (i.e., past medical history or family history) that might steer the decisions to a particular type of repair and away from another.

This chapter on the surgical treatment of pelvic organ prolapse is up-to-date, as it reviews the FDA notifications and subsequent withdrawal of vaginally placed mesh for the treatment of pelvic organ prolapse from the US market. The data on autologous grafts and biological materials are also reviewed. The results seem to suggest that there is room to improve and develop materials and/or modify techniques or teaching so that surgical outcomes can continue to improve. One graft that surgeons have continued to rely on is abdominally placed mesh. Even prior to the withdrawal of vaginally placed mesh, abdominally placed mesh, at the time of sacrocolpopexy, had been used with increasing frequency [102]. The authors highlighted rates of sacrocolpopexy mesh "erosions," occurring in up to 10% of patients. We will see over time, as technique utilization changes, how prevalence of complications changes, for better or for worse.

As medical professionals, we try to make decisions using the highest-quality data available. Large randomized comparative studies are costly. Further, treatment durability data require long periods of time to mature. Techniques, tools, and materials are constantly changing. This means that we are often left to make clinical decision with data that has inherent limitations. Newer goals of surgical correction emerge such as uterine preservation [103]. We will see techniques described and investigated to achieve these goals [104–106]. If the interest in uterine preservation grows, we will require more data on appropriate preoperative screening/risk assessment along with long-term outcome data to counsel our patients appropriately.

We are lucky to have comprehensive reviews like this chapter to lay out what we know, and see what questions remain unanswered. The diversity of treatment options makes counseling extremely complex, but if we aim to utilize shared decision making, the data generated by this cycle of questions and answers allow the patient to contribute to selection of the surgical approach that works best for their case.

References

1. DeLancey JOL. Anatomie aspects of vaginal eversion after hysterectomy. Am J Obstet Gynecol [Internet]. 1992;166(6):1717–28. Available from: https://linkinghub.elsevier.com/retrieve/pii/000293789291562O.
2. Barber MD, Maher C. Epidemiology and outcome assessment of pelvic organ prolapse. Int Urogynecol J [Internet]. 2013;24(11):1783–90. Available from: http://www.ncbi.nlm.nih.gov/pubmed/24142054.
3. Jelovsek JE, Maher C, Barber MD. Pelvic organ prolapse. Lancet [Internet]. 2007;369(9566):1027–38. Available from: https://linkinghub.elsevier.com/retrieve/pii/S0140673607604620.
4. Vergeldt TFM, Weemhoff M, IntHout J, Kluivers KB. Risk factors for pelvic organ prolapse and its recurrence: a systematic review. Int Urogynecol J [Internet]. 2015;26(11):1559–73. Available from: http://www.ncbi.nlm.nih.gov/pubmed/25966804.
5. Jack GS, Nikolova G, Vilain E, Raz S, Rodríguez LV. Familial transmission of genitovaginal prolapse. Int Urogynecol J Pelvic Floor Dysfunct [Internet]. 2006;17(5):498–501. Available from: http://www.ncbi.nlm.nih.gov/pubmed/16365693.
6. Cartwright R, Kirby AC, Tikkinen KAO, Mangera A, Thiagamoorthy G, Rajan P, et al. Systematic review and metaanalysis of genetic association studies of urinary symptoms and prolapse in women. Am J Obstet Gynecol [Internet]. 2015;212(2):199.e1–24. Available from: http://www.ncbi.nlm.nih.gov/pubmed/25111588.
7. Ward RM, Velez Edwards DR, Edwards T, Giri A, Jerome RN, Wu JM. Genetic epidemiology of pelvic organ prolapse: a systematic review. Am J Obstet Gynecol [Internet]. 2014;211(4):326–35. Available from: http://www.ncbi.nlm.nih.gov/pubmed/24721264.
8. Barber MD, Brubaker L, Nygaard I, Wheeler TL, Schaffer J, Chen Z, et al. Defining success after surgery for pelvic organ prolapse. Obstet Gynecol [Internet]. 2009;114(3):600–9. Available from: http://www.ncbi.nlm.nih.gov/pubmed/19701041.
9. Maher C, Feiner B, Baessler K, Haya N, Brown J. Surgery for women with apical vaginal prolapse (Review). Summary of findings for the main comparison. Cochrane Database Syst Rev. 2016;(10):1–196.
10. Hendrix SL, Clark A, Nygaard I, Aragaki A, Barnabei V, McTiernan A. Pelvic organ prolapse in the Women's health initiative: gravity and gravidity. Am J Obstet Gynecol [Internet]. 2002;186(6):1160–6. Available from: http://www.ncbi.nlm.nih.gov/pubmed/12066091.
11. Amin K, Lee U. Surgery for anterior compartment vaginal prolapse. Urol Clin North Am [Internet]. 2018;46(1):61–70. Available from: https://doi.org/10.1016/j.ucl.2018.08.008.
12. Halpern-Elenskaia K, Umek W, Bodner-Adler B, Hanzal E. Anterior colporrhaphy: a standard operation? Systematic review of the technical aspects of a common procedure in randomized controlled trials. Int Urogynecol J. 2018;29(6):781–8.
13. Kelly HA, Dumm WM. Urinary incontinence in women, without manifest injury to the bladder. 1914. Int Urogynecol J Pelvic Floor Dysfunct [Internet]. 1998;9(3):158–64. Available from: http://www.ncbi.nlm.nih.gov/pubmed/9745976.
14. Anger JT, Scott VCS, Kiyosaki K, Khan AA, Sevilla C, Connor SE, et al. Quality-of-care indicators for pelvic organ prolapse: development of an infrastructure for quality assessment. Int Urogynecol J [Internet]. 2013;24(12):2039–47. Available from: http://www.ncbi.nlm.nih.gov/pubmed/23644812.
15. Eilber KS, Alperin M, Khan A, Wu N, Pashos CL, Clemens JQ, et al. Outcomes of vaginal prolapse surgery among female Medicare beneficiaries: the role of apical support. Obstet Gynecol [Internet]. 2013;122(5):981–7. Available from: http://www.ncbi.nlm.nih.gov/pubmed/24104778.
16. Olsen A, Smith V, Bergstrom J, Colling J, Clark A. Epidemiology of surgically managed pelvic organ prolapse and urinary incontinence. Obstet Gynecol [Internet]. 1997 Apr [cited 2019 Apr 2];89(4):501–6. Available from: http://linkinghub.elsevier.com/retrieve/pii/S0029784497000586.
17. Weber AM, Walters MD, Piedmonte MR, Ballard LA. Anterior colporrhaphy: a randomized trial of three surgical techniques. Am J Obstet Gynecol [Internet]. 2001;185(6):1299–304; discussion 1304–6. Available from: http://www.ncbi.nlm.nih.gov/pubmed/11744900.

18. Chmielewski L, Walters MD, Weber AM, Barber MD. Reanalysis of a randomized trial of 3 techniques of anterior colporrhaphy using clinically relevant definitions of success. Am J Obstet Gynecol [Internet]. 2011;205(1):69.e1–8. Available from: http://www.ncbi.nlm.nih.gov/pubmed/21545996.
19. Bergman I, Söderberg MW, Kjaeldgaard A, Ek M. Does the choice of suture material matter in anterior and posterior colporrhaphy? Int Urogynecol J [Internet]. 2016;27(9):1357–65. Available from: http://www.ncbi.nlm.nih.gov/pubmed/26935306.
20. Song H-S, Choo GY, Jin L-H, Yoon S-M, Lee T. Transvaginal cystocele repair by purse-string technique reinforced with three simple sutures: surgical technique and results. Int Neurourol J [Internet]. 2012;16(3):144–8. Available from: http://www.ncbi.nlm.nih.gov/pubmed/23094221.
21. Lowder JL, Park AJ, Ellison R, Ghetti C, Moalli P, Zyczynski H, et al. The role of apical vaginal support in the appearance of anterior and posterior vaginal prolapse. Obstet Gynecol [Internet]. 2008;111(1):152–7. Available from: http://www.ncbi.nlm.nih.gov/pubmed/18165404.
22. Elmér C, Altman D, Engh ME, Axelsen S, Väyrynen T, Falconer C, et al. Trocar-guided transvaginal mesh repair of pelvic organ prolapse. Obstet Gynecol [Internet]. 2009;113(1):117–26. Available from: http://www.ncbi.nlm.nih.gov/pubmed/19104367.
23. Simon M, Debodinance P. Vaginal prolapse repair using the Prolift kit: a registry of 100 successive cases. Eur J Obstet Gynecol Reprod Biol [Internet]. 2011;158(1):104–9. Available from: http://www.ncbi.nlm.nih.gov/pubmed/21636208.
24. Souders CP, Eilber KS, McClelland L, Wood LN, Souders AR, Steiner V, et al. The truth behind transvaginal mesh litigation. Female Pelvic Med Reconstr Surg [Internet]. 2017 Jun [cited 2019 Apr 2];24(1):1. Available from: http://www.ncbi.nlm.nih.gov/pubmed/28657986.
25. Urogynecologic Surgical Mesh Implants | FDA [Internet]. [cited 2019 May 26]. Available from: https://www.fda.gov/medical-devices/implants-and-prosthetics/urogynecologic-surgical-mesh-implants.
26. Altman D, Väyrynen T, Engh ME, Axelsen S, Falconer C, Nordic Transvaginal Mesh Group. Anterior colporrhaphy versus transvaginal mesh for pelvic-organ prolapse. N Engl J Med [Internet]. 2011;364(19):1826–36. Available from: http://www.ncbi.nlm.nih.gov/pubmed/21561348.
27. Sivaslioglu AA, Unlubilgin E, Dolen I. A randomized comparison of polypropylene mesh surgery with site-specific surgery in the treatment of cystocoele. Int Urogynecol J Pelvic Floor Dysfunct [Internet]. 2008;19(4):467–71. Available from: http://www.ncbi.nlm.nih.gov/pubmed/17901910.
28. Vollebregt A, Fischer K, Gietelink D, van der Vaart CH. Primary surgical repair of anterior vaginal prolapse: a randomised trial comparing anatomical and functional outcome between anterior colporrhaphy and trocar-guided transobturator anterior mesh. BJOG [Internet]. 2011;118(12):1518–27. Available from: http://www.ncbi.nlm.nih.gov/pubmed/21864325.
29. El-Nazer MA, Gomaa IA, Ismail Madkour WA, Swidan KH, El-Etriby MA. Anterior colporrhaphy versus repair with mesh for anterior vaginal wall prolapse: a comparative clinical study. Arch Gynecol Obstet [Internet]. 2012;286(4):965–72. Available from: http://www.ncbi.nlm.nih.gov/pubmed/22648445.
30. de Tayrac R, Cornille A, Eglin G, Guilbaud O, Mansoor A, Alonso S, et al. Comparison between trans-obturator trans-vaginal mesh and traditional anterior colporrhaphy in the treatment of anterior vaginal wall prolapse: results of a French RCT. Int Urogynecol J [Internet]. 2013;24(10):1651–61. Available from: http://www.ncbi.nlm.nih.gov/pubmed/23512113.
31. Maher C, Feiner B, Baessler K, Christmann-Schmid C, Haya N, Brown J. Surgery for women with anterior compartment prolapse. Cochrane Database Syst Rev [Internet]. 2016;11:CD004014. Available from: http://www.ncbi.nlm.nih.gov/pubmed/27901278.
32. Jonsson Funk M, Visco AG, Weidner AC, Pate V, Wu JM. Long-term outcomes of vaginal mesh versus native tissue repair for anterior vaginal wall prolapse. Int Urogynecol J [Internet]. 2013;24(8):1279–85. Available from: http://www.ncbi.nlm.nih.gov/pubmed/23400940.
33. Chung DE, James M, Sui W, Theofanides MC, Onyeji I, Matulay J. Safety of mesh for vaginal cystocele repair: analysis of national patient characteristics and complications. J Urol [Internet]. 2017;198(3):632–7. Available from: https://doi.org/10.1016/j.juro.2017.04.015.
34. Glazener CM, Breeman S, Elders A, Hemming C, Cooper KG, Freeman RM, et al. Mesh, graft, or standard repair for women having primary transvaginal anterior or posterior compartment prolapse surgery: two parallel-group, multicentre, randomised, controlled trials (PROSPECT). Lancet [Internet]. 2017;389(10067):381–92. Available from: https://doi.org/10.1016/S0140-6736(16)31596-3.
35. Morling JR, McAllister DA, Agur W, Fischbacher CM, Glazener CMA, Guerrero K, et al. Adverse events after first, single, mesh and non-mesh surgical procedures for stress urinary incontinence and pelvic organ prolapse in Scotland, 1997-2016: a population-based cohort study. Lancet (London, England) [Internet]. 2017;389(10069):629–40. Available from: http://www.ncbi.nlm.nih.gov/pubmed/28010993.
36. Nazemi TM, Kobashi KC. Complications of grafts used in female pelvic floor reconstruction: mesh erosion and extrusion. Indian J Urol [Internet]. 2007 Apr [cited 2019 Apr 2];23(2):153–60. Available from: http://www.ncbi.nlm.nih.gov/pubmed/19675793.
37. Rudnicki M, Laurikainen E, Pogosean R, Kinne I, Jakobsson U, Teleman P. Anterior colporrhaphy compared with collagen-coated transvaginal mesh for anterior vaginal wall prolapse: a randomised con-

trolled trial. BJOG [Internet]. 2014;121(1):102–10; discussion 110-1. Available from: http://www.ncbi.nlm.nih.gov/pubmed/24118844.

38. Rudnicki M, Laurikainen E, Pogosean R, Kinne I, Jakobsson U, Teleman P. A 3-year follow-up after anterior colporrhaphy compared with collagen-coated transvaginal mesh for anterior vaginal wall prolapse: a randomised controlled trial. BJOG [Internet]. 2016;123(1):136–42. Available from: http://www.ncbi.nlm.nih.gov/pubmed/26420345.
39. Gandhi S, Goldberg RP, Kwon C, Koduri S, Beaumont JL, Abramov Y, et al. A prospective randomized trial using solvent dehydrated fascia lata for the prevention of recurrent anterior vaginal wall prolapse. Am J Obstet Gynecol [Internet]. 2005;192(5):1649–54. Available from: http://www.ncbi.nlm.nih.gov/pubmed/15902172.
40. Menefee SA, Dyer KY, Lukacz ES, Simsiman AJ, Luber KM, Nguyen JN. Colporrhaphy compared with mesh or graft-reinforced vaginal paravaginal repair for anterior vaginal wall prolapse: a randomized controlled trial. Obstet Gynecol [Internet]. 2011;118(6):1337–44. Available from: http://www.ncbi.nlm.nih.gov/pubmed/22067717.
41. Dahlgren E, Kjølhede P, RPOP-PELVICOL Study Group. Long-term outcome of porcine skin graft in surgical treatment of recurrent pelvic organ prolapse. An open randomized controlled multicenter study. Acta Obstet Gynecol Scand [Internet]. 2011;90(12):1393–401. Available from: http://www.ncbi.nlm.nih.gov/pubmed/21895613.
42. Cormio L, Mancini V, Liuzzi G, Lucarelli G, Carrieri G. Cystocele repair by autologous rectus fascia graft: the pubovaginal cystocele sling. J Urol [Internet]. 2015;194(3):721–7. Available from: http://www.ncbi.nlm.nih.gov/pubmed/25837536.
43. Angulo A, Kligman I. Retroperitoneal sacrocolpopexy for correction of prolapse of vaginal vault. Surg Gynecol Obstet [Internet]. 1989;169(4):319–23. Available from: http://www.ncbi.nlm.nih.gov/pubmed/2528833.
44. Chen Z, Wong V, Wang A, Moore KH. Nine-year objective and subjective follow-up of the ultra-lateral anterior repair for cystocele. Int Urogynecol J Pelvic Floor Dysfunct. 2014;25(3):387–92.
45. P Mallipeddi, N Kohli, AC Steele, RG Owens, MM Karram. Vaginal paravaginal repair in the surgical treatment of anterior vaginal wall prolapse. Prim Care Update Ob Gyns [Internet]. 1998;5(4):199–200. Available from: http://www.ncbi.nlm.nih.gov/pubmed/10838380.
46. Young SB, Daman JJ, Bony LG. Vaginal paravaginal repair: one-year outcomes. Am J Obstet Gynecol [Internet]. 2001;185(6):1360–6; discussion 1366-7. Available from: http://www.ncbi.nlm.nih.gov/pubmed/11744910.
47. Hosni MM, El-Feky AEH, Agur WI, Khater EM. Evaluation of three different surgical approaches in repairing paravaginal support defects: a comparative trial. Arch Gynecol Obstet [Internet]. 2013;288(6):1341–8. Available from: http://www.ncbi.nlm.nih.gov/pubmed/23797932.
48. Richardson AC, Lyon JB, Williams NL. A new look at pelvic relaxation. Am J Obstet Gynecol [Internet]. 1976;126(5):568–73. Available from: http://www.ncbi.nlm.nih.gov/pubmed/984127.
49. Richardson AC, Edmonds PB, Williams NL. Treatment of stress urinary incontinence due to paravaginal fascial defect. Obstet Gynecol [Internet]. 1981;57(3):357–62. Available from: http://www.ncbi.nlm.nih.gov/pubmed/7465150.
50. Bedford ND, Seman EI, O'Shea RT, Keirse MJNC. Long-term outcomes of laparoscopic repair of cystocoele. Aust N Z J Obstet Gynaecol. 2015;55(6):588–92.
51. Richardson AC. The rectovaginal septum revisited: its relationship to rectocele and its importance in rectocele repair. Clin Obstet Gynecol [Internet]. 1993;36(4):976–83. Available from: http://www.ncbi.nlm.nih.gov/pubmed/8293598.
52. Madsen LD, Nüssler E, Kesmodel US, Greisen S, Bek KM, Glavind-Kristensen M. Native-tissue repair of isolated primary rectocele compared with nonabsorbable mesh: patient-reported outcomes. Int Urogynecol J [Internet]. 2017;28(1):49–57. Available from: http://www.ncbi.nlm.nih.gov/pubmed/27379892.
53. Mellgren A, Anzén B, Nilsson BY, Johansson C, Dolk A, Gillgren P, et al. Results of rectocele repair. A prospective study. Dis Colon Rectum [Internet]. 1995;38(1):7–13. Available from: http://www.ncbi.nlm.nih.gov/pubmed/7813350.
54. Abramov Y, Gandhi S, Goldberg RP, Botros SM, Kwon C, Sand PK. Site-specific rectocele repair compared with standard posterior colporrhaphy. Obstet Gynecol [Internet]. 2005;105(2):314–8. Available from: http://www.ncbi.nlm.nih.gov/pubmed/15684158.
55. Mowat A, Maher D, Baessler K, Haya N, Maher C. Surgery for women with posterior compartment prolapse (Review). Summary of findings for the main comparison. 2018;(3).
56. Raz S. Atlas of vaginal reconstructive surgery [Internet]. New York: Springer New York; 2015. Available from: http://link.springer.com/10.1007/978-1-4939-2941-2.
57. Maher C, Baessler K. Surgical management of pelvic organ prolapse in women. Maher C, Baessler K. Surgical management of pelvic organ prolapse in women. Cochrane Collab. 2010;25–30. Cochrane Collab. 2013;(4):25–30.
58. Paraiso MFR, Barber MD, Muir TW, Walters MD. Rectocele repair: a randomized trial of three surgical techniques including graft augmentation. Am J Obstet Gynecol [Internet]. 2006;195(6):1762–71. Available from: http://www.ncbi.nlm.nih.gov/pubmed/17132479.
59. Sung VW, Rardin CR, Raker CA, Lasala CA, Myers DL. Porcine subintestinal submucosal graft augmentation for rectocele repair: a randomized controlled trial. Obstet Gynecol [Internet]. 2012;119(1):125–

33. Available from: http://www.ncbi.nlm.nih.gov/pubmed/22183220.
60. American Urogynecologic Society | Choosing Wisely [Internet]. [cited 2019 Apr 2]. Available from: http://www.choosingwisely.org/societies/american-urogynecologic-society/.
61. Alas AN, Anger JT. Role of apical support defect: correction in women undergoing vaginal prolapse surgery. Curr Opin Obstet Gynecol [Internet]. 2014;26(5):386–92. Available from: http://www.ncbi.nlm.nih.gov/pubmed/25136761.
62. Walters MD, Ridgeway BM. Surgical treatment of vaginal apex prolapse. Obstet Gynecol [Internet]. 2013 Feb 1 [cited 2019 Apr 3];121(2 Pt 1):354–74. Available from: http://www.ncbi.nlm.nih.gov/pubmed/23344287.
63. Serati M, Braga A, Bogani G, Leone Roberti Maggiore U, Sorice P, Ghezzi F, et al. Iliococcygeus fixation for the treatment of apical vaginal prolapse: efficacy and safety at 5 years of follow-up. Int Urogynecol J [Internet]. 2015;26(7):1007–12. Available from: http://www.ncbi.nlm.nih.gov/pubmed/25653034.
64. Suh DH, Jeon MJ. Risk factors for the failure of iliococcygeus suspension for uterine prolapse. Eur J Obstet Gynecol Reprod Biol [Internet]. 2018;225:210–3. Available from: https://doi.org/10.1016/j.ejogrb.2018.05.001.
65. Barber MD, Brubaker L, Burgio KL, Richter HE, Nygaard I, Weidner AC, et al. Comparison of 2 transvaginal surgical approaches and perioperative behavioral therapy for apical vaginal prolapse: the OPTIMAL randomized trial. JAMA [Internet]. 2014;311(10):1023–34. Available from: http://www.ncbi.nlm.nih.gov/pubmed/24618964
66. Jelovsek JE, Barber MD, Norton P, Brubaker L, Gantz M, Richter HE, et al. Effect of uterosacral ligament suspension vs sacrospinous ligament fixation with or without perioperative behavioral therapy for pelvic organ vaginal prolapse on surgical outcomes and prolapse symptoms at 5 years in the OPTIMAL randomized clinical trial. JAMA. 2018;319(15):1554–65.
67. Detollenaere RJ, den Boon J, Stekelenburg J, IntHout J, Vierhout ME, Kluivers KB, van Eijndhoven HW. Sacrospinous hysteropexy versus vaginal hysterectomy with suspension of the uterosacral ligaments in women with uterine prolapse stage 2 or higher: multicentre randomised non-inferiority trial. BMJ. 2015;351:h3717
68. Lo TS, Pue LB, Hung TH, Wu PY, Tan YL. Long-term outcome of native tissue reconstructive vaginal surgery for advanced pelvic organ prolapse at 86 months: hysterectomy versus hysteropexy. J Obstet Gynaecol Res. 2015;41(7):1099–107.
69. Clemons JL, Weinstein M, Guess MK, Alperin M, Moalli P, Gregory WT, et al. Impact of the 2011 FDA transvaginal mesh safety update on AUGS members' use of synthetic mesh and biologic grafts in pelvic reconstructive surgery. Female Pelvic Med Reconstr Surg [Internet]. 19(4):191–8. Available from: http://www.ncbi.nlm.nih.gov/pubmed/23797515.
70. Zhu Q, Shu H, Du G, Dai Z. Impact of transvaginal modified sacrospinous ligament fixation with mesh for the treatment of pelvic organ prolapse-before and after studies. Int J Surg [Internet]. 2018;52(February):40–3. Available from: https://doi.org/10.1016/j.ijsu.2018.02.021.
71. Gutman RE, Nosti PA, Sokol AI, Sokol ER, Peterson JL, Wang H, et al. Three-year outcomes of vaginal mesh for prolapse: a randomized controlled trial. Obstet Gynecol [Internet]. 2013;122(4):770–7. Available from: http://www.ncbi.nlm.nih.gov/pubmed/24084533.
72. Halaska M, Maxova K, Sottner O, Svabik K, Mlcoch M, Kolarik D, et al. A multicenter, randomized, prospective, controlled study comparing sacrospinous fixation and transvaginal mesh in the treatment of posthysterectomy vaginal vault prolapse. Am J Obstet Gynecol [Internet]. 2012;207(4):301.e1–7. Available from: http://www.ncbi.nlm.nih.gov/pubmed/23021692.
73. Svabik K, Martan A, Masata J, El-Haddad R, Hubka P. Comparison of vaginal mesh repair with sacrospinous vaginal colpopexy in the management of vaginal vault prolapse after hysterectomy in patients with levator ani avulsion: a randomized controlled trial. Ultrasound Obstet Gynecol [Internet]. 2014;43(4):365–71. Available from: http://www.ncbi.nlm.nih.gov/pubmed/24615948.
74. Gutman RE, Rardin CR, Sokol ER, Matthews C, Park AJ, Iglesia CB, et al. Vaginal and laparoscopic mesh hysteropexy for uterovaginal prolapse: a parallel cohort study. Am J Obstet Gynecol [Internet]. 2017;216(1):38.e1–38.e11. Available from: http://www.ncbi.nlm.nih.gov/pubmed/27596620.
75. Ginath S, Garely AD, Condrea A, Vardy MD. Mesh erosion following abdominal sacral colpopexy in the absence and presence of the cervical stump. Int Urogynecol J Pelvic Floor Dysfunct. 2013;24(1):113–8.
76. Tan-Kim J, Menefee SA, Luber KM, Nager CW, Lukacz ES. Prevalence and risk factors for mesh erosion after laparoscopic-assisted sacrocolpopexy. Int Urogynecol J [Internet]. 2011 Feb [cited 2019 Apr 3];22(2):205–12. Available from: http://www.ncbi.nlm.nih.gov/pubmed/20842494.
77. Maloney JC, Dunton CJ, Smith K. Repair of vaginal vault prolapse with abdominal sacropexy. J Reprod Med [Internet]. 1990;35(1):6–10. Available from: http://www.ncbi.nlm.nih.gov/pubmed/2405156.
78. Culligan PJ, Blackwell L, Goldsmith LJ, Graham CA, Rogers A, Heit MH. A randomized controlled trial comparing fascia lata and synthetic mesh for sacral colpopexy. Obstet Gynecol [Internet]. 2005;106(1):29–37. Available from: http://www.ncbi.nlm.nih.gov/pubmed/15994614.
79. Nygaard I, Brubaker L, Zyczynski HM, Cundiff G, Richter H, Gantz M, et al. Long-term outcomes

following abdominal sacrocolpopexy for pelvic organ prolapse. JAMA [Internet]. 2013;309(19):2016–24. Available from: http://www.ncbi.nlm.nih.gov/pubmed/23677313.

80. Wu YM, Reid J, Chou Q, MacMillan B, Leong Y, Welk B. Association between method of pelvic organ prolapse repair involving the vaginal apex and reoperation: a population-based, retrospective cohort study. Int Urogynecol J. 2019;30(4):537–44.
81. Linder BJ, Gershman B, Bews KA, Glasgow AE, Occhino JA. A national contemporary analysis of perioperative outcomes for vaginal vault prolapse: minimally invasive sacrocolpopexy versus nonmesh vaginal surgery. Female Pelvic Med Reconstr Surg [Internet]. 2019; Available from: http://www.ncbi.nlm.nih.gov/pubmed/30628947;25:342.
82. Schlunt Eilber K, Rosenblum N, Gore J, Raz S, Rodríguez LV. Perineocele: symptom complex, description of anatomic defect, and surgical technique for repair. Urology. 2006;67(2):265–8.
83. Glavind K, Kempf L. Colpectomy or Le Fort colpocleisis – a good option in selected elderly patients. Int Urogynecol J Pelvic Floor Dysfunct [Internet]. 2005;16(1):48–51; discussion 51. Available from: http://www.ncbi.nlm.nih.gov/pubmed/15322743.
84. Krissi H, Aviram A, Eitan R, From A, Wiznitzer A, Peled Y. Risk factors for recurrence after Le Fort colpocleisis for severe pelvic organ prolapse in elderly women. Int J Surg [Internet]. 2015;20:75–9. Available from: http://www.ncbi.nlm.nih.gov/pubmed/26079498.
85. Toz E, Apaydın N, Uyar İ, Okay G, Kocakaya B, Özcan A. Outcomes of vaginal hysterectomy and constricting colporrhaphy with concurrent levator myorrhaphy and high perineorrhaphy in women older than 75 years of age. Clin Interv Aging. 2015;10:1009.
86. Lavelle ES, Giugale LE, Winger DG, Wang L, Carter-Brooks CM, Shepherd JP. Prolapse recurrence following sacrocolpopexy vs uterosacral ligament suspension: a comparison stratified by pelvic organ prolapse quantification stage. Am J Obstet Gynecol [Internet]. 2018;218(1):116.e1–5. Available from: https://doi.org/10.1016/j.ajog.2017.09.015.
87. Maher CF, Feiner B, DeCuyper EM, Nichlos CJ, Hickey KV, O'Rourke P. Laparoscopic sacral colpopexy versus total vaginal mesh for vaginal vault prolapse: a randomized trial. Am J Obstet Gynecol [Internet]. 2011 Apr 1 [cited 2019 Apr 5];204(4):360.e1–e7. Available from: https://www.sciencedirect.com/science/article/pii/S0002937810022702?via%3Dihub.
88. Maher CF, Qatawneh AM, Dwyer PL, Carey MP, Cornish A, Schluter PJ. Abdominal sacral colpopexy or vaginal sacrospinous colpopexy for vaginal vault prolapse: A prospective randomized study. Am J Obstet Gynecol [Internet]. 2004 Jan 1 [cited 2019 Apr 5];190(1):20–6. Available from: https://www.sciencedirect.com/science/article/pii/S000293780301086X?via%3Dihub.
89. Coolen A-LWM, van Oudheusden AMJ, Mol BWJ, van Eijndhoven HWF, Roovers J-PWR, Bongers MY. Laparoscopic sacrocolpopexy compared with open abdominal sacrocolpopexy for vault prolapse repair: a randomised controlled trial. Int Urogynecol J [Internet]. 2017 Oct 17 [cited 2019 Apr 5];28(10):1469–79. Available from: http://link.springer.com/10.1007/s00192-017-3296-5.
90. Rondini C, Braun H, Alvarez J, Urzúa MJ, Villegas R, Wenzel C, et al. High uterosacral vault suspension vs Sacrocolpopexy for treating apical defects: a randomized controlled trial with twelve months follow-up. Int Urogynecol J [Internet]. 2015 Aug 25 [cited 2019 Apr 5];26(8):1131–8. Available from: http://link.springer.com/10.1007/s00192-015-2666-0.
91. Ow LL, Lim YN, Lee J, Murray C, Thomas E, Leitch A, et al. RCT of vaginal extraperitoneal uterosacral ligament suspension (VEULS) with anterior mesh versus sacrocolpopexy: 4-year outcome. Int Urogynecol [Internet]. 2018 Nov 30 [cited 2019 Apr 5];29(11):1607–14. Available from: http://link.springer.com/10.1007/s00192-018-3687-2.
92. Tate SB, Blackwell L, Lorenz DJ, Steptoe MM, Culligan PJ. Randomized trial of fascia lata and polypropylene mesh for abdominal sacrocolpopexy: 5-year follow-up. Int Urogynecol J [Internet]. 2011 Feb 27 [cited 2019 Apr 5];22(2):137–43. Available from: http://link.springer.com/10.1007/s00192-010-1249-3.
93. Deprest J, Ridder D De, Roovers J-P, Werbrouck E, Coremans G, Claerhout F. Medium term outcome of laparoscopic sacrocolpopexy with xenografts compared to synthetic grafts. J Urol [Internet]. 2009 Nov 1 [cited 2019 Apr 5];182(5):2362–8. Available from: https://www.sciencedirect.com/science/article/pii/S0022534709017728.
94. To V, Hengrasmee P, Lam A, Luscombe G, Lawless A, Lam J. Evidence to justify retention of transvaginal mesh: comparison between laparoscopic sacral colpopexy and transvaginal Elevate™ mesh. Int Urogynecol J. 2017;28(12):1825–32.
95. Dietz V, van der Vaart CH, van der Graaf Y, Heintz P, Schraffordt Koops SE. One-year follow-up after sacrospinous hysteropexy and vaginal hysterectomy for uterine descent: a randomized study. Int Urogynecol J [Internet]. 2010 Feb 16 [cited 2019 Apr 5];21(2):209–16. Available from: http://link.springer.com/10.1007/s00192-009-1014-7.
96. Persu C, Chapple CR, Cauni V, Gutue S, Geavlete P. Pelvic Organ Prolapse Quantification System (POP-Q) - a new era in pelvic prolapse staging. J Med Life [Internet]. 2011[cited 2019 May 26];4(1):75–81. Available from: http://www.ncbi.nlm.nih.gov/pubmed/21505577.
97. Cvach K, Dwyer P. Surgical management of pelvic organ prolapse: abdominal and vaginal approaches. World J Urol. 2012;30(4):471–7.
98. Jones HW, Rock JA, editors. Te Linde's operative gynecology. 8th ed: Wolters Kluwer Health; PA, Philadelphia, 2015.
99. Nygaard I, Bradley C, Brandt D; Women's Health Initiative. Pelvic organ prolapse in older women:

prevalence and risk factors. Obstet Gynecol. 2004;104(3):489–97.
100. Chow D, Rodríguez LV. Epidemiology and prevalence of pelvic organ prolapse. Curr Opin Urol. 2013;23(4):293–8.
101. Slade, E, Daly, C, Mavranezouli, I, Dias, S, Kearney, R, Hasler, E, Carter, P, Mahoney, C, Macbeth, F, Delgado Nunes, V. Primary surgical management of anterior pelvic organ prolapse: a systematic review, network meta-analysis and cost-effectiveness analysis. BJOG. 2020;127:18–26.
102. Slopnick EA, Petrikovets A, Sheyn D, et al. Surgical trends and patient factors associated with the treatment of apical pelvic organ prolapse from a national sample. Int Urogynecol J. 2019;30:603–9. https://doi.org/10.1007/s00192-018-3769-1.
103. Meriwether KV, Balk EM, Antosh DD, Olivera CK, Kim-Fine S, Murphy M, Grimes CL, Sleemi A, Singh R, Dieter AA, Crisp CC, Rahn DD. Uterine-preserving surgeries for the repair of pelvic organ prolapse: a systematic review with meta-analysis and clinical practice guidelines. Int Urogynecol J. 2019;30(4):505–22.
104. Milani R, Manodoro S, Cola A, Bellante N, Palmieri S, Frigerio M. Transvaginal uterosacral ligament hysteropexy versus hysterectomy plus uterosacral ligament suspension: a matched cohort study. Int Urogynecol J. 2019 Dec 17.
105. Transvaginal uterosacral hysteropexy resulted in similar objective and subjective cure rates, and patient satisfaction, without differences in complication rates, compared with vaginal hysterectomy. However, postoperative cervical elongation may lead to higher central recurrence rates and need for reoperation.
106. Sussman RD, Peyronnet B, Brucker BM. The current state and the future of robotic surgery in female pelvic medicine and reconstructive surgery. Turk J Urol. 2019;45(5):331–9.

Addressing Recurrent Pelvic Organ Prolapse: Unique Challenges of Recurrent Prolapse

16

Payton Schmidt and Dee E. Fenner

Case Scenario

An 82-year-old female with history significant for mild cognitive impairment, hypothyroidism, polymyalgia rheumatica, and prolapse status post a total vaginal hysterectomy 20 years prior presented with 7 years of recurrent prolapse symptoms. On examination, her POP-Q was significant for Aa-1, Ba-1, C-7, D X, Bp +4, Ap +3, GH 2.5/4, PB 3.5, TVL 9. She was initially managed with a Gellhorn pessary, but due to discomfort, she elected to proceed with surgical management. She desired the ability to have intercourse in the future. She underwent an uncomplicated sacrospinous ligament suspension, anterior and posterior colporrhaphy, and cystoscopy. She was very satisfied with the results of her surgery and had excellent pelvic support at her 6-week postoperative check.

Treatment of recurrent pelvic organ prolapse (POP) can often be challenging. Approximately 30% of women will undergo reoperation for recurrent prolapse [1, 2], costing approximately $295.5 million and $450.6 million in Medicare and non-Medicare reimbursement rates, respectively [1]. Recurrent POP, as defined by the International Urogynecologic Association (IUGA) Research and Development Committee Opinion, is "recurrent, direct or indirect POP reaching or going below the level of the hymen (POP-Q≥stage 2b) for objective recurrence and having symptoms attributed to recurrent POP for subjective recurrence" [1]. Indirect POP refers to an uncorrected or new defect, while direct refers to the repaired compartment. The incidence of recurrent POP varies, as it is dependent on how it is defined (anatomical based on vaginal examination, symptoms, or reoperation rate), and the true incidence is likely to remain unclear due to many women not seeking further treatment. Given that women with recurrent prolapse are at higher risk for recurrence after subsequent surgeries, treatment needs to be tailored to each individual patient based on careful assessment of the risks and benefits of all options. In this chapter, we will review the diagnosis and management strategies for addressing recurrent pelvic organ prolapse.

Electronic Supplementary Material The online version of this chapter (https://doi.org/10.1007/978-3-030-54839-1_16) contains supplementary material, which is available to authorized users.

Commentary by Howard B. Goldman, Cleveland Clinic, Glickman Urologic and Kidney Institute, Cleveland, OH, USA

P. Schmidt (✉) · D. E. Fenner
University of Michigan, Department of Obstetrics and Gynecology, Ann Arbor, MI, USA
e-mail: payton@med.umich.edu

K. C. Kobashi, S. D. Wexner (eds.), *Female Pelvic Medicine*,
https://doi.org/10.1007/978-3-030-54839-1_16

Why Does Recurrent Pelvic Organ Prolapse Occur?

Understanding pelvic organ prolapse first requires one to understand the principles of normal pelvic support. Normal pelvic organ support is provided by the interaction between the levator ani muscles and pelvic connective tissues. DeLancey described three levels of support (Fig. 16.1): Level 1 – the upper third of the vagina and cervix are supported by the cardinal and uterosacral ligaments; Level 2 – the middle third of the vagina is supported by the arcus tendineous fascia pelvis and fascia of the levator ani; and Level 3 – the lower third fuses with the perineal membrane, the perineal body, and the levator ani muscles [3]. Prolapse is due to failure of this intricate system that connects the muscles, ligaments, and organs with the bony attachments to the pelvis.

The levator ani muscles and pelvic connective tissue are two complementary mechanisms critical for pelvic organ support [4, 5]. Muscle or connective tissue failure are strongly correlated with pelvic organ prolapse [5]. Levator ani muscle injury is associated with higher rates of primary [5] and recurrent prolapse [6]. Women with longer cardinal ligaments are at higher risk of prolapse [5]. Clinical and biomechanical finite element analysis studies have shown that muscle and connective tissue failures (levator and apical ligament impairments) can result in anterior and/or posterior compartment failure [4, 7]. Furthermore, transperineal ultrasound shows that descent of cystoceles and rectoceles primarily reflect failed apical support [4, 7] – highlighting the importance of Level 1 apical support at the time of prolapse repair.

Prolapse in the anterior, posterior, or apical compartment depends on the presence of anterior, posterior, levator, and/or apical support impairments. Additionally, it has been shown that the interaction of prolapse with opposing compartments affects the development of rectoceles

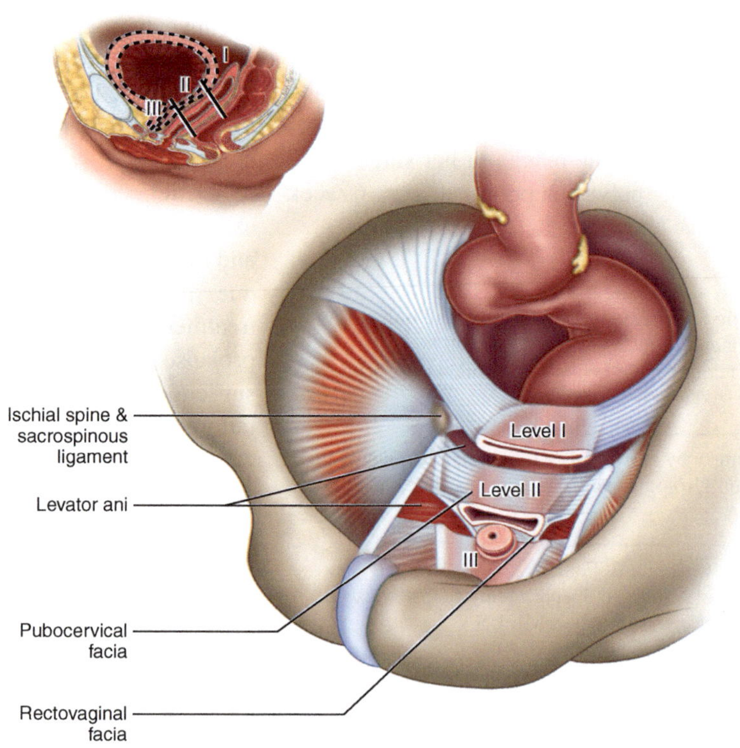

Fig. 16.1 Level of pelvic support [3]. (Courtesy of John O. L. DeLancey, MD)

or cystoceles [7]. This is highlighted by the "organ competition theory," whereby two vaginal walls compete for the limited opening (genital hiatus) [7]. This is seen clinically when a woman undergoes repair for cystocele and has a recurrence in the posterior compartment. It is therefore important to consider all the components of pelvic support when addressing recurrent pelvic organ prolapse – both for surgical planning and patient counseling. If proceeding with surgical treatment, the goal of surgical management of prolapse should be to perform all indicated surgical repairs necessary to restore normal pelvic organ support between the muscles and connective tissues.

Table 16.1 Risk factors for pelvic organ prolapse

Risk factors for recurrent pelvic organ prolapse
Greater age
Levator avulsion injury
Greater POP-Q Ba score
Enlarged genital hiatus
Family history of pelvic organ prolapse
Personal history of pelvic organ prolapse
Failure to correct all compartments at the time of previous surgery
Multiple previous surgeries for pelvic organ prolapse
BMI ≥ 30
Chronic obstructive pulmonary disease
Chronic constipation
Chronic heavy lifting
Connective tissue disorder (Ehlers-Danlos syndromes)

What Are Risk Factors Associated with Recurrent Pelvic Organ Prolapse?

Assessment of risk factors for recurrence helps identify possible causes of the recurrence, weigh risks and benefits of treatment options, and counsel patients on expected outcomes. Preoperative risk factors for recurrent prolapse include greater age, presence of levator avulsion injury, greater POP-Q Ba, enlarged genital hiatus, family history of pelvic organ prolapse, personal history of pelvic organ prolapse, and failure to correct all compartments at the time of previous surger(ies) [1, 8]. The more often a patient has undergone previous pelvic floor reconstructive surgery, the greater is her risk for recurrent prolapse and need for repeat surgery to treat it [9]. Failure to correct all compartments at the time of surgery, including undetected opposing compartment defects due to "organ competition," is also associated with surgical failure [1, 7]. Table 16.1 shows a summary of risk factors for recurrent pelvic organ prolapse.

Various reconstructive surgeries have differing reported rates of prolapse recurrence. Abdominal sacrocolpopexy is considered to have lower risk for recurrence, with rates of approximately 34% 7 years after surgery [10]. A longitudinal cohort study by Jelovsek et al. found that, in comparison to abdominal sacrocolpopexy, patients were at higher risk of recurrence if they underwent native tissue repair with uterosacral ligament or sacrospinous ligament suspension, but experienced unchanged outcomes if they underwent colpocleisis [8].

How Do You Diagnose Recurrent Pelvic Organ Prolapse?

When a patient presents with recurrent pelvic organ prolapse, it is important to do a comprehensive history and physical examination to identify any risk factors for recurrence. Symptoms and level of bother should be assessed to help guide treatment options. Assessing the patient's medical comorbidities can help counsel on expectations based on risk of recurrence, as well as guide discussions regarding treatment options by weighing risks and benefits. Review of surgical history can identify risks for recurrence, as well as guide future surgical treatment options. Operative reports, when available, should be reviewed. Examination will help determine if there was a direct or indirect recurrence, which can help establish if it was a failure of the surgery or a new prolapse occurrence. Imaging studies are often not necessary; however, ultrasound can identify hiatal ballooning and levator avulsion injury. MRI, especially dynamic MRI, can assess for levator injury and extent of pelvic organ prolapse. MRI can also identify if there was a

Table 16.2 Suggested imaging for workup of recurrent pelvic organ prolapse

Imaging	Indication
Cystoscopy	Concern for mesh erosion
Endoscopy	Concern for fistula
Ultrasound, transperineal	Hiatal ballooning, levator avulsion injury
MRI, dynamic	Levator injury, extent of pelvic organ prolapse, evaluate for mesh approximation

surgical failure, such as seeing if a mesh is still approximated to the sacrum after a sacrocolpopexy. Other imaging procedures can be performed to rule out other complications of prolapse surgery. Table 16.2 shows suggested imaging and relevant indications for the workup of recurrent pelvic organ prolapse.

What Are Treatment Options for Pelvic Organ Prolapse?

Treatment options should be discussed with patients and be in line with their expectations and goals for care. Options include expectant management, pessary use, pelvic floor physical therapy (PFPT), behavioral modifications, and surgical management. At this time, conservative options such as pessary, PFPT, and behavioral modifications have not been shown to be particularly effective for recurrent prolapse. While there is no evidence for vaginal pessaries, PFPT, smoking cessation, avoidance of heavy lifting, or weight loss in the treatment of recurrent POP [1, 2], one might consider conservative therapy for a mild degree of prolapse – where presumably, the risk outweighs the benefit – if the patient is a poor surgical candidate or elects not to proceed with repeat surgery. Surgical options should be chosen based on the expected durability, recovery time, risk of immediate and delayed postoperative complications, and desire for future vaginal intercourse.

When proceeding with surgical management, the surgeon should consider where there are anatomic defects. Surgical treatments are categorized by either reconstructive or obliterative approaches. To date, there are few randomized controlled trials evaluating different surgical approaches for correction of recurrent POP. Recurrence is often cited as a reason to use mesh (either vaginally or abdominally) due to lower risk of recurrence reported in the primary prolapse literature. However, this does not take into account the higher risk of both perioperative complications (bleeding, surgical site infections) [11] and long-term postoperative complications (mesh erosions and pain) [12]. Decision regarding route and type of surgery must be dependent on patient preference, the surgeon's clinical judgement, a balance of risks and benefits, and any available evidence regarding different proposed approaches.

Treatment of Recurrent Apical Prolapse

For apical prolapse, Level 1 support needs to be re-established. Surgical approaches to re-establish support at the level of the cardinal and uterosacral ligaments include uterosacral ligament suspension, McCall's culdoplasty, sacrospinous ligament suspension, ileococcygeus fixation, sacrocolpopexy, or the use of vaginal mesh kits. An obliterative approach includes colpocleisis (total for posthysterectomy patients and LeFort colpocleisis for those with uterus in situ).

Treatment of Recurrent Apical Prolapse: Vaginal Approach – Native Tissue

Native tissue vaginal surgical approaches include uterosacral ligament suspension (USLS), sacrospinous ligament suspension (SSLS), McCall's culdoplasty, or ileococcygeus fixation. There is no available data looking at the impact of these approaches on outcomes for surgery performed for recurrent pelvic organ prolapse alone. Morgan et al. evaluated USLS in a meta-analysis, and showed that anatomic success rates for this procedure were 81.2%, 98.3%, and 87.4% for anterior, apical, and posterior compartments, respectively [13]. Failure rates (i.e., recurrence) by compartment for SSLS are reported to be 6.9–27.5%, 1.5–5.7%, and 0–3.9% for anterior, apical, and posterior prolapse, respectively [14]. McCall's culdoplasty used in 19 women with vault prolapse resulted in no recurrences [2]. Ileococcygeus fixation was reported to have a 91% success rate in 50 patients after mean follow-up of 21 months [15]. Based on available data, uterosacral and sacrospinous ligament suspensions are effective native-tissue options. We recommend the SSLS be performed using the Michigan Four-Wall technique (see Video 16.1).

Treatment of Recurrent Apical Prolapse: Vaginal Mesh

Considerable attention has been paid to the use of vaginal mesh for prolapse surgery. One study investigating unilateral SSLS with mesh interposition and extension into the anterior and posterior wall, as indicated based on the presence of anterior or posterior prolapse, for recurrent prolapse showed no recurrence of apical prolapse, with a mean follow-up of 2.9 years [16]. However, over the last 15 years of investigation into transvaginal mesh, it is unclear if the risks outweigh the benefit of lower recurrence. In a 5-year follow-up study investigating the use of transvaginal mesh, mesh erosions occurred in 16.6% of cases, caused dyspareunia in 13.3% of cases, and resulted in reoperation in 5.5% of cases [12]. As a result, the Society of Gynecologic Surgeons released a clinical practice guideline that recommends against the use of transvaginal mesh [17].

Treatment of Recurrent Apical Prolapse: Abdominal Approach

Sacrocolpopexy, via either open abdominal or laparoscopic (with or without robotic assistance) approaches, is a durable surgical treatment option for prolapse. Abdominal sacrocolpopexy (ASC) resulted in no recurrence of prolapse in women with triple compartment pelvic organ prolapse [18]. Minimally invasive techniques – via laparoscopy, with or without robotic assistance – to perform sacrocolpopexy have also shown good outcomes for recurrent prolapse. There were no additional recurrences after 16 women with recurrence after transvaginal mesh underwent laparoscopic sacrocolpopexy (LSC) [19]. Additionally, repeat LSC appears to be a reasonable option, as shown in the study by Mearini et al., that found no recurrences with a mean follow-up of 41 months in women who had had a recurrence after LSC who underwent repeat LSC [20]. Overall, objective success rates reported for sacrocolpopexy used in recurrent prolapse cases range from 84% to 100% [1].

Treatment of Recurrent Apical Prolapse: Summary

In a large cohort study of women with either primary or recurrent prolapse, Jelovsek et al. reported odds ratios for prolapse recurrence after various procedures [8]. In comparison to abdominal sacrocolpopexy, which was considered the referent in this study, the odds ratios (confidence interval) for recurrence of prolapse after USLS, SSLS, and colpocleisis were 9.4 (5.3–16.9), 9.4 (5.3–16.9), and 1.13 (0.51–2.53), respectively. However, the odds of one or more serious adverse events were 0.43 (0.29–0.62), 0.47 (0.30–0.74), and 0.33 (0.18–0.59), respectively. In addition, overall health status improvement favored USLS and SSLS (1.684 (1.07–2.65) and 1.805 (1.06–3.09), respectively). Colpocleisis was not statically different with regard to overall health improvement status [8]. This study did not differentiate abdominal and laparoscopic technique for sacrocolpopexy; therefore, these calculations should be interpreted with these limitations in mind. Given the above findings, native tissue vaginal repairs – either reconstructive or obliterative – should be considered, given reasonable outcomes when weighing the risk of recurrence and the benefits of overall health improvement and lower complication rates.

Treatment of Anterior Prolapse

History of anterior prolapse is a risk factor for recurrent POP; therefore, anterior prolapse is a distinct problem to manage. Many studies have investigated different procedures to repair recurrent anterior wall prolapse, including native-tissue anterior colporrhaphy, anterior colporrhaphy with porcine or polypropyelene mesh, and anterior colporrhaphy with paravaginal repair. In a study by Dahlgren et al., recurrence rates were the same when using porcine skin graft with anterior colporrhaphy versus native tissue anterior colporrhaphy [57% vs. 62%, OR (95% CI) 1.24 (0.52–2.91)] [21]. Recurrence rates were higher in women who underwent a native tissue anterior colporrhaphy than those who underwent transvaginal mesh (TVM), with recurrence rates at 12 months reported as 55.1% versus 7.8%, $p < 0.001$, respectively. However, there was an 8% mesh erosion rate in the TVM group [22]. When comparing permanent, polypropylene mesh versus porcine mesh, there was no significant difference in anterior wall recurrence (28.1% vs. 43.6%, $p = 0.06$, respectively); however, mesh erosions were more common with permanent TVM (6.3% vs. 0%, $p = 0.02$). In comparing the effectiveness of anterior colporrhaphy – alone or in combination with paravaginal repairs – in women with recurrent prolapse, those in the anterior colporrhaphy group had a longer time to anatomic recurrence (median 41 vs. 12 months, $p = 0.022$) [23]. Based on this information, native tissue repair with anterior repair is a reasonable, safe option. If there is concomitant prolapse in other compartments, however, an anterior colporrhaphy should be paired with other indicated procedures. Mesh can be considered for recurrent prolapse of the anterior compartment after discussion of its risks and benefits with the patient.

Treatment of Posterior Prolapse

Treatment of posterior prolapse includes posterior colporrhaphy, with or without permanent or biologic graft materials. In comparing posterior colporrhaphy with and without porcine graft use, recurrent prolapse 3 years after surgery was more common in the native tissue repair group (17% vs. 40%), OR 0.3 (CI 0.09–0.97). Women who had a repair using porcine graft had a 4.4% minor mesh erosion rate and three developed vaginal stenosis, with one requiring reoperation. The authors concluded that use of porcine graft did not provide advantages over native tissue repair [21]. Transvaginal mesh with polypropylene mesh has also been investigated. Withagen et al. showed that there were lower failure rates in women who had repairs using TVM than in those who underwent native tissue repair for posterior compartment prolapse (7.7% vs. 24.5%, $p = 0.003$, respectively). However, there were no differences in symptom decrease or improvement in quality of life [22]. Based on these studies, recurrence rates could be decreased with the use of mesh, but the small improvements likely do not outweigh the risks. We therefore recommend native tissue posterior colporrhaphy, with any additional indicated procedures based on other compartment failures. Mesh studies do not support the use of mesh for treatment of posterior compartment prolapse.

Summary

Recurrent pelvic organ prolapse is a unique and challenging clinical scenario for the urogynecologist. While the use of transvaginal mesh may decrease recurrence rates, the high complication rates that occur in the years following surgery may not be worth the small benefits in anatomic outcomes. If transvaginal mesh is being considered, its use in repairs for anterior compartment prolapse has the most robust evidence for lower recurrence rates. Native tissue repairs with anterior and/or posterior repairs have higher recurrence rates, but low complication rates and good outcomes in quality-of-life and symptom improvement. The need for apical suspension should always be evaluated and addressed as indicated. Sacrocolpopexy is a durable surgical option that has much fewer complications related to mesh erosions than those seen with transvaginal mesh. In a patient who is young, relatively healthy, and an optimal surgical candidate, sacrocolpopexy is a good option. Vaginal repairs with uterosacral ligament and sacrospinous ligament suspensions are safe and reasonable options for correction of recurrent prolapse, with lower impact on morbidity than abdominal procedures. Ultimately, when addressing recurrent pelvic organ prolapse, the surgeon should always weigh the risks and benefits of all proposed interventions and ensure that treatment options are in line with patient expectations.

Commentary

Howard B. Goldman

Recurrence after pelvic organ prolapse repair is not an uncommon occurrence. Drs. Schmidt and Fenner do an excellent job reviewing risk factors, evaluation, and management options of such recurrences. A few important points they noted to prevent recurrence are highlighted.

It is unusual to have significant prolapse, particularly involving the anterior compartment, without associated apical prolapse. Accordingly, it is critical that apical prolapse be identified and addressed, as failure to do so almost certainly dooms the isolated anterior repair to failure. This points to the challenge of an effective anterior compartment repair. This compartment appears to be the most likely to recur, particularly when stage 3 or greater.

Opposing compartment defects should also be identified. As the authors note, mild prolapse in one compartment may enlarge to fill the space occupied by an opposing larger prolapse after the larger one is repaired. Thus, prolapse of any significance should be repaired if one is embarking on the repair of any symptomatic prolapse.

The importance of a colpocleisis or some other obliterative procedure – perhaps a levator myorrhaphy in those without any significant posterior prolapse – in the woman who has no plans for future sexual activity should not be understated. These procedures have high success rates, low complication rates, and are not difficult to perform. For the appropriate patient, an obliterative procedure is ideal as either the primary or secondary operation.

There is an inherent recurrence rate after prolapse repair. Future advances in regenerative medicine may hold the promise of reducing or preventing prolapse and its recurrence. Only time will tell.

References

1. Ismail S, Duckett J, Rizk D, Sorinola O, Kammerer-Doak D, Contreras-Ortiz O, et al. Recurrent pelvic organ prolapse: International Urogynecological Association Research and Development Committee opinion. Int Urogynecol J. 2016;27(11):1619–32.
2. Toh VV, Bogne V, Bako A. Management of recurrent vault prolapse. Int Urogynecol J. 2012;23(1):29–34.
3. DeLancey JO. Anatomic aspects of vaginal eversion after hysterectomy. Am J Obstet Gynecol. 1992;166(6 Pt 1):1717–24; discussion 24-8.
4. Reid RI. Repair of recurrent prolapse. Best Pract Res Clin Obstet Gynaecol. 2011;25(2):175–96.
5. DeLancey JO. What's new in the functional anatomy of pelvic organ prolapse? Curr Opin Obstet Gynecol. 2016;28(5):420–9.
6. Model AN, Shek KL, Dietz HP. Levator defects are associated with prolapse after pelvic floor surgery. Eur J Obstet Gynecol Reprod Biol. 2010;153(2):220–3.
7. Luo J, Chen L, Fenner DE, Ashton-Miller JA, DeLancey JO. A multi-compartment 3-D finite element model of rectocele and its interaction with cystocele. J Biomech. 2015;48(9):1580–6.
8. Jelovsek JE, Chagin K, Lukacz ES, Nolen TL, Shepherd JP, Barber MD, et al. Models for predicting recurrence, complications, and health status in women after pelvic organ prolapse surgery. Obstet Gynecol. 2018;132(2):298–309.
9. Denman MA, Gregory WT, Boyles SH, Smith V, Edwards SR, Clark AL. Reoperation 10 years after surgically managed pelvic organ prolapse and urinary incontinence. Am J Obstet Gynecol. 2008;198(5):555.e1–5.
10. Nygaard I, Brubaker L, Zyczynski HM, Cundiff G, Richter H, Gantz M, et al. Long-term outcomes following abdominal sacrocolpopexy for pelvic organ prolapse. JAMA. 2013;309(19):2016–24.
11. Caveney M, Haddad D, Matthews C, Badlani G, Mirzazadeh M. Short-term complications associated with the use of transvaginal mesh in pelvic floor reconstructive surgery: results from a multi-institutional prospectively maintained dataset. Neurourol Urodyn. 2017;36(8):2044–8.
12. Ubertazzi EP, Soderini HFE, Saavedra Sanchez AJM, Fonseca Guzman C, Pavan LI. Long-term outcomes of transvaginal mesh (TVM) in patients with pelvic

organ prolapse: a 5-year follow-up. Eur J Obstet Gynecol Reprod Biol. 2018;225:90–4.
13. Margulies RU, Rogers MA, Morgan DM. Outcomes of transvaginal uterosacral ligament suspension: systematic review and metaanalysis. Am J Obstet Gynecol. 2010;202(2):124–34.
14. Morgan DM, Larson K. Uterosacral and sacrospinous ligament suspension for restoration of apical vaginal support. Clin Obstet Gynecol. 2010;53(1):72–85.
15. Maher CF, Murray CJ, Carey MP, Dwyer PL, Ugoni AM. Iliococcygeus or sacrospinous fixation for vaginal vault prolapse. Obstet Gynecol. 2001;98(1):40–4.
16. Lo TS, Horng SG, Huang HJ, Lee SJ, Liang CC. Repair of recurrent vaginal vault prolapse using sacrospinous ligament fixation with mesh interposition and reinforcement. Acta Obstet Gynecol Scand. 2005;84(10):992–5.
17. Murphy M, Society of Gynecologic Surgeons Systematic Review G. Clinical practice guidelines on vaginal graft use from the society of gynecologic surgeons. Obstet Gynecol. 2008;112(5):1123–30.
18. Gilleran JP, Zimmern P. Abdominal mesh sacrocolpopexy for recurrent triple-compartment pelvic organ prolapse. BJU Int. 2009;103(8):1090–4.
19. Iglesia CB, Hale DS, Lucente VR. Laparoscopic sacrocolpopexy versus transvaginal mesh for recurrent pelvic organ prolapse. Int Urogynecol J. 2013;24(3):363–70.
20. Mearini L, Nunzi E, Di Biase M, Costantini E. Laparoscopic management of vaginal vault prolapse recurring after pelvic organ prolapse surgery. Urol Int. 2016;97(2):158–64.
21. Dahlgren E, Kjolhede P. Long-term outcome of porcine skin graft in surgical treatment of recurrent pelvic organ prolapse. An open randomized controlled multicenter study. Acta Obstet Gynecol Scand. 2011;90(12):1393–401.
22. Withagen MI, Milani AL, de Leeuw JW, Vierhout ME. Development of de novo prolapse in untreated vaginal compartments after prolapse repair with and without mesh: a secondary analysis of a randomised controlled trial. BJOG. 2012;119(3):354–60.
23. Morse AN, O'Dell KK, Howard AE, Baker SP, Aronson MP, Young SB. Midline anterior repair alone vs anterior repair plus vaginal paravaginal repair: a comparison of anatomic and quality of life outcomes. Int Urogynecol J Pelvic Floor Dysfunct. 2007;18(3):245–9.

17 High-Grade Prolapse

Philip Toozs-Hobson and Amallia Brair

Case Scenario

A 67-year-old diabetic woman, who has had 3 children by normal vagina birth, presents with feeling a bulge coming down in her vagina. She also complained of evacuatory difficulties with her bowels but no urinary symptoms. In the past, she has had a total abdominal hysterectomy at the age of 40 due to fibroids and a posterior vaginal repair at the age of 50. She is sexually active and would prefer surgery as conservative measures have failed.

On Examination

Her pelvic organ prolapse quantification (POPQ) was as follows:

−2	−2	+2
4	3	8 cm
0	+1	–

Commentary by Una Lee, Virginia Mason Medical Center, Department of Urology, Seattle, WA, USA

P. Toozs-Hobson (✉)
Birmingham Women's and Children's NHS Foundation Trust, Department of Urogynecology, Birmingham, UK
e-mail: p.toozs-hobson@nhs.net

A. Brair
Birmingham Women's and Children's NHS Foundation Trust, Department of Pelvic Floor Medicine, Birmingham, UK

There is stage 3 vault prolapse and stage 2 posterior vaginal wall prolapse.

Bimanual vaginal examination revealed no masses.

Prevalence

The exact prevalence of pelvic organ prolapse is hard to conclude, since many women do not seek medical advice; however, it has been predicted that about half of parous women have some degree of prolapse and approximately 10–20% of these go on to seek medical advice [1].

Clinical Assessment

In this woman, the risk factors accounting for her prolapse are as follows:

1. Post-menopausal status: The lack of oestrogen may affect the connective tissues, making them weaker and thus attributing to her prolapse.
2. Parity: Having had three pregnancies puts strain on the pelvic floor muscles, hence weakening them. Additionally, the mode of delivery, with the first vaginal delivery being the most significant, plays an essential role in causing prolapse.
3. Previous Surgery Hysterectomy: A total hysterectomy involves division of the supporting

K. C. Kobashi, S. D. Wexner (eds.), *Female Pelvic Medicine*,
https://doi.org/10.1007/978-3-030-54839-1_17

ligaments, including the uterosacral and cardinal ligaments, thereby compromising the main support, which may in turn contribute to the development of her vault prolapse. Previous posterior repair recurrent prolapse after previous repair is a risk factor for further prolapse.
4. Underlying collagen type.
5. Obesity: Increased pressure in the abdomen can increase the risk of prolapse.
6. Lifestyle:
   (a) *Smoking* can lead to chronic cough, which increases the pressure in the abdomen and pelvis.
   (b) *Constipation* can result in straining, which increases pressure on the pelvic floor muscles.
   (c) *Occupation.* Certain jobs, particularly those requiring heavy lifting, can be very detrimental to the pelvic floor.
   (d) *Diet.* An unhealthy diet can lead to obesity and constipation, which, as described above, may in turn result in an extra load on the pelvic floor muscles.
7. Co-morbidities: In the long term, diabetes may lead to neuropathy. When it affects nerves that control involuntary functions of the body, it is known as autonomic neuropathy. Autonomic neuropathy affecting the bowel may cause constipation or diarrhoea, both of which may lead to straining that can cause evacuatory difficulties and strain on the pelvic floor support.

Management

Prolapse is usually accompanied by other symptoms such as urinary, bowel or sexual problems. Here, no urinary symptoms of concern have been revealed. There are two schools of thought. Some clinicians would advocate for doing urodynamics before prolapse surgery, mainly for the purpose of counselling patients; however, urodynamics is not in itself predictive of the outcome of the prolapse surgery.

Conservative measures include doing nothing, pelvic floor exercises, or a pessary. In this case, ring pessaries would be best, since she is sexually active. However, there are many types of pessaries, and increasingly, patients are self-managing their pessaries, thereby widening their choices and giving them the ability to remove their pessary prior to intercourse if this is an issue. Advice about bowel emptying and using appliances includign foot stool to change anorectal angle. We have not outlined the role of quality of life assessment as this is outside the remit of this chapter but should be considered in all patients.

Surgery Since both central and posterior compartment prolapses are present, there are different techniques that can be used to address her pelvic floor anatomy. Not uncommonly, one procedure may be adequate to fix the problem. In this case colpocliesis is not considered as the patient wishes to remain sexually active.

Surgical Options for Fixing the Vault of the Vagina

There are several surgical options, two of which involve using mesh. As a general rule, mesh should be avoided in patients with pre-existing chronic pelvic or vaginal pain, history of allergy, diabetes or immunosuppression.

Infracoccygeal Vaginal Vault Mesh Suspension

The infracoccygeal vault suspension with mesh involves using a thin band of mesh inserted through the ischiorectal fossa via an incision in each buttock. This mesh strip is then stitched to the vault of the vagina to support the apex. The procedure can be performed via either a posterior or an anterior approach to access the sacrospinous ligament. In the above patient, a posterior approach would be preferable, since she also has posterior compartment prolapse, and often the posterior vaginal wall prolapse would correct itself after fixing the vault. Accordingly, a formal posterior repair is frequently not necessary following support of the apex. The vaginal procedure typically results in a shorter hospital stay and is associated with fewer complications than the abdominal techniques. The use of a thin band of mesh provides extra support with exposure of mesh into the vagina occurring very rarely. Additionally, the location of the necessary incision allows the mesh to be attached to the vagina without the incision overlying the mesh. This is important in minimizing the risk of mesh extrusion given that a common cause of mesh extrusion is failure of the incision to heal over the mesh.

The National Institute for Health and Care Excellence (NICE), which is a body of the Department of Health in the United Kingdom that publishes guidelines, states that there is currently insufficient evidence regarding the effectiveness of this procedure and that more research is needed [2]. Practitioners using this technique are advised to perform a continuous audit to review their results.

Our unit contributed to the NICE evaluation over a 4-year period to evaluate the outcome of the infracoccygeal vault suspension, and the early results were promising. Eighty-seven percent of patients reported a successful outcome at 3-month follow-up; however, long-term follow-up is mandatory for proper assessment of the procedure.

Sacrocolpopexy (SCP)

Sacrocolpopexy (SCP) is a second operation that uses mesh that is placed via an abdominal approach that can be performed either laparoscopically or through an open abdominal incision. The SCP involves suspension of the vault of the vagina to the sacral promontory using a bridge of mesh. This technique attempts to restore the vagina to its original axis and position by reproducing the support of the uterosacral and cardinal ligaments. This technique does require a level of expertise, and much depends on the training, preference and experience of the surgeon.

This technique can also be offered as an alternative to hysterectomy in women when uterine preservation is requested and is called a sacrohysteropexy. The uterus is suspended to the sacrum by stitching one end of the mesh onto the cervix and the other end of the mesh onto the sacrum.

NICE has recognized the efficacy of this procedure and has thus approved its use under special criteria [3].

Sacrospinous Ligament Fixation (SSLF)

Sacrospinous ligament fixation (SSLF) involves suspension of the vaginal vault to stitches placed into the sacrospinous ligament to provide level one support. One major advantage of this procedure is that it is performed vaginally, so in theory, it affords a lower risk of complications and potentially a quicker recovery. A further advantage of the vaginal approach is that it can be done under spinal/regional anaesthesia. Sacrospinous fixation can also be used in the presence of the uterus for treatment of uterocervical prolapse or procidentia. In such a case, the stitches are placed into the cervix rather than through the vaginal wall. Despite all of the advantages of an SSLF, this procedure cannot be performed in a short vagina (less than approximately 6 cm), since the ischial spine cannot be reached and palpated to guide placement of the stitches into the sacrospinous ligament. In such cases, the infracoccygeal vaginal vault mesh suspension described above can be used.

A specific drawback of the SSLF is the potential for postoperative buttock pain which occurs in 10–15% of patients and typically resolves by 6 weeks post-operatively, the incidence and severity of this may be reduced if a Capio device is used which limits the depth of the bite of tissue incorporated in the stitch. Pain relief, anti-inflammatory agents, and reassurance are usually all that is needed [4]. Another potential complication is post-operative gluteal pain which can radiate down the posterior surface of the leg due to a pudendal nerve injury. In such a case, re-operation with removal of the offending sutures should be performed. If placement of new stitches is considered, they should be placed more medially or on the contralateral side [4]. One of the potential downsides of a sacrospinous ligament fixation compared to the other two surgical procedures discussed above is the post-operative development of a cystocoele over the long term.

Surgical Options for Repairing the Posterior Wall of the Vagina

In many cases, posterior vaginal wall prolapse may correct itself with vault fixation though a re-do posterior repair can be done concomitant with an infracoccygeal vaginal vault mesh suspension. The role of vaginally placed mesh in pelvic surgery remains controversial, and the role in the posterior compartment has been questioned. Careful and critical evaluation of the pros and cons of its use posteriorly should be discussed and documented, particularly in light of the PROSPECT data [5]. If an enterocoele is present, it can be repaired using Moscowitz technique.

One point of note to discuss when counselling the patient is the difference between anatomy and physiology; as such, correcting a defect may not correct function, so any evacuatory bowel problem may not improve if there is an associated physiological problem such as a neuropathy due to diabetes mellitus. In such cases a proctogram or dynamic MRI of the plevis may be required to assess function along with anorectal manometry.

Surgical Complications

The current standard of consent in the UK is to discuss risks, benefits and alternatives. The process should be clearly documented and should include a discussion supplemented by appropriate written information (generic and specific in the form of a letter) and signing of a consent. Consent should be re-confirmed on the day of surgery. In an ideal situation, the surgeon should be able to discuss his/her own data (or that of their unit); as such, the use of a formal database to record experience can be helpful. General risks include those which may occur due to any surgery: bleeding, infection, increased risk of developing a blood clot, (DVT/PE) injury to adjacent structures (visceral injury), pain (generalized and dyspareunia), failure to achieve satisfactory result and the need for further surgery or immediate conversion to laparotomy. More specific complications depend on the type of surgery being performed, although there are a few drawbacks to any prolapse surgery such as developing de novo urinary symptoms or worsening of existing ones, vaginal scarring or shortening, dyspareunia, failure to achieve the desired result or even recurrence of the prolapse with the attendant risk of revision surgery to remove mesh. Patients shoud be aware mesh implants are designed as permenant and may not be able to be removed in their entirety. Where possible, assessment of the risk should also be documented, both in absolute terms and related to whether there is an increased risk based on the patient. Patients should be carefully informed and counselled with regard to potential complications if mesh is being considered and that real long-term data is still evolving. Exposure or erosion of the mesh into nearby structures, such as the vagina, urethra, bladder or, in rare circumstances, the bowel, may occur. Chronic pelvic or vaginal pain, fistula formation or sexual problems may develop. The use of mesh was based on its use in hernia surgery, where the extra support for weak tissues is thought to reduce recurrence. As such, mesh has been considered by many as a second-line measure but can be utilized as a first-line option in rare situations, such as in patients with collagen disorders or post trauma where the bony supports become defective.

If laparoscopy is to be used, patients need to know about the potential for visceral injury (bladder, bowel, blood vessel, ureteric), incisional hernia at the site of trocar insertion into the abdominal wall and post-operative shoulder pain or other problems related to pneumoperitoneum.

Table 17.1 compares the three procedures.

Prolapse Prevention

In order to prevent recurrence of prolapse, patients should try to maintain a healthy BMI, since extra weight can put strain on the pelvic floor muscles and weaken them. Smokers should quit smoking, since this can lead to a chronic cough, which in turn may lead to extra pressure on the pelvic floor muscles. The same applies for chronic constipation, which should be addressed with proper diet and evaluation by gastroenterology when necessary. Lifting of heavy objects should be avoided as much as possible, and when unavoidable, the woman should lift in a sitting position and purposefully tighten her pelvic floor muscles during lifting.

Table 17.1 Comparing the three procedures

Type of procedure	Infracoccygeal vaginal vault mesh suspension	Sacrocolpopexy	Sacrospinous ligament fixation
Use of mesh	Yes	Yes	No
Approach	Vaginal	Abdominal	Vaginal
Anaesthesia	General or spinal	General	General or spinal
Duration of operation	Relatively short	Relatively long compared to vaginal procedures	Relatively short
Contraindications	Patients with chronic pain	Patients with chronic pain	Short vagina
Specific complications		Laparoscopic complications	Buttock pain, cystocoele, urinary stress incontinence
Pain	Less	More (since abdominal incision is required)	Less
Vaginal axis after the procedure	Remains the same	Remains the same	Changes
Approval by NICE	No	Yes	Yes

Commentary

Una Lee

This chapter on high-grade pelvic prolapse by Phillip Toozs Hobson and Amallia Brair concisely reviews prevalence, risk factors, conservative and surgical management options, surgical complications and prevention. High-grade prolapse is a particularly challenging clinical scenario because it reflects a severe loss of native support and has been associated with a higher rate of recurrence over time. Pelvic prolapse is an intimate condition in which education and counselling is critical to patient's understanding, expectations and treatment satisfaction. A patient-centred approach is important to capture the patient's perspective and meet their needs.

Patients often ask why prolapse occurs and how they can prevent it from worsening. The chapter clearly outlines the risk factors that contribute to the pathophysiology of prolapse, of which the top three listed include: childbirth injury, the post-menopausal state and hysterectomy. Prevention of prolapse is also on patients' minds as women want to pro-actively prevent worsening or recurrence of prolapse. Patients can be counselled on maintaining a healthy weight, stopping smoking and using proper form when lifting, and can also be informed that prolapse can also worsen or recur due to biologic factors that are beyond their control. Counselling patients on the potential risk of prolapse recurrence over time is part of a thorough informed consent process and can help patients have realistic expectations of this disease.

In this case, the patient is a 67-year-old woman with history of prior hysterectomy and prior rectocele repair. Her prolapse symptoms include vaginal bulge and difficulty evacuating bowels. Eliciting a patient's pelvic floor symptoms explicitly allows one to address their symptoms with directed treatment. Women with female pelvic floor disorders often have concerns that may or may not related to their pelvic prolapse, and these concerns can be treated separate from the prolapse. For example educating patients on the differences between urinary incontinence and prolapse is an important distinction.

In her case, she has one of the most common symptoms associated with pelvic organ prolapse: vaginal bulge symptoms. Patients describe the feeling of a bulge or ball that may worsen later in the day or with activity and is bothersome due to its constant or intermittent presence. The absence of vaginal bulge symptoms has been shown to be the prolapse symptom most likely to be associated with patient-reported treatment success [6]. Also, in her case, she has difficulty evacuating her bowels. This symptom has been shown to improve or resolve in two-thirds of women after rectocele repair, with 11% developing new symptoms and 50% having one or more persistent symptoms [7]. It would be important to ask her about whether she splints, where she splints and for how long she has needed to splint to evacuate her bowels, as a longer history of splinting is associated with persistent splinting post-operatively [8]. Normal post-operative vaginal support is associated with a reduced risk of incomplete bowel emptying [7]. "Support" can be improved in women with attenuated tissues through surgical reconstruction that aims to create additional support. The three levels of support described by Delancey are fundamental surgical principles in prolapse repair.

On her exam, the post-hysterectomy vaginal vault is 3 cm beyond the hymen, and the posterior vaginal wall is bulging 1 cm beyond the hymen. She is a candidate for surgical repair that aims to restore her vaginal and pelvic floor anatomy, while minimizing risk of complications. A combination of surgical techniques can be utilized to both address the vaginal vault and the posterior compartment. Addressing the vault with an abdominal or vaginal approach apical procedure would likely improve her vaginal bulge symptoms tremendously. Support for the vaginal apex is an essential component of a durable surgical repair for women with advanced prolapse [9]. For her bowel symptoms, a directed exam and clinical history could help determine if she would benefit from a transvaginal rectocele repair with or without perineorrhaphy in addition to an apical procedure.

The use of transvaginal mesh in the posterior compartment has been associated with an unacceptably high rate of complications including erosion and pain, and therefore is not recommended. Sacrocolpopexy mesh has been associated with a lower rate of complications, but still has a known risk of mesh erosion into the vagina, bowel and bladder, as well as pelvic pain and dyspareunia. Native tissue rectocele repair also has a known risk of pain, dyspareunia and recurrence, but the complications associated with native tissues rectocele repair will not be mesh-specific complications.

For an individual patient, the most important outcome of her prolapse surgery is the relief of her symptoms and improvement in her quality of life, while at the same time, avoiding long-term surgical complications. Every patient and surgeon desires to restore normal and natural pelvic floor anatomy in a durable, safe manner and therefore restore vaginal, urinary, bowel, sexual, and general function and support. The authors of the chapter discuss the significance of counselling patients on the difference between anatomy and physiology, and even when the anatomy is restored, bowel dysfunction or symptoms may persist. As surgeons and physicians, we recognize that there are limitations to our reconstructive (restorative and/or compensatory) surgical techniques and the pathophysiology of the pelvic floor is complex. Given the multi-dimensional nature of prolapse, we can do better in listening to and educating patients, as well as counselling patients with realistic expectations of what can and what cannot be achieved through surgery. To quote Dr. Francis Peabody, "The secret of the care of the patient is in caring for the patient" [10]. Listening to the patient's specific prolapse symptoms and counselling them with a thorough informed consent is key to meeting the needs of women with pelvic prolapse.

References

1. Beck RP. Pelvic relaxation prolapse. In: Kase NG, Weingold AB, editors. Principles and practice of clinical gynaecology. New York: Wiley; 1983. p. 677–85.
2. https://www.nice.org.uk/guidance/ipg581/resources/infracoccygeal-sacropexy-using-mesh-to-repair-vaginal-vault-prolapse-pdf-1899872163618757
3. https://www.nice.org.uk/guidance/ipg583/chapter/1-Recommendations#.Wqu5DIaOi30
4. Rock J, Jones H. Te Linde's operative gynaecology. 9th ed. Philadelphia: Lippincott Williams and Wilkins; 2003. p. 1009.
5. Ma Glazener C, Breeman S, Elders A, et al. Mesh, graft, or standard repair for women having primary transvaginal anterior or posterior compartment prolapse surgery: two parallel-group, multicentre, randomised, controlled trials (PROSPECT). Lancet. 2017;389(10067):381–92.
6. Barber MD, Brubaker L, Nygaard I, et al. Defining success after surgery for pelvic organ prolapse. Obstet Gynecol. 2009;114:600.
7. Gustilo-Ashby AM, Paraiso MF, Jelovsek JE, et al. Bowel symptoms 1 year after surgery for prolapse:

further analysis of a randomized trial of rectocele repair. Am J Obstet Gynecol. 2007;197:76 e1.
8. Sung VW, Rardin CR, Raker CA, et al. Changes in bowel symptoms 1 year after rectocele repair. Am J Obstet Gynecol. 2012;207:423 e1.
9. Toozs-Hobson P, Boos K, Cardozo L. Management of vaginal vault prolapse. Br J Obstet Gynaecol. 1998;105:13.
10. Peabody FW. The care of the patient. JAMA. 1927;88:877.

Part V

Addressing Unique Complications and Situations

18 Voiding Dysfunction or Urinary Retention Following Pelvic Floor Reconstruction

Dena Moskowitz, Una Lee, and Alvaro Lucioni

Case Scenario

A 62-year-old gravida two, para two, woman who had undergone hysterectomy many years prior presented with symptomatic pelvic organ prolapse (POP) to an outside institution. Review of her records indicated that she denied urinary incontinence but did report increased urinary frequency with small volume voids. Initial examination revealed stage 2 prolapse with the leading edge in the anterior compartment. Post void residual by straight catheterization was 200 mL. A urodynamic study was performed with the prolapse reduced and showed a stable bladder with a capacity of 480 mL, no SUI, and complete bladder emptying with a peak flow of 28.6 mL/s and a detrusor pressure (Pdet) at peak flow of 31 cm H_2O.

She subsequently underwent a repair of her POP with anterior and posterior colporrhaphy, sacrospinous ligament fixation, and cadaveric fascia reinforcement of the apex and anterior wall. Midline placating sutures were used to perform the anterior repair, and the sacrospinous ligaments were identified bilaterally and accessed via the anterior vaginal incision for suture placement using a Capio device. A dermal biologic graft was placed and sutured to the apex, along the anterior vaginal wall to the level of the distal vagina, reinforcing the anterior repair. The posterior repair was carried out in a native tissue fashion by using midline plicating sutures.

Postoperatively, she was unable to void and a bladder catheter was placed. She passed a voiding trial in the office 1 week later and continued to do well until approximately 4 weeks after surgery when she returned to the office describing a sensation of incomplete bladder emptying. Post void residual was 775 mL. Examination showed no recurrence of her prolapse, and she was started on clean intermittent catheterization.

A workup for her urinary retention was pursued when it persisted to 8 weeks postoperatively. Cystourethroscopy was normal. She was started on an alpha-blocker, in an effort to facilitate voiding. Urodynamic testing was performed and showed a normal capacity, stable bladder, and pressure flow analysis showed a peak flow of 15.3 mL/s with a Pdet at peak flow of 45 cm H_2O and a PVR of 400 mL. Although many would agree that this pressure and flow are indicative of obstruction in a female patient, this was not recognized by her surgeon. She underwent a stage 1 trial of sacral neuromodulation for 2 weeks for a diagnosis of nonobstructive urinary retention, with no benefit.

Commentary by Alexander Gomelsky, LSU Health – Shreveport, Department of Urology, Shreveport, LA, USA

D. Moskowitz · U. Lee · A. Lucioni (✉)
Virginia Mason Medical Center, Department of Urology, Seattle, WA, USA
e-mail: alvaro.lucioni@virginiamason.org

K. C. Kobashi, S. D. Wexner (eds.), *Female Pelvic Medicine*,
https://doi.org/10.1007/978-3-030-54839-1_18

On repeat examination 7 months postoperatively, there was felt to be a band of tissue in the midvagina that was perhaps causing a physical obstruction of the bladder neck. She was taken back to the operating room at 8 months postoperatively to excise the biological graft anteriorly. This was completed by opening the anterior vaginal wall, identifying the graft, and dissecting it down to the insertion points on the sacrospinous ligaments bilaterally. She noted some improvement in her symptoms with spontaneous morning voids of 150 mL but still was otherwise completely dependent on catheterization.

The patient presented initially to our clinic at 3 months after the removal of the biologic graft (11 months after initial prolapse repair). Examination showed stage 2 apical and posterior wall prolapse with no prolapse of the anterior wall, perhaps because the support of the apex had been taken down by the most recent surgery; yet, the anterior wall plication sutures were still intact. Cystourethroscopy demonstrated elevation of the urethra, and urodynamic studies demonstrated no detrusor pressure generated during attempted voiding. This was in contrast to her most recent study, which demonstrated higher pressure voiding (Pdet Qmax 45 cm H_2O) and was perhaps due to loss of bladder contractility over time given the nearly 1-year time span from her initial surgery. Fluoroscopy demonstrated funneling of the bladder neck, but no proximal urethral dilation to indicate obstruction at that level. EMG showed appropriate silencing during attempt to void.

Based on her history, examination findings, and UDS, it was determined that she had bladder neck obstruction from her initial prolapse repair. She then underwent an extensive transvaginal urethrolysis. The urethra was noted to be densely adherent to the pubic bone and a circumferential release was performed. Postoperatively, she was able to void and decreased her self-catheterization from four times to two times daily. She was pleased with her result and did not wish to pursue any further treatment. She was not symptomatic from her prolapse, and accordingly, her recurrent apical prolapse was not addressed.

Discussion

Multiple types of voiding dysfunction can occur after surgery for pelvic organ prolapse (POP), the most common of which is stress urinary incontinence (SUI), seen in greater than 50% of women undergoing abdominal sacrocolpopexy [1]. Other types of voiding dysfunction ranging from irritative voiding symptoms (25%) to difficulty voiding (10%) can also occur [2]. The exact prevalence is difficult to define due to variations in definitions between large studies. Up to one-third of women with stage 2 POP will have incomplete emptying and/or overactive bladder (OAB) symptoms prior to undergoing treatment [3]. In many women, obstructive voiding symptoms will resolve with prolapse reduction [4]; however, it is also possible to develop de novo urinary retention as a result of surgical reconstruction for POP, even without a concomitant anti-incontinence procedure [5]. Urinary retention after POP repair is usually transient. Here, the authors describe a patient with persistent urinary retention after POP repair, requiring surgical correction.

Pathophysiology

While the incidence and mechanism of unmasking occult SUI after prolapse repair is well described, the onset of de novo urinary retention or other voiding dysfunction is not. The mechanism behind the development of de novo SUI following POP repair is thought to be the unkinking of the urethra that occurs with reduction of the prolapse that was previously protective against the SUI. Using this reasoning, one would correctly expect that a large number of women with irritative voiding symptoms prior to surgery would be cured of this after POP repair, and this could possibly be due to relief of obstruction [6, 7]. Consistent with this, a small retrospective cohort showed that relief of OAB symptoms can be predicted by preoperative Pdet at maximal flow. It was determined that long-standing obstruction contributed to these symptoms [8].

Conversely, surgical correction of POP has been thought to be the cause of outlet obstruction in some patients. The most widely accepted etiology of postoperative urinary retention after POP repair is an anatomical kinking of the urethra due to surgical technique that can mimic a Kelley plication. In our patient described in the case scenario, the bladder neck was hypersuspended, suggestive of a potential etiology of obstruction. Obstruction after anterior colporrhaphy is not widely reported, and multiple studies contradict this as a mechanism for voiding difficulties after anterior repair. Lakeman et al. prospectively performed urodynamic investigation in women before and after anterior colporrhaphy and demonstrated that the surgery did not induce outlet obstruction [9]. Additionally, Kitta et al. demonstrated a temporary decrease in bladder contractility index after anterior repair with no change in obstructive parameters [10]. Taken together, these findings would suggest that in the majority of patients with urinary retention after anterior repair, obstructive symptoms are not due to an anatomical finding and are not usually persistent. Nevertheless, in performing anterior colporrhaphy, it is important to avoid plicating sutures too close to the bladder neck to prevent obstruction.

Similarly, anatomical obstruction does not explain the prevalence of voiding dysfunction in women with isolated posterior compartment defects or the high occurrence of urinary retention that occurs after isolated posterior compartment repairs. Cole et al. describe a population of patients with an isolated rectocele or posterior enterocele. They found an elevated post void residual (PVR) in 48% of women and more than half with high voiding pressures at maximal flow [11]. Book et al. [12] describe a population of patients who underwent surgery for symptomatic posterior compartment prolapse and compared urinary retention rates to those undergoing procedures for SUI. They found significantly more patients who underwent posterior colporrhaphy failed their voiding trials than patients who had a suburethral sling. The authors postulate that the dissection involved in this type of pelvic floor surgery results in pain and impaired relaxation of the pelvic floor musculature. Of note, all of the patients in this series demonstrated only transient urinary retention. Accordingly, it is reasonable to assume that this pelvic floor muscle guarding could, at least in part, also be responsible for urinary retention seen after apical, and/or anterior compartment repairs.

Finally, pelvic floor muscle dysfunction is common in women with prolapse, and the levator ani muscles play a particularly important role in pelvic support. Deficiency of these muscles correlates to the severity of prolapse [13]. Though somewhat counterintuitive, these muscles have also been shown to assist in both urinary bladder and bowel evacuation [14]. Consistent with this is the finding of Ghafar et al. that urogenital hiatus size and decreased levator ani contraction strength are predictive factors for emptying disorders after POP repair [15]. Overall, the presence of persistent voiding dysfunction after POP repair is multifactorial with potential contributors including anatomic obstruction, muscle guarding, and weakness of the pelvic floor musculature.

Role of Urodynamics

Urodynamic testing can be useful not only in the determination of the cause of retention after POP repair, but also in the prediction of voiding dysfunction. Patient counseling prior to surgery is important, and patients with longstanding low-grade obstruction may be more prone to developing OAB symptoms after surgery, a major contributor to dissatisfaction [16]. Several studies have demonstrated that low Pdet at maximal flow (<10 cm H_2O) and high preoperative post void residual volume were significant predictors of postoperative voiding dysfunction [5, 8]. Although these are not the only factors at play, they can be used in combination with patient-specific factors such as prolapse severity, genital hiatus size, and type of surgery to counsel patients if the clinician believes they are at higher than average risk of resultant urinary retention after POP repair [8, 17].

Identification of bladder outlet obstruction through urodynamic evaluation in women is an area of ongoing study but can be useful in delineating the causes of voiding dysfunction and urinary retention after POP repair. Although there are no specific criteria to diagnose anatomic bladder outlet obstruction, it is generally accepted that obstructed women have a lower peak flow rate ($\leq$12 mL/s), higher Pdet at maximal flow ($\geq$20 cm H_2O), and higher PVR [18–20]. The use of nomograms specifically designed to identify outlet obstruction in women can be particularly useful [21]. Compared to EMG alone, supplemental fluoroscopic images can help distinguish between anatomical obstruction and dysfunctional voiding [22].

Used alone, urodynamic evaluation is not specific enough to identify anatomic obstruction requiring surgical intervention after POP repair. Application of nomograms to determine obstruction, while a useful tool, can suggest obstruction in patients who are completely asymptomatic and obviously do not warrant intervention [23]. Accordingly, the clinician should use the comprehensive clinical picture of history, patient symptoms, physical examination, fluoroscopic images, and urodynamic parameters to decide which patients would benefit from further treatment.

Management

Preoperative counseling is paramount in managing incomplete emptying after prolapse repair. Women with high stage prolapse, a large genital hiatus, low Pdet at maximal flow, diabetes mellitus, elevated PVR, and concurrent midurethral sling placement may be at higher risk of postoperative urinary retention and should be prepared for the possibility of at least temporary difficulty with emptying after surgery [5, 15, 17]. There is high variability in the management of postoperative catheterization between surgeons due to lack of specific guidelines [24]. The authors typically use an indwelling catheter for the first night postoperatively in women undergoing transabdominal POP repair, or in vaginal repairs that involve hysterectomy. Catheters are removed at the end of surgery for patients undergoing outpatient vaginal prolapse repairs.

When women do have urinary retention after POP repair, the initial treatment is to initiate bladder drainage with either transurethral catheterization or self-intermittent catheterization. A randomized controlled trial between the two strategies showed that clean intermittent catheterization is favorable over transurethral catheterization due to a lower risk of developing urinary tract infection and a shorter period of incomplete emptying requiring catheterization for drainage [25]. Adequate pain control and treatment of constipation is helpful in facilitating the resolution of short-term urinary retention. There is no standard PVR cut-off value to define when catheterization should be initiated. Women who are voiding, asymptomatic, without neurogenic diagnosis, and have PVR less than 300 mL are considered low risk and can be monitored conservatively, particularly if they have had an elevated post void residual preoperatively [26].

In most cases of urinary retention after POP repair, there is spontaneous resolution within the first week [15, 17, 25]. In women with urinary retention that does not resolve within the first week postoperatively, an evaluation should be performed to identify the cause. A thorough history can identify obstructive symptoms in patients who are still voiding and careful attention should be paid to symptoms of urinary hesitancy, intermittency, weak stream, and positional maneuvers used to void. Physical examination will identify anatomic causes of obstruction including a hypersuspended bladder neck and anterior vaginal wall.

Cystourethroscopy may be helpful to identify an abnormal angle of the urethra and bladder neck. The presence of trabeculation may indicate a long-standing obstruction. Urodynamics, particularly with fluoroscopic imaging, can help identify cases of obstruction of the bladder neck versus those of voiding dysfunction [22]. Patients with voiding dysfunction can be treated with physical therapy, biofeedback, medical therapy to aid in bladder neck relaxation (alpha-blockers, such as tamsulosin), and medications to assist in striated sphincter relaxation (muscle relaxants, such as baclofen).

In nonobstructive urinary retention, sacral neuromodulation is an effective treatment. Studies have demonstrated its efficacy for nonrelaxation of the striated sphincter, seen in Fowler's syndrome [27]. Long-term data has shown promising results in the restoration of spontaneous voiding in patients with and without pelvic pain [28–30]. Prior to initiating a trial of sacral neuromodulation, patients should be counseled that the battery will require surgical replacement, likely within 5 years of implantation, and that they will not be able to have an MRI performed below the neck with the device in place.

Cases of anatomic obstruction should be managed surgically, with specific focus on the cause of obstruction. The most likely anatomic explanation for postoperative obstruction is suspension of the bladder neck or plication of the anterior vaginal wall distally, causing urethral and bladder neck obstruction. In the very early postoperative period, this can be treated by release of the plicating sutures. Later in the course, urethrolysis may be necessary to restore mobility of the bladder neck and urethra and allow normal voiding to occur. Patients undergoing urethrolysis require careful counseling about the risk of urinary incontinence after the procedure.

Summary

In this patient scenario, urinary retention was caused by anatomical obstruction due to distal plication sutures from an anterior colporrhaphy. Her risk factors for urinary retention after POP repair included a baseline elevated post void residual (200 mL) and preoperative obstructive symptoms, though it should be acknowledged that both of these could have been related to her prolapse. The surgery was likely not considered as a significant cause of her urinary retention by her original surgeon, since she did not undergo a sling concomitant with her original pelvic prolapse repair. It is noteworthy that her initial postoperative urodynamic study was significant for obstruction; however, the study performed in our clinic was equivocal. Nevertheless, taken together with her physical examination findings, history, and cystourethroscopy, the etiology of her urinary retention was clear and led to her successful surgical treatment.

Commentary

Alexander Gomelsky

Urinary dysfunction is a diagnostic and therapeutic challenge following any pelvic reconstructive surgery. It may manifest in purely storage symptoms (e.g., urinary frequency, urgency, and urgency urinary incontinence), purely voiding symptoms (e.g., hesitancy, straining to void, elevated postvoid residual (PVR), and urinary retention), or a combination of storage and voiding symptoms. Furthermore, the constellation of symptoms may be similar to the patient's preoperative status, worsened after surgery, or appear de novo in previously asymptomatic women. These symptoms are frequently bothersome and may cause a significant imposition on a woman's postoperative quality of life, even in those women with postoperative resolution of their initial stress urinary incontinence (SUI) or pelvic organ prolapse (POP).

Owing to the many constellations of symptoms and postoperative findings, diagnosis and effective treatment is not typically straightforward. The only (relatively) clear scenario is urinary retention after a midurethral sling. If a woman develops impaired emptying and elevated PVR after MUS placement, it is due to excess tension on the sling. While repeating voiding trials after a brief period of indwelling catheterization or beginning clean intermittent catheterization (CIC) is reasonable in the immediate postoperative period (and up to 2–4 weeks), sling incision should be performed if these symptoms persist.

The diagnosis and treatment of postoperative voiding difficulty after POP repair is more challenging. These patients should be separated into two groups: those who underwent a concomitant anti-incontinence procedure and those who did not. In the setting of a sling, retention due to sling obstruction should be first on the differential diagnosis, followed by impaired bladder function due to narcotics, anesthesia, and/or delayed return of bowel function, and pelvic floor spasm/ failure of relaxation with voiding. In those without sling placement, the latter factors should be considered as primary causes of urinary retention. The authors of the chapter describe another, less common surgical category: women who underwent POP repair using an augmentation graft with subsequent scarring and urinary retention. As with all women considered for pelvic surgery, a close inspection of preoperative, perioperative, and postoperative factors is imperative in ensuring a successful outcome.

First, prevention and anticipation of postoperative problems is imperative. As the authors correctly point out, the urodynamic definition of obstruction in women is incomplete; however, urodynamics, especially with the use of fluoroscopy, are extremely helpful to define a baseline prior to surgery. Hence, detrusor function, both during filling and emptying, can be documented. I will frequently institute a trial of temporary POP reduction with a pessary in the group of women with both POP and significant storage and emptying symptoms. Being able to reevaluate preoperative symptoms in this patient population achieves several purposes. First, occult SUI may be more easily demonstrated, which may enhance the patient's understanding of the concept of occult SUI. Second, an improvement in storage and emptying while the POP is reduced allows for more confidence while counseling the patient regarding postoperative expectations after POP repair. Conversely, if storage and emptying symptoms persist or are unchanged with POP reduction, then there is a strong likelihood that these symptoms may persist after corrective POP surgery and adjunctive treatments may be necessary.

Second, the choice of corrective POP procedure may play a role in the status of postoperative storage and emptying symptoms. The authors correctly point out that repairs of both, the anterior and posterior compartments, may be associated with failure of pelvic floor relaxation and subsequent short-term voiding difficulty. It is also important to note that the use of interposition grafts may, in itself, be associated with additional changes. An acute inflammatory reaction will ensue regardless of adjunct material and eventual incorporation of the interposition material varies. Furthermore, the additional dissection required to reach and expose the attachment points for the graft (e.g. arcus tendineus fascia pelvis and sacrospinous ligament) may ultimately be associated with more scarring.

Third, prompt recognition and management of postoperative complications is imperative. No fault can be found with the authors' approach in this patient. Conservative measures such as behavioral modification, CIC, nonnarcotic pain control, and enhancing return of bowel function will optimize bladder emptying in the short term. The use of postoperative pelvic floor muscle training may be useful and, although the evidence is sparse in this population, a brief trial of alpha-adrenergic blocker or a percutaneous sacral nerve evaluation is a low-risk, high-reward option. The use of urodynamic evaluation is likewise appropriate, especially when a preoperative study is available for comparison. Cystoscopy should be performed in all of these patients to define postoperative anatomy and eliminate urinary tract injury as a causative factor. Since any de novo voiding symptoms that do not respond to observation and conservative measures ultimately have to be attributed to the original surgery, the decision to pursue additional surgery is a reasonable one. A less-morbid option like a takedown of the previous repair is a good start, proceeding to full urethrolysis if unsuccessful.

The final take-away point is that, even in expert hands, long-term or permanent voiding and storage dysfunction is a distinct possibility despite correct diagnosis and uneventful surgery. This is humbling for the surgeon and further underscores the need for extensive preoperative counseling, even when "routine" procedures are planned. Finally, in the face of postoperative complications, continuing close counseling and maintaining clear lines of communication with the patient and their family cannot be overemphasized.

References

1. Brubaker L, Cundiff GW, Fine P, Nygaard I, Richter HE, Visco AG, et al. Abdominal sacrocolpopexy with Burch colposuspension to reduce urinary stress incontinence. N Engl J Med. 2006;354(15):1557–66.
2. Pham T, Kenton K, Mueller E, Brubaker L. New pelvic symptoms are common after reconstructive pelvic surgery. Am J Obstet Gynecol. 2009;200(1):88 e1–5.
3. Slieker-ten Hove MC, Pool-Goudzwaard AL, Eijkemans MJ, Steegers-Theunissen RP, Burger CW, Vierhout ME. The prevalence of pelvic organ prolapse symptoms and signs and their relation with bladder and bowel disorders in a general female population. Int Urogynecol J Pelvic Floor Dysfunct. 2009;20(9):1037–45.
4. Romanzi LJ, Chaikin DC, Blaivas JG. The effect of genital prolapse on voiding. J Urol. 1999;161(2):581–6.
5. Lo TS, Shailaja N, Hsieh WC, Uy-Patrimonio MC, Yusoff FM, Ibrahim R. Predictors of voiding dysfunction following extensive vaginal pelvic reconstructive surgery. Int Urogynecol J. 2017;28(4):575–82.
6. Basu M, Duckett J. The association of changes in opening detrusor pressure with the resolution of overactive bladder symptoms after repair of pelvic organ prolapse. NeurourolUrodyn. 2011;30(4):595–8.
7. Basu M, Wise B, Duckett J. Urgency resolution following prolapse surgery: is voiding important? Int Urogynecol J. 2013;24(8):1309–13.
8. Fletcher SG, Haverkorn RM, Yan J, Lee JJ, Zimmern PE, Lemack GE. Demographic and urodynamic factors associated with persistent OAB after anterior compartment prolapse repair. NeurourolUrodyn. 2010;29(8):1414–8.
9. Lakeman MM, Hakvoort RA, Van de Weijer EP, Emanuel MH, Roovers JP. Anterior colporrhaphy does not induce bladder outlet obstruction. Int Urogynecol J. 2012;23(6):723–8.
10. Kitta T, Mitsui T, Kanno Y, Chiba H, Moriya K, Nonomura K. Postoperative detrusor contractility temporarily decreases in patients undergoing pelvic organ prolapse surgery. Int J Urol. 2015;22(2):201–5.
11. Cole EE, Kaufman MR, Scarpero HM, Dmochowski RR. The effects of isolated posterior compartment defects on lower urinary tract symptoms and urodynamic findings. BJU Int. 2006;97(5):1024–6.
12. Book NM, Novi B, Novi JM, Pulvino JQ. Postoperative voiding dysfunction following posterior colporrhaphy. Female Pelvic Med Reconstr Surg. 2012;18(1):32–4.
13. Rostaminia G, White D, Hegde A, Quiroz LH, Davila GW, Shobeiri SA. Levator ani deficiency and pelvic organ prolapse severity. Obstet Gynecol. 2013;121(5):1017–24.
14. Shafik A, El-Sibai O. Effect of levator ani muscle contraction on urethrovesical and anorectal pressures and role of the muscle in urination and defecation. Urology. 2001;58(2):193–7.
15. Ghafar MA, Chesson RR, Velasco C, Slocum P, Winters JC. Size of urogenital hiatus as a potential risk factor for emptying disorders after pelvic prolapse repair. J Urol. 2013;190(2):603–7.
16. Mahajan ST, Elkadry EA, Kenton KS, Shott S, Brubaker L. Patient-centered surgical outcomes: the impact of goal achievement and urge incontinence on patient satisfaction one year after surgery. Am J Obstet Gynecol. 2006;194(3):722–8.
17. Hakvoort RA, Dijkgraaf MG, Burger MP, Emanuel MH, Roovers JP. Predicting short-term urinary retention after vaginal prolapse surgery. NeurourolUrodyn. 2009;28(3):225–8.
18. Nitti VW, Tu LM, Gitlin J. Diagnosing bladder outlet obstruction in women. J Urol. 1999;161(5):1535–40.
19. Groutz A, Blaivas JG, Chaikin DC. Bladder outlet obstruction in women: definition and characteristics. NeurourolUrodyn. 2000;19(3):213–20.
20. Lemack GE, Zimmern PE. Pressure flow analysis may aid in identifying women with outflow obstruction. J Urol. 2000;163(6):1823–8.
21. Blaivas JG, Groutz A. Bladder outlet obstruction nomogram for women with lower urinary tract symptomatology. NeurourolUrodyn. 2000;19(5):553–64.
22. Brucker BM, Fong E, Shah S, Kelly C, Rosenblum N, Nitti VW. Urodynamic differences between dysfunctional voiding and primary bladder neck obstruction in women. Urology. 2012;80(1):55–60.
23. Massolt ET, Groen J, Vierhout ME. Application of the Blaivas-Groutz bladder outlet obstruction nomogram in women with urinary incontinence. NeurourolUrodyn. 2005;24(3):237–42.
24. Hakvoort RA, Burger MP, Emanuel MH, Roovers JP. A nationwide survey to measure practice variation of catheterisation management in patients undergoing vaginal prolapse surgery. Int Urogynecol J Pelvic Floor Dysfunct. 2009;20(7):813–8.
25. Hakvoort RA, Thijs SD, Bouwmeester FW, Broekman AM, Ruhe IM, Vernooij MM, et al. Comparing clean intermittent catheterisation and transurethral indwelling catheterisation for incomplete voiding after vaginal prolapse surgery: a multicentre randomised trial. BJOG. 2011;118(9):1055–60.
26. Stoffel JT, Peterson AC, Sandhu JS, Suskind AM, Wei JT, Lightner DJ. AUA White Paper on Nonneurogenic Chronic Urinary Retention: consensus definition, treatment algorithm, and outcome end points. J Urol. 2017;198(1):153–60.
27. Goodwin RJ, Swinn MJ, Fowler CJ. The neurophysiology of urinary retention in young women and its treatment by neuromodulation. World J Urol. 1998;16(5):305–7.
28. Dasgupta R, Wiseman OJ, Kitchen N, Fowler CJ. Long-term results of sacral neuromodulation for women with urinary retention. BJU Int. 2004;94(3):335–7.
29. Aboseif S, Tamaddon K, Chalfin S, Freedman S, Mourad MS, Chang JH, et al. Sacral neuromodulation in functional urinary retention: an effective way to restore voiding. BJU Int. 2002;90(7):662–5.
30. Aboseif S, Tamaddon K, Chalfin S, Freedman S, Kaptein J. Sacral neuromodulation as an effective treatment for refractory pelvic floor dysfunction. Urology. 2002;60(1):52–6.

19 Addressing Pelvic Floor Disorders in Patients with Neurogenic Bladder

Deborah S. Hess and Gary E. Lemack

Introduction

Pelvic floor disorders are highly prevalent among parous women, with rates of pelvic organ prolapse and incontinence being estimated at between 30% and 94%. Nearly one-eighth of these women require surgical repair [1, 2]. Women with a variety of neurologic conditions remain susceptible to various pelvic floor disorders. Neurologic conditions that commonly affect the bladder, such as multiple sclerosis, Parkinson's disease (PD), and spinal cord injury (SCI), are the primary focus of this chapter.

Case Scenario 1

A 63-year-old woman with relapsing remitting multiple sclerosis, G3P2 with a history of one vaginal delivery and one cesarean section is evaluated for urinary incontinence. She is wearing 4–6 pads per day, changing them when they are soaked through. She often leaks with a sense of urgency but also admits to leaking with cough, sneeze, and laugh. She has a postvoid residual today in the clinic of 40cc. On examination, she is found to have POP-Q stage 2 cystocele and stage 1 vault prolapse. She is not bothered by her bulge. She underwent urodynamic testing both with and without packing that revealed some detrusor overactivity (DO) with leakage at capacity of 350cc, normal compliance, and no stress incontinence. She was counseled on options for management of stress and urge incontinence. Given both her urodynamic findings and the fact that she is more bothered by urgency than stress, we first recommended dietary changes, the use of urge suppression techniques, timed voiding, and medical management. Regarding her pelvic organ prolapse, we discussed management options including expectant management, pessary as well as surgical repair. Given her low (or lack of) bother, she has elected for expectant management. Because bladder function can change over time in patients with MS and because she was placed on an OAB agent, which can cause some degree of voiding dysfunction, she is followed back periodically to monitor her urinary symptoms and her postvoid residual urine.

Commentary by W. Stuart Reynolds, Vanderbilt University Medical Center, Department of Urology, Nashville, TN, USA

D. S. Hess
Wilmington Health, Department of Urology, Wilmington, NC, USA

G. E. Lemack (✉)
University of Texas Southwestern Medical Center, Department of Urology, Dallas, TX, USA
e-mail: gary.lemack@utsouthwestern.edu

K. C. Kobashi, S. D. Wexner (eds.), *Female Pelvic Medicine*, https://doi.org/10.1007/978-3-030-54839-1_19

Multiple Sclerosis

Overview

Multiple sclerosis (MS) is a multifocal, demyelinating, chronic inflammatory condition of the central nervous system. Its incidence increases after age 18 and peaks between 20 and 40 years of age. Women are younger than men at the time of diagnosis and affected nearly twice as commonly [3]. The vast majority of patients with MS will report lower urinary tract symptoms if queried, though many may not seek urological care. The most frequently reported urologic symptoms among these patients include urgency and urge incontinence; however, disorders of voiding dysfunction are also prevalent among women with MS, and stress urinary incontinence (SUI) clearly can occur in women of this age group with MS.

Stress Incontinence

In the general population, the prevalence of stress urinary incontinence (SUI) has been shown to range from 17% to 41% [4]. In the MS population, the reported prevalence has varied from 16% to 55.9%, with a prevalence of 31.4% found in a recent study of 400 women [5–7]. In a study of 280 women with MS at a tertiary care neurogenic bladder clinic, SUI was noted in 45 women by condition-specific questionnaire or physical examination (16%) [5]. This is lower than expected as the prevalence of SUI in an age-matched non-neurogenic population is estimated to be closer to 50% [8]. The authors postulated that the lower prevalence in this population is likely to be multifactorial. In part, they thought that a tertiary care center may be more likely to see women who have already been primarily treated elsewhere. An additional explanation was that patients with MS have a neurogenically enhanced vesicourethral unit, either from lesions in the cervical spinal cord, which would impact bladder and external urethral sphincter function, or from increased tone or spasticity of the pelvic floor musculature, leading to increased outlet resistance [5]. Murphy et al. found the prevalence of SUI among the MS population to be more comparable to the non-neurogenic population. Reported risk factors that also affect the non-neurogenic population included birth weight >4 kg, pelvic organ prolapse (POP), and multiple pregnancies. They also reported risk factors specific to MS including a lower expanded disability status scale (EDSS) score, relapsing remitting form of MS (RRMS), urge incontinence, a larger volume at 'strong desire to void', and anticholinergic use [6].

Evaluation and Management of SUI in MS Population

Workup for stress incontinence, particularly for those women contemplating surgical intervention, may be more extensive than in the non-neurogenic population. Questionnaire data can be obtained to quantify the severity and bother of SUI; however, there are no widely used quality-of-life questionnaires specific to the MS patient [9]. The UDI-6 has been used to objectively evaluate SUI, and question 3 (urinary leakage related to physical activity, laughing, or coughing) has been specifically shown to be associated with SUI in this patient population [5]. The American Urological Association/Society of Urodynamics, Female Pelvic Medicine and Urogenital Reconstruction and Female Urology guidelines for surgical treatment of female SUI state that surgical management for SUI may be offered to patients with neurological conditions with SUI after appropriate evaluation and counseling and emphasize that additional evaluation beyond the focused workup of history, physical, SUI demonstration, postvoid residual, and urinalysis should be offered for these patients. Both SUFU/AUA and the European Association of Urology recommend a low threshold for additional testing with urodynamics (UDS) in this population [10]. In particular, testing for concurrent detrusor overactivity (DO) or detrusor sphincter dyssynergia (DSD) might influence surgical decision-making with regard to SUI treatment. Those with severe DO might be considered to be at elevated risk for persistent urgency and urge incontinence after SUI treatment, while those with DESD are likely to be at risk for impaired bladder emptying following intervention and should be prepared to perform CIC.

During the workup for SUI, a thorough physical exam, including a focused neurological exam and pelvic exam, should be performed. As MS patients are more likely to catheterize, it is important to evaluate on exam for leakage as well as urethral erosion, particularly in those with chronic indwelling Foley catheters.

Various management options exist for SUI in the MS population, though in general, a more conservative approach, at least initially, is recommended by the authors, due to concerns about long-standing voiding dysfunction that can occur following surgery in this population. In the previously referenced study, of the 280 women with MS, 16% were noted to have SUI, of whom only 11% went on to have surgical intervention: 2 transurethral injections and 4 slings/suspensions. One patient was successfully managed with pelvic floor muscle training [5]. Management, as described in this study, can include any of the management options offered to non-neurogenic patients: pelvic floor physical therapy, injection therapy, or surgery. Owing to concerns about voiding dysfunction following sling surgery in neurogenic patients, the European Association of Urology guidelines do recommend that patients with neurogenic SUI be able to perform self-catheterization before pursuing surgical intervention [10].

Voiding Dysfunction, Urgency, and Urge Incontinence in MS Population

Voiding dysfunction is highly prevalent in the MS population, with over 90% of patients reporting or experiencing some form of voiding dysfunction or incontinence [11]. Axonal damage in the pons and spinal cord can lead to altered innervation of the lower urinary tract and can cause detrusor sphincter dyssynergia (DSD), detrusor overactivity (DO), and detrusor hypocontractility [11]. DSD is commonly diagnosed during the voiding phase of urodynamic studies with the use of EMG or, preferably, fluoroscopy during voiding [12]. The prevalence of DSD in MS patients is approximately 20–25%, with cervical lesions being specifically associated with development of DSD [12, 13]. While MS patients are unlikely to experience upper tract deterioration as a result of their voiding dysfunction, those with severe DSD, poor compliance, or inadequately managed retention should have their upper tracts monitored regularly. Repeated videourodynamics may also be necessary in select patients, particularly those with a change in lower urinary tract symptoms (LUTSs) (i.e., worsening incontinence), more frequent UTIs, or worsening postvoid residual findings.

There are few options for the management of voiding dysfunction and DSD in the MS population. The efficacy of alpha-blockers for management of DSD has been examined. In a non-placebo-controlled study of 28 patients (20 female and 8 male) with MS, Stankovich et al. showed that tamsulosin improved quality of life in 96% of patients, decreased PVR and involuntary detrusor contractions, and increased flow rate and bladder capacity [14]. Although the data on efficacy of alpha-blockers in this population are limited, the use of tamsulosin is rather benign, given its minimal side-effect profile and may, therefore, be of value for symptomatic voiding dysfunction. Injection of onabotulinum toxin A (Botox – 100 U) into the external sphincter has also been shown to improve voiding parameters, specifically in the spinal cord injury population with DSD. This has been shown to improve voiding pressures and PVR [12]. The mainstay of management for the MS population with DSD or other voiding dysfunction remains clean intermittent catheterization (CIC), with the option for indwelling catheters in those who are unable to perform or do not have a caretaker to perform CIC. In patients with severe MS and voiding dysfunction, a suprapubic tube may be the only option in the setting of poor dexterity and upper tract threats. A catheterizable channel may be an option for patients with reasonable dexterity but those unable to perform CIC via urethra.

More common than DSD are urgency and urge incontinence in the MS population. As previously discussed, the prevalence of lower urinary tract symptoms among this population has been reported to be as high as 90%, with the majority of these patients experiencing some urgency or urge incontinence. In general, we advocate a noninvasive initial approach to diagnostic evaluation of MS patients with urgency and urge incontinence (symptom assessment, exam, urinalysis, and PVR) before starting noninvasive treatments. Additional measures such as videourodynamics may be appropriate in patients who do not respond to initial therapies or those with elevated PVR.

When considering treatment, it is important to assess not only the degree of symptom severity, but also the degree of bother, as no potential treatment is entirely benign. The mainstay of treatment for these patients is anticholinergics. We do recommend that these medications be used with caution as these patients are prone to developing constipation, in which case mirabegron may be preferred. Additionally, all overactive bladder (OAB) medications carry a (low) risk of urinary retention, which may be elevated in the setting of DSD or detrusor underactivity. Patients with voiding dysfunction and simultaneous urgency/urge incontinence who already perform CIC are prime candidates for refractory OAB treatments such as onabotulinum toxin A, as they are already catheterizing and have eliminated the risk of retention.

Regarding third-line therapy, the use of onabotulinum toxin A and sacral neuromodulation have been evaluated in the MS population. In studies with both MS and spinal cord injury (SCI) patients, the majority of patients treated with onabotulinum toxin A experienced significant improvement in symptoms [11, 15]. Sacral neuromodulation may also be used, especially if the patient has significant DO; however, these studies are small and require further evaluation.

Pelvic Organ Prolapse: Prevalence

Pelvic organ prolapse (POP) is very common among the general female population, affecting nearly 50% of parous women [1]. Among the MS population, it has been shown to have a lower prevalence. At a tertiary care neurogenic bladder clinic, among the MS population, the prevalence of POP was 9%, with most patients asymptomatic. By compartment, the prolapse was 9% posterior, 35% anterior, and 56% anterior and posterior. There was no difference in age, BMI, or MS subtype between MS patients with and without prolapse, though patients with POP did have a higher mean parity. Of these patients, only 26% proceeded with surgical repair [5]. Massot et al. found that among the 363 patients with MS seen at their center, 9 (2.5%) had POP. The incidence among patients with SUI was 4.4%, while it was 1.6% among those without SUI ($p = 0.146$) [7].

Evaluation and Management of POP in MS Population

Workup for POP in the MS population is similar to that in the non-neurogenic population. Patients should first be questioned about the presence of a bothersome bulge, as Dillon et al. found that the majority of MS patients with POP were asymptomatic [5]. Given that typically the indication for surgical intervention for POP is the presence of POP-specific symptoms, establishing symptoms and severity is an important first step. Confirmatory diagnosis can be made on physical exam and quantified using the POP-Q system. Options for management in the small population of symptomatic patients include those that are nonoperative and operative as described in earlier chapters. Patients' ability to undergo any kind of surgical management should be taken into account when recommending management options. A pessary can be used either as initial management, to determine patient satisfaction with a possible future surgical repair and presence or absence of concomitant SUI, or as definitive management. We do recommend the use of concurrent topical estrogen cream and weekly removal and washing when using pessaries in this scenario. A unique indication for surgical intervention among MS (and SCI) patients on CIC is POP severe enough that it impedes the ability to self-catheterize.

Parkinson's Disease

Overview

Parkinson's disease (PD) is a progressive neurodegenerative condition. The diagnosis is primarily clinical, based on history and exam, with signs and symptoms classically including hypokinesia, bradykinesia, rigidity, and rest tremor. It affects 100–180 per 100,000 with a rising prevalence with age [16]. While lower urinary tract symptoms (LUTSs) are more common in this patient population, stress incontinence and pelvic organ prolapse rates are comparable to that of the general population. The reported prevalence of LUTS in patients with PD ranges from 38% to 71% [17–19]. The severity of LUTS has been shown to increase with progression of PD [20]. In a 2003 study of 61 patients with idiopathic Parkinson's disease, the prevalence of LUTS among PD patients was 39.3% compared to 10.8% in the control group (made up of 74 spouses, family and caretakers), with the most common irritative symptoms being nocturia, frequency, and urinary incontinence among the PD patients [18]. Storage symptoms are more commonly reported in these patients than voiding symptoms [21]. Urinary incontinence can be seen in 28% of women with PD [22], and a study of 50 PD patients reported the incontinence distribution among both men and women with PD as 26% urge and 10% stress, with all SUI patients being female (22.7%) [23].

Evaluation and Management of SUI in PD Population

Given the high prevalence of overactive bladder and urge incontinence, it is important to obtain additional testing if there is concern for concomitant stress incontinence in these patients; therefore, urodynamics may be appropriate, particularly in a woman with mixed urinary incontinence [24, 25]. The American Urological Association/Society of Urodynamics and Female Urology guidelines recommend periodic postvoid residual measurements in these patients to monitor for disease progression. Urodynamics may be performed as part of the initial management; however, the role of follow-up urodynamics is less clear, since upper tract deterioration is generally uncommon in these patients [25]. More common urodynamic findings in these patients include DO and reduced bladder capacity for storage abnormalities, and detrusor underactivity for voiding phase abnormalities. The prevalence of DO in this patient population can be as high as 45–93%, and a bladder capacity less than 200 mL is seen in nearly half of these patients [21]. If symptomatic stress incontinence is demonstrated on urodynamic testing, treatment may be offered to these patients, though certainly, their functional status, risk factors for surgery, and ability to perform intermittent catheterization should be considered in surgical decision making.

Perioperative considerations include challenges associated with disruption of their medication schedule, reduced mobility, and medication interaction and side effects. Additionally, PD patients are more prone to immobility, dysphagia, respiratory dysfunction, urinary retention, and psychiatric symptoms [26]. Recommendations for perioperative management of the PD population to reduce risk include minimizing nothing-by-mouth status duration, avoiding drug interactions and medications that can worsen parkinsonism, frequent assessment of swallowing ability, use of incentive spirometry, avoidance of indwelling Foley catheters while monitoring postvoid residuals, and aggressive physical therapy. These should all be considerations when planning a surgical intervention in this population [26].

Evaluation and Management of Pelvic Organ Prolapse in PD Population

The presence of POP in the female PD population has not been widely studied. Initial evaluation should include a pelvic exam with quantification using the POP-Q system in symptomatic patients. While there is no reason to suspect that aging women with PD, particularly those who are multiparous, would not be at risk for POP, overall, the likelihood of their requiring intervention would seem to be lower based on diminished physical activity as the PD progresses. With regard to management of POP in the PD population, it is not unlike that in the non-neurogenic population. If considering a surgical intervention, we recommend attention to the previously mentioned perioperative considerations.

Evaluation and Management of Urgency and Urge Urinary Incontinence (UUI) in the PD Population

Initial evaluation should include a symptom assessment, pelvic exam, and PVR to ensure that the patient is not retaining, even though the risk of retention does not appear to be significantly increased in this population of women. As with SUI, UDS may prove useful; however, it is not always required. As explained by Brucker et al., the treatment of urgency and UUI in PD patients should focus on optimizing quality of life while minimizing morbidity from the treatment. Immobility, bradykinesia, and cognitive decline can all have a significant effect on management of LUTS. Care must be taken to not negatively impact overall quality of life while trying to treat these voiding symptoms [21]. Behavioral modification can prove very useful in this population as detrimental side effects are minimized. This would include bladder training, fluid and diet management, biofeedback training, and patient education. With regard to medication, PD medications can impact a patient's LUTS. Levodopa has an unclear effect on LUTS in PD; however, it has been shown to initially exacerbate urinary symptoms in some studies, followed by a resulting improvement in urinary symptoms over time. The mainstay of medical management remains anticholinergic medications; however, one should be wary of using these in patients with cognitive decline or memory loss as well as significant constipation. Medications evaluated in this population include Oxybuynin, Trospium, Solifenacin, and Mirabegron. From this list, Trospium is a quaternary ammonium derivative with less blood-brain barrier penetration and, therefore, in theory, fewer cognitive adverse events. Mirabegron, while not widely studied in this population, has not been shown to result in any cognitive adverse events and has no anticholinergic side effects (which are common with other anti-Parkinson medications), and may, therefore, be preferable [21].

Third-line therapy includes both intravesical onabotulinum toxin A injection and sacral neuromodulation. Neither of these is widely studied in this population; however, use of third-line therapies is again influenced by overall impact on quality of life and morbidity. Onabotulinum toxin A has been shown to be effective and safe in small populations of PD patients with LUTS. Similarly, neuromodulation has been studied in smaller studies of PD patients and shown to improve DO and capacity [21], though long-term studies are lacking.

Ultimately, many of these patients are managed with incontinent solutions such as pads or diapers to minimize mobility concerns. Secondary mobility issues often limit the effectiveness of many of the therapies that can be offered. In these patients, perineal care and hygiene should be addressed as well. In rare circumstances with concomitant wounds and poor healing, one may consider suprapubic tube (SPT); however, this should be in the setting of UTI precautions and counseling.

Case Scenario 2

A 41-year-old female with a history of T6 spinal cord injury (T6 ASIA A status post T5–8 fusion) from a distant dirt bike accident presents with symptomatic bladder prolapse. She is G1P1 by vaginal delivery and had a trans-vaginal hysterectomy 3 years ago. She failed a pessary trial with an outside provider.

She initially managed her bladder with clean intermittent catheterization but had difficulty catheterizing with her leg spasms and did not desire a catheterizable channel, so now has an indwelling suprapubic catheter. She had prior videourodynamics demonstrating a diminished bladder capacity with detrusor overactivity at 150 mL and dyssynergic sphincter activity and grade 1 vesicoureteral reflux. No leakage was noted with a pack in place and Valsalva maneuver.

On exam in clinic, her POP-Q was reported as Aa +3; Ba +10; C +10; D n/a; Ap +3; Bp +10; gh 4; pb 3; tvl 10, consistent with procidentia. Treatment options for pelvic organ prolapse were discussed including observation, pessary, and surgery. She preferred a surgical management. Given the absence of pelvic muscle tone and severity of prolapse, she was counseled to undergo a robotic sacrocolpopexy.

Spinal Cord Injury

Overview

Spinal cord injury in the United States is estimated to affect between 24 and 77 per million people, or 12–20,000 new cases per year [27]. These patients often have multiple health problems, of which bladder-related issues have been cited as among the most important [28]. Women have been shown to comprise approximately one-quarter of the traumatic and approximately half of the nontraumatic SCI population [29]. For the first 6–8 weeks, patients with suprasacral injuries may experience spinal shock and present with detrusor areflexia. Following this initial period, some women may have return of spontaneous voiding; however, many develop incontinence. Baseline UDS following resolution of spinal shock is recommended; this can either be at the time of return of bladder function or, if no return of bladder function, after approximately 3–6 months. Electromyography (EMG) and fluoroscopic images are recommended as well during UDS [30]. Fluoroscopic images are highly recommended to evaluate both the upper tracts as well as the outlet, assessing for sphincteric dysfunction. Monitoring for autonomic dysreflexia during UDS, especially in patients with an injury above T6, is imperative.

Evaluation and Management of Urinary Incontinence in SCI Population

Evaluation of UI in SCI patients includes a physical exam as well as urodynamic studies, preferably with EMG and fluoroscopy as described above. SCI patients have been shown to be at increased risk for UI, which may be due to multiple factors. Detrusor overactivity, poor compliance, detrusor external sphincter dyssynergia (DESD), and even intrinsic sphincteric deficiency (ISD) may be present (particularly in patients with low thoracic or lumbar lesions), and level of the injury is not always predictive of urodynamic findings, particularly in patients with lower thoracic and upper lumbar injures. One study of SCI patients secondary to vascular (iatrogenic) causes demonstrated the variability of findings that can be noted in this scenario [31]. In a study of 609 women with SCI, 49% experienced incontinence: 27% daily, 13% weekly, and 9% monthly. There was an increased rate of incontinence among wheelchair-bound patients and those women who were living alone. Incontinence was associated with decreased quality of life in these women [29]. Management, therefore, should be strongly considered both for improvement in quality of life as well as minimizing leakage onto the perineal skin to prevent skin or wound breakdown. Management can include pubovaginal fascial slings (for those with ISD), and less commonly bulking agents, and artificial sphincters. We typically would advocate for fascial slings in the scenario of ISD, in part because it may not be entirely tension-free, and in part because it is hypothesized that repeat catheterization through a mesh sling may put the patient at greater risk for urethral erosion. Options for management of impaired compliance and refractory detrusor overactivity, both of which can lead to significant incontinence, are covered in other aspects of the textbook.

Urethral Erosion in SCI Patients

SCI patients, particularly tetraplegics, are frequently managed with indwelling urethral catheters. Long-term indwelling urethral catheters put these patients at risk for urethral erosion. This can lead to ISD and, in turn, continuous incontinence. Often, this leakage persists even following SPT placement. Continuous leakage puts these patients at risk for perineal skin breakdown. Some of these patients, therefore, require an outlet procedure for management of severe ISD. Methods of management advocated include bladder neck closure versus a tight pubovaginal or spiral sling in patents with sufficient urethral length. Patients undergoing bladder neck closure can be managed by SPT alone (tetraplegics) or a catheterizable channel/augmentation cystoplasty (in the appropriately selected paraplegic patient).

Evaluation and Management of POP in SCI Population

Spinal cord injury patients remain subject to POP; however, there is little literature available regarding the prevalence of POP in SCI patients. While most women are treated for POP based on symptomatic vaginal bulge, many SCI patients may lack this sensation. POP may, therefore, be diagnosed on physical exam and not at the time of the history. If there is indeed POP present without sensation, some scenarios in which to consider management include vaginal bleeding due to advanced prolapse or difficulty with catheterization. Management may include both nonsurgical (pessary) and surgical repair. We do recommend the use of vaginal estrogen cream in conjunction with a pessary to prevent skin breakdown and ulceration.

Commentary

W. Stuart Reynolds

While lower urinary tract dysfunction, such as neurogenic overactive bladder and incomplete emptying or retention, is frequently encountered in caring for patients with neurologic diseases, pelvic floor disorders are less appreciated in many of these patients. This chapter does an excellent job of reviewing pelvic floor disorders in a number of neurologic diseases, highlighting important nuances that make treating these disorders challenging at times. There is also a general lack of information or clinical data on many important aspects of these disorders in these populations, including on prevalence, impact on the patient, and optimal management strategies.

Changing demographics means increased prevalence of some disorders [32, 33], and providers will likely see an increasing number of men and women with neurologic diseases and concomitant pelvic floor disorders in their practices. Being able to recognize these disorders and provide meaningful management will increasingly become important. In many situations, a multidisciplinary approach to care of patients with neurologic diseases may be necessary or advantageous. The diversity of neurologic manifestations and variable range of physical impairment typically require a highly individualized approach to manage lower urinary tract dysfunction and pelvic floor disorders. Pathophysiologic changes inherent to the underlying condition likely affect outcomes of traditional treatment modalities – for example, in a woman with neurologic disease, should we expect the same outcomes for a transvaginal, native tissue pelvic organ prolapse repair or suspension? What would be the impacts of increased weight-bearing for self-transfer on pelvic floor musculature or on outcomes of a procedure? How would pelvic floor muscle paralysis impact on a such a repair? Lastly, bowel dysfunction is also common in patients with neurologic diseases. Management of concurrent neurogenic bowel disorders in neurogenic patients often falls to the pelvic floor provider. As is nicely highlighted in this chapter, for all scenarios, the medical literature is deficient and further study is needed to help direct management of pelvic floor disorders in neurogenic patients.

References

1. Maher C, Feiner B, Baessler K, Schmid C. Surgical management of pelvic organ prolapse in women. Cochrane Database Syst Rev. 2013;(4):CD004014.
2. Olsen AL, Smith VJ, Bergstrom JO, Colling JC, Clark AL. Epidemiology of surgically managed pelvic organ prolapse and urinary incontinence. Obstet Gynecol. 1997;89(4):501–6.
3. Kamm CP, Uitdehaag BM, Polman CH. Multiple sclerosis: current knowledge and future outlook. Eur Neurol. 2014;72(3–4):132–41.
4. Gasquet I, Tcherny-Lessenot S, Gaudebout P, Bosio Le Goux B, Klein P, Haab F. Influence of the severity of stress urinary incontinence on quality of life, health care seeking, and treatment: a national cross-sectional survey. Eur Urol. 2006;50(4):818–25.
5. Dillon BE, Seideman CA, Lee D, Greenberg B, Frohman EM, Lemack GE. A surprisingly low prevalence of demonstrable stress urinary incontinence and pelvic organ prolapse in women with multiple sclerosis followed at a tertiary neurogenic bladder clinic. J Urol. 2013;189(3):976–9.
6. Murphy AM, Bethoux F, Stough D, Goldman HB. Prevalence of stress urinary incontinence in women with multiple sclerosis. Int Neurourol J. 2012;16(2):86–90.
7. Massot C, Khenioui H, Agnani O, Guyot M-A, Hautecoeur P, Donze C. Stress urinary incontinence in women with multiple sclerosis. Int Neurourol J. 2016;20(3):224–31.
8. Markland AD, Richter HE, Fwu C-W, Eggers P, Kusek JW. Prevalence and trends of urinary incontinence in adults in the United States, 2001 to 2008. J Urol. 2011;186(2):589–93.
9. Welk B, Morrow SA, Madarasz W, Potter P, Sequeira K. The conceptualization and development of a patient-reported neurogenic bladder symptom score. Res Rep Urol. 2013;5:129–37.
10. Groen J, Pannek J, Castro Diaz D, Del Popolo G, Gross T, Hamid R, et al. Summary of European Association of Urology (EAU) guidelines on neuro-urology. Eur Urol. 2016;69(2):324–33.
11. Corcos J. A urological challenge: voiding dysfunction in multiple sclerosis. Can Urol Assoc J. 2013;7(9–10 Suppl 4):S181–2.
12. Stoffel JT. Detrusor sphincter dyssynergia: a review of physiology, diagnosis, and treatment strategies. Transl Androl Urol. 2016;5(1):127–35.
13. Araki I, Matsui M, Ozawa K, Takeda M, Kuno S. Relationship of bladder dysfunction to lesion site in multiple sclerosis. J Urol. 2003;169(4):1384–7.
14. Stankovich EI, Borisov VV, Demina TL. [Tamsulosin in the treatment of detrusor-sphincter dyssynergia of the urinary bladder in patients with multiple sclerosis]. Urologiia. 2004;(4):48–51.
15. Khan S, Game X, Kalsi V, Gonzales G. Long-term effect on quality of life of repeat detrusor injections of botulinum neurotoxin-A for detrusor overactivity in patients with multiple scl... - PubMed - NCBI [Internet]. [cited 2019 Feb 2]. Available from: https://www.ncbi.nlm.nih.gov/pubmed/21334639.
16. National Collaborating Centre for Chronic Conditions (UK). Parkinson's disease: National clinical guideline for diagnosis and management in primary and secondary care [Internet]. London: Royal College of Physicians (UK); 2006 [cited 2018 Jun 19]. (National Institute for Health and Clinical Excellence: Guidance). Available from: http://www.ncbi.nlm.nih.gov/books/NBK48513/.
17. Sakakibara R, Tateno F, Nagao T, Yamamoto T, Uchiyama T, Yamanishi T, et al. Bladder function of patients with Parkinson's disease. Int J Urol. 2014;21(7):638–46.
18. Campos-Sousa RN, Quagliato E, da Silva BB, de Carvalho RM, Ribeiro SC, de Carvalho DFM. Urinary symptoms in Parkinson's disease: prevalence and associated factors. Arq Neuropsiquiatr. 2003;61(2B):359–63.
19. Sakakibara R, Panicker J, Finazzi-Agro E, Iacovelli V, Bruschini H, Parkinson's Disease Subcomittee, The Neurourology Promotion Committee in The International Continence Society. A guideline for the management of bladder dysfunction in Parkinson's disease and other gait disorders. Neurourol Urodyn. 2016;35(5):551–63.
20. Magerkurth C, Schnitzer R, Braune S. Symptoms of autonomic failure in Parkinson's disease: prevalence and impact on daily life. Clin Auton Res. 2005;15(2):76–82.
21. Brucker BM, Kalra S. Parkinson's disease and its effect on the lower urinary tract: evaluation of complications and treatment strategies. Urol Clin North Am. 2017;44(3):415–28.
22. Winge K. Lower urinary tract dysfunction in patients with parkinsonism and other neurodegenerative disorders. Handb Clin Neurol. 2015;130:335–56.
23. Jost WH, Schimrigk K. [Urinary incontinence in patients with Parkinson syndrome]. Wien Klin Wochenschr. 1996;108(10):296–302.
24. Collins CW, Winters JC, American Urological Association, Society of Urodynamics Female Pelvic Medicine and Urogenital Reconstruction. AUA/SUFU adult urodynamics guideline: a clinical review. Urol Clin North Am. 2014;41(3):353–62, vii.
25. Winters JC, Dmochowski RR, Goldman HB, Herndon CDA, Kobashi KC, Kraus SR, et al. Urodynamic studies in adults: AUA/SUFU guideline. J Urol. 2012;188(6, Supplement):2464–72.
26. Katus L, Shtilbans A. Perioperative management of patients with Parkinson's disease. Am J Med. 2014;127(4):275–80.
27. Ma VY, Chan L, Carruthers KJ. Incidence, prevalence, costs, and impact on disability of common conditions requiring rehabilitation in the United States: stroke, spinal cord injury, traumatic brain injury, multiple sclerosis, osteoarthritis, rheumatoid arthritis, limb loss, and back pain. Arch Phys Med Rehabil. 2014;95(5):986–995.e1.
28. Bloemen-Vrencken JHA, Post MWM, Hendriks JMS, De Reus ECE, De Witte LP. Health problems of per-

sons with spinal cord injury living in the Netherlands. Disabil Rehabil. 2005;27(22):1381–9.
29. Elmelund M, Klarskov N, Biering-Sørensen F. Prevalence of urinary incontinence in women with spinal cord injury. Spinal Cord. 2018;56(12):1124–33.
30. Harris CJ, Lemack GE. Neurourologic dysfunction: evaluation, surveillance and therapy. Curr Opin Urol. 2016;26(4):290–4.
31. Gomelsky A, Lemack GE, Weld KJ, Dmochowski RR. Urodynamic patterns following ischemic spinal cord events. J Urol. 2003;170(1):122–5.
32. Wallin MT, Culpepper WJ, Campbell JD, Nelson LM, Langer-Gould A, Marrie RA, Cutter GR, Kaye WE, Wagner L, Tremlett H, Buka SL, Dilokthornsakul P, Topol B, Chen LH, LaRocca NG; US Multiple Sclerosis Prevalence Workgroup. The prevalence of MS in the United States: a population-based estimate using health claims data. Neurology. 2019;92(10):e1029–e1040.
33. Ascherio A, Schwarzschild MA. The epidemiology of Parkinson's disease: risk factors and prevention. Lancet Neurol. 2016;15(12):1257–72.

20 Mesh Complications in the Female Lower Urinary Tract

Jessica J. Rueb, Samir Derisavifard, and Sandip Vasavada

Abbreviations

IUGA	International Urogynecological Association
ICS	International Continence Society
MUS	Midurethral sling
POP	Pelvic organ prolapse

Cases Scenarios

Case Scenario 1

Urinary tract erosion: A 52-year-old woman's five recurrent culture documented urinary tract infections within 12 months after placement of a synthetic midurethral sling. Her urinary force of stream was initially slow but is otherwise similar to preoperative flow rates. She undergoes a cystoscopy for evaluation of the recurrent infections and is found to have a mesh perforation inside her urethra.

Case Scenario 2

Vaginal extrusion: A 65-year-old woman with a 50-pack year smoking history has complaints of vaginal spotting 3 years after a vaginal mesh placement for anterior vaginal wall prolapse. Her partner describes occasional pain with vaginal sexual relations. She has a pelvic examination, which demonstrates a 2.0-cm vaginal mesh extrusion in the midline of the anterior wall with a stage 1 vaginal anterior vaginal wall prolapse.

Case Scenario 3

Pain with or without erosion or extrusion: A 49-year-old woman complains of vaginal and groin pain 6 months after undergoing a transobturator vaginal sling. She developed pain immediately after the surgery, and this has not improved much in the subsequent months. She is an avid runner and cannot run due to the pain. Additionally, intercourse is painful.

Commentary by Amanda S. J. Chung, The University of Sydney, Sydney, NSW, Australia
Royal North Shore Hospital, St Leonards, NSW, Australia
Concord Repatriation General Hospital, Concord, NSW, Australia
Macquarie University Hospital, Department of Urology, Sydney, NSW, Australia

J. J. Rueb · S. Derisavifard
Cleveland Clinic, Glickman Urological and Kidney Institute, Cleveland, OH, USA

S. Vasavada (✉)
Cleveland Clinic, Department of Urology, Cleveland, OH, USA
e-mail: vasavas@ccf.org

K. C. Kobashi, S. D. Wexner (eds.), *Female Pelvic Medicine*,
https://doi.org/10.1007/978-3-030-54839-1_20

Case Scenario 4

Fistula involving mesh: A 61-year-old woman is 1 year after a midurethral synthetic sling and describes new-onset urge and stress incontinence and recurrent urinary tract infections. She has not improved with anticholinergics. Her exam shows suburethral tenderness, slight urine pooling in the vagina, and microscopic hematuria on urinalysis. Her cystoscopy shows a mesh perforation in the midurethra and a fistulous communication into the vagina.

Overall Management Concepts

Vaginal mesh complications can be simple or debilitating, so the managing surgeon should be familiar with all aspects of the mesh placement and its removal or revision. If one is inexperienced or does not manage the complication properly, the patient may require multiple additional interventions, and this may be the starting point for continued pain, incontinence, fistula formation, or other issues that have been postulated to be the genesis of the national mesh litigation. It is the authors' belief that since the mesh was placed vaginally, the mesh complication can and should be managed vaginally and proper use of vaginal reconstructive principles can effectively manage the problem without creating additional issues. The consent process is an important step in the management of patients with mesh-related problems as some cases may require staged reconstruction or result in the need for additional interventions should mesh erosion/exposure recur or should the patient have persistent or new pain.

Case Scenario 1

Urinary tract erosion: A 52-year-old woman presents with recurrent urinary incontinence following a midurethral sling 5 years prior. The patient states following her surgery, her incontinence worsened. She has associated symptoms of urinary urgency, frequency, and recurrent urinary tract infections. Upon exam, she has tenderness along the anterior vaginal wall with no evidence of mesh extrusion in the vagina. Cystoscopy shows urethral erosion of mesh.

Presentation

In the above scenario, the patient has experienced what is commonly referred to as a "mesh erosion" into the urethra. The incidence of true mesh erosions is very low (<1%), and in fact much of what was referred to as mesh erosion is thought to represent missed urinary tract perforation during mesh placement [1]. Thus, the International Urogynecological Association (IUGA)/International Continence Society (ICS) recommends use of the term "perforation" with regard to these complications [2]. Risk factors for mesh perforation following midurethral sling (MUS) include diabetes, trocar perforation, and bleeding [3]. Symptoms of mesh perforation following any type of mesh surgery can be quite variable. The patient can present with recurrent urinary tract infections, hematuria, dysuria, obstructive voiding symptoms, irritative voiding symptoms, pain, urinary calculi, or urinary fistula [4]. Symptoms can present even years later; therefore, physicians must maintain a high index of suspicion in these cases.

Evaluation

In addition to a careful history and a thorough physical exam, the key to diagnosis of a mesh perforation is through cystoscopic exam of the bladder and urethra. Use of flexible cystoscope or a rigid cystoscope with both a 30-degree and 70-degree lens is advisable. When an exam is insufficient, studies such as translabial ultrasound may significantly increase the accuracy of locating mesh [5].

Options for Treatment

A mesh perforation within the lower urinary tract can be removed through several approaches. Holmium laser treatment of the intraluminal mesh is a minimally invasive option with less risk of recurrent stress urinary incontinence in the setting of an MUS. Lee et al. reported the need for a second procedure in 22% of patients following MUS mesh perforation and 50% of those following POP mesh perforation. Thus, all endoscopic approached cases require follow-up with cystoscopy to evaluate for recurrence [6]. A vaginal repair is an approach often undertaken by pelvic surgeons. This approach allows for the possibility of placing an interposition graft such as a Martius flap for a large defect or performing a concomitant fascial sling at the time of repair. Shah et al. reported complete resolution of mesh complication with the transvaginal approach and a 71% continence rate with a concomitant fascial sling [7]. Additionally, some surgeons may elect a robotic approach for a mesh perforation into the bladder [8].

Case Scenario 2

Vaginal extrusion: A 65-year-old woman who underwent placement of a midurethral sling 3 years ago presents for evaluation of new-onset bloody vaginal discharge. She reports weeks of vaginal spotting, especially when wiping. She denies any associated pain, recurrent stress urinary incontinence, or any voiding complaints. She also remarks that her husband sometimes finds intercourse uncomfortable, reporting a sandpaper-like sensation on penetration. She herself has no dyspareunia and is unsure if it is a coincidental finding with the discharge or if the two are related.

Presentation

In this situation, the provided history suggests vaginal exposure of the previously placed MUS sling mesh, now more formally referred to as mesh "extrusion" [2]. This terminology infers movement of the mesh out of the vaginal wall in a delayed process whereby the mesh becomes exposed over time. This differs from a mesh "perforation" as previously discussed whereby the mesh enters a viscus structure like the urethra, bowel, or bladder. The incidence of this complication ranges between 0% and 8.1% for midurethral slings [9]. A Cochrane Review suggests a risk of extrusion slightly higher with the transobturator versus the retropubic approach (24 vs. 21 per 1000 pts) [10]. Higher extrusion rates were noted with the predecessors (ObTape® and UraTape®) of our current mesh iterations because of a closed tight weave that prevented adequate tissue ingrowth and scarring [11]. These are no longer in use.

Risk factors for mesh extrusion include medical comorbidities as well as surgical technical considerations. A history of tobacco use, diabetes, previous incontinence, pelvic organ prolapse, or bariatric surgery has been shown to independently predict sling mesh extrusion, primarily because these conditions compromise wound healing [12, 13]. Additionally, many postmenopausal women suffer from vaginal atrophy that manifests as less robust, poorly perfused vaginal epithelial tissue that theoretically may be another culpable factor accelerating vaginal mesh extrusion. Anecdotally, some surgeons pretreat patients with vaginal atrophy with topical estrogen cream to rejuvenate the vaginal epithelium before sling placement with the expectation that it stimulates angiogenesis and better wound contraction, thereby preventing extrusion [14]. However, a review by the Society of Gynecologic Surgeons has found no credible evidence that vaginal estrogen use reduces surgical complications of pelvic surgeries [15]. Intraoperative placement of the sling in the appropriate tissue plane between the periurethral fascia and the vaginal wall is a paramount requisite to minimizing the risk of mesh extrusion [16]. At the time of hydrodissection, mucosal blanching with injection infers a superficial plane, whereas a lack of tissue distension suggests one that is too deep. Extending the area of hydrodissection lateral to the vaginal sulci can further assist in elevating the vaginal wall off of the pubic bone for optimal mesh placement.

Evaluation

If a mesh exposure is presumed, a focused history should establish the presence of vaginal bleeding or discharge, pelvic or groin pain, dyspareunia, or "hispareunia" as it is known colloquially if pain is reported by a male sexual partner. Any mesh palpation on self-exam, voiding dysfunction, or urinary tract infections should also be noted. Additionally, a thorough pelvic exam is required. Inspection with a half speculum may reveal nonspecific granulation tissue or visible exposed mesh along the anterior vaginal wall overlying the midurethra. The anterior vaginal wall should be palpated along the course of the sling. Cystoscopy can be considered if the patient is unable to tolerate a pelvic exam secondary to pain or if the history suggests concomitant mesh perforation as well.

Options for Treatment

Considerations for treatment include the location and size of the mesh extrusion as well as the surrounding tissue quality. Observation and expectant management is a reasonable first-line option if a patient is asymptomatic [17]. Other conservative approaches include topical estrogen cream use or mesh excision in the office. A 6–12-week trial of hormone cream may effectively eliminate mesh extrusion in patients with less than 5 mm of exposure. That being said, it has been shown that up to 60% of patients who are initially managed conservatively do proceed with surgical intervention for definitive management [18].

Surgical excision should begin with injecting lidocaine with epinephrine circumferentially into the vaginal mucosa around the site of mesh extrusion. The epithelized edges of the vaginal mucosa should then be excised sharply in order to provide a fresh edge for closure. The visible, exposed portion of the mesh should also be excised sharply with scissors. Subsequently, the defect should be primarily closed. In cases with more extensive mesh exposure, partial or total sling excision may be required. If continence preservation is a goal, advancement of vaginal skin flaps over the exposed mesh has been shown to be a viable option [8, 19].

Case Scenario 3

Pain with or without erosion or extrusion: A 49-year-old woman complains of vaginal and groin pain 6 months after undergoing a transobturator vaginal sling. She developed pain immediately after the surgery, and this has not improved much in the subsequent months. She is an avid runner and cannot run due to the pain. Additionally, intercourse is painful.

Presentation

In this scenario, a patient, who is of an athletic build, has developed significant pain that is not improving with time after placement of a transobturator mesh sling. It is unclear if this patient developed the pain due to the mesh itself creating some reaction in the muscular tissues or a small neural injury in the groin space that is creating the unrelenting pain. Regardless, one should point map to accurately identify the offending site(s) of pain. Presumably, the pain would be over the groin level at the point of skin perforation during sling placement, suburethrally, or anywhere along the expected course of the sling. That said, suburethral pain may indicate a different problem than just the groin pain (e.g., evaluation for suspect bladder outlet obstruction, urethral mesh perforation, etc.). If the pain is localized to one or both groins, again, point mapping of the precise site of the pain is important so as to manage the exact site. Determining if this is global "pelvic pain" versus pelvic floor dysfunction and levator spasm versus a true mesh-related pain scenario is important. One must assure that the approach to patient management is tailored to their needs, and a clear expectation management plan should be put in place in advance of any interventions. While one usually takes for granted that the mesh-related pain is a phenomenon uniquely associated with transobturator mesh placement, it can occur in the setting of retropubically placed mesh; however, the pain issues in the latter are much less frequent and often occur in the setting of suburethral problems such as perforations, exposures, or obstruction.

Evaluation

A detailed history and physical evaluation should help determine a course of action to aid in the patient's symptoms. Pain proximate in timing to the sling placement should be a tip-off to the likely source for the pain, and subsequent examination should be beneficial in guiding therapy. As mentioned, pain point mapping should be performed in the office and documented to determine appropriate planning of the next steps. The use of cystoscopy is important to assure no urethral mesh perforation is evident, and a careful pelvic exam or vaginoscopy can reveal mesh exposure. Urodynamics can be done adjunctively if bladder outlet obstruction is suspected; however, again if problems developed since the sling placement, urodynamics results are unlikely to change the outcomes of therapy except to determine if suburethral mesh is to be excised. Imaging can be helpful if abscess formation occurs or adjacent organ involvement is suspected, but routine imaging is usually not necessary. Some authors have postulated a role for preoperative translabial ultrasound to identify the sling and better determine its location and any other characteristics of the sling (malposition, twisting, perisling fluid, etc.) [5].

Options for Treatment

The usual course of action once one identifies the site of pain is to start with conservative management measures before more invasive mesh removal approaches are initiated. This may entail liberal use of nonsteroidal anti-inflammatory medications, physical therapy to the affected site(s) and/or trigger point injections. At this time, there is no consensus on the composition of the trigger point injection medication. Options include lidocaine, bupivacaine, ropivicaine, with or without concurrent triamcinolone [20]. In our practice, the injectable medication chosen is provider dependent, but again, this is not necessarily data driven as to the best regimen. If these approaches fail after adequate trials, then one may consider tailored mesh removal. It is the opinion of the authors that the entire mesh need not be removed at the initial setting unless point pain mapping demonstrates bilateral groin pain and suburethral pain from the mesh. Often, the pain is localized to one groin and release of the tension from that area may be sufficient to manage the problem. This entails a vaginal incision, exposure and dissection of the sling followed by lysing or cutting the sling as it enters the transobturator space. An adequate margin of mesh should be removed to ensure no mesh is present near the incisional closures to avoid later mesh extrusions. If this is not sufficient or pain point mapping reveals the pain to be more localized to the groin itself (exit incisions and inner thigh), one can proceed with a formal groin dissection to remove the mesh [21]. This should be performed by an experienced surgeon who is familiar with the anatomy of this space as it is not commonly exposed during most female pelvic surgeries. In this case, a combined vaginal and groin approach is utilized to excise as much mesh as possible in the area localized to the pain. Again, most patients, at least at the initial setting, do not need the entire mesh excised (bilateral groin excisions). Studies have shown improvement in global response pain scores in this subset of patients [22]. Postoperative groin drain placement is necessary, and supportive measures for pain should be considered. Adjunctive physical therapy should be offered to patients suboptimally improved with just the surgical excision of the mesh.

Case Scenario 4

Fistula involving mesh: A 61-year-old woman is 1 year after a midurethral synthetic sling and describes new-onset urge and stress incontinence and recurrent urinary tract infections. She has not improved with anticholinergics. Her exam shows suburethral tenderness, slight urine pooling in the vagina, and microscopic hematuria on urinalysis.

Her cystoscopy shows a mesh perforation in the midurethra and a fistulous communication into the vagina.

Presentation

Fistula formation after mesh placement is uncommon but is often related to mesh perforation into the viscus (urethra, bladder, or bowel). Urinary perforation will often result in findings such as hematuria, pain, recurrent infections, urgency, frequency, or obstructive voiding symptoms. Bowel perforation may yield fecal leakage into the vaginal lumen and abscess formation, but this would usually be related to prolapse mesh placed in the posterior compartment with resultant bowel complications from perforation. Otherwise, many of the same concepts will be considered as in scenario A with the patient with mesh perforation into the urethra.

Evaluation

Similar to scenario A, evaluation should be targeted toward identification of the mesh location and assurance that no obstruction or other problem is coexistent. Once the mesh is identified as the offending source, further detailed evaluation is mostly beneficial for optimal operative planning. The use of cystoscopy (our center is biased to flexible cystoscopy to facilitate retroflexed bladder views), including other forms of imaging such as translabial ultrasonography or magnetic resonance imaging (MRI), is helpful. In this patient, she has microscopic hematuria and this should render cystoscopy imperative. A complete upper tract evaluation should also be performed to rule out any upper tract source of microhematuria.

Options for Treatment

Urethral Fistula

In these cases, the management is similar to what is described in the first case. Smoking cessation should be discussed in advance of surgery for those patients who are smokers as smoking is a known risk factor when it comes to the development of complications, and to improve wound healing. Attention should be paid to removal of mesh adjacent to the reconstruction to avoid any foreign body being near the repair to optimize healing. Furthermore, flap development should be considered prospectively as one may need to employ this after the mesh removal. A labial-based Martius flap may be very beneficial in the scenario of a urethral fistula, as the urethra tends to be a high-pressure zone and some experts believe that this fact may put a reconstructed urethra at higher risk for development of an urethrovaginal fistula. A urethral Foley catheter is necessary for optimal healing and should be left in place for a minimum of 2 weeks. A voiding cystourethrogram can be utilized to ensure complete closure.

Bladder Fistula

In the case of a bladder fistula, similar principles of mesh removal are employed with mesh adjacent to the closure being excised. The obvious problem in this area becomes the proximity of the ureters to the reconstruction. One should consider prophylactic ureteral catheter placement or stenting in at-risk patients. The consideration to an indwelling stent is that if a small almost microscopic incision is inadvertently created in the ureter, one may not notice it; yet, it may heal over an indwelling stent left in for a few weeks. Again, flap usage after primary reconstruction with absorbable sutures may be helpful to aid in healing and prevent fistula recurrence. A catheter should be left indwelling for 2–3 weeks to assure resolution. A voiding cystourethrogram can be utilized in this scenario as well to ensure closure at the time of the bladder removal.

Rectal Fistula

This scenario may occur in the face of vaginal mesh augmentation of a posterior or apical repair. One may see a patient with this complication as they have vaginal discharge, often copious, and possibly an infected mesh. Again, mesh removal with adjacent mesh excision to avoid mesh from being near the reconstruction is required. Some of these cases may require complete mesh excision and reconstruction. The assistance of a colorectal surgeon may be beneficial to help with bowel wall reconstruction. These patients do not have to undergo colonic diversion and can be managed primarily with vaginal mesh excision and reconstruction in layers again with use of a posteriorly harvested Martius labial fat pad graft.

Summary

These described scenarios are due to the unique complications associated with the placement of vaginal mesh. In the United States, the use of vaginally placed mesh *for prolapse* has been discontinued and is not available for the practitioners use. Still, some patients come back after having mesh placed several years ago, often with the described predisposing factors such as smoking history and have symptoms. Mesh issues should be evaluated with the goal to identify and characterize the level of symptom prior to any intervention with appropriate patient expectations being set in advance of any therapy.

Commentary

Amanda S. J. Chung

In this chapter, the authors have provided an excellent and thoughtful description of vaginal mesh complications, evaluation, clinical principles, and management options in the structure of four representative clinical vignettes:

- Urinary tract perforation of mesh, with note made of the difference between erosion and perforation
- Vaginal extrusion of mesh
- Pain without erosion or extrusion
- Fistula involving mesh

The authors are to be particularly commended on their considered approach to what can be highly emotionally charged and potentially litigious mesh complication scenarios.

The authors rightly acknowledge the presence of unique complications that can surround vaginal mesh implantation for the therapy of POP and SUI, and therefore the importance of the premesh implantation workup and counselling including appropriate consent process. Additionally, the authors highlight the need for appropriate follow-up and the importance of the implanting surgeon to be well versed on such mesh complications and their management following mesh implantation [23].

In the evaluation of all mesh complication clinical scenarios, a thorough history and careful examination is important, including cystoscopic and vaginal examination, to confirm whether the mesh is indeed implicated in the current clinical condition or whether it is simply an "innocent bystander." This is particularly important in the climate of much hype and fear of mesh in some continents in recent years. Once thorough evaluation has been completed, the principles of management include the usual course of action, which include starting with more conservative management measures before more invasive mesh removal or revision measures are undertaken. A proportion of mesh complications can respond well to conservative treatment measures. An important tenet of care is to avoid creating further harm and thereby avoid compounding the initial clinical problems as much as is possible [24].

Indeed, no two mesh complications are exactly the same, and appreciation of subtleties and attention to detail are an asset to surgeons managing these difficult clinical problems. Furthermore, multidisciplinary co-operation, particularly in complex multiorgan cases, is valuable and such collegial relationships are highly desirable and to be fostered for the best care of our patients [25].

References

1. Nitti VW. Complications of midurethral slings and their management. Can Urol Assoc J. 2016;6(5-S2):120.
2. Haylen B, Freeman R, Swift S, Dwyer P, Lee J, Rizk D, et al. An International Urogynecological Association (IUGA)/International Continence Society (ICS) joint terminology and classification of the complications

related directly to the insertion of prostheses (meshes, implants, tapes) and grafts in female pelvic flo. Neurourol Urodyn. 2011;30(Jan 2011):2–12.
3. Cohen SA, Goldman HB. Mesh perforation into a viscus in the setting of pelvic floor surgery—presentation and management. Curr Urol Rep. 2016;17(9):1–7.
4. Winters C, Fitzgerald M, Barber M. The use of synthetic mesh in female pelvic reconstructive surgery. BJU Int. 2006;98(s1):70–6.
5. Staack A, Vitale J, Ragavendra N, Rodríguez LV. Translabial ultrasonography for evaluation of synthetic mesh in the vagina. Urology. 2014;83(1):68–74.
6. Lee CH, Ku JY, Lee K, Lee JZ, Shin DG. Clinical application of a transurethral holmium laser excision of exposed polypropylene mesh at lower urinary tract: single surgeon experience with long-term follow-up. Female Pelvic Med Reconstr Surg. 2018;24(1):26–31.
7. Shah K, Nikolavsky D, Gilsdorf D, Flynn BJ. Surgical management of lower urinary mesh perforation after mid-urethral polypropylene mesh sling: mesh excision, urinary tract reconstruction and concomitant pubovaginal sling with autologous rectus fascia. Int Urogynecol J Pelvic Floor Dysfunct. 2013;24(12):2111–7.
8. Macedo FIB, O'Connor J, Mittal VK, Hurley P. Robotic removal of eroded vaginal mesh into the bladder. Int J Urol. 2013;20(11):1144–6.
9. Abbott S, Unger CA, Evans JM, Jallad K, Mishra K, Karram MM, et al. Evaluation and management of complications from synthetic mesh after pelvic reconstructive surgery: a multicenter study. Am J Obstet Gynecol [Internet]. 2014;210(2):163.e1–8. Available from: https://doi.org/10.1016/j.ajog.2013.10.012.
10. Ford AA, Rogerson L, Cody JD, Aluko P, Ogah JA. Mid-urethral sling operations for stress urinary incontinence in women. Cochrane Database Syst Rev [Internet]. 2017 Jul 31 [cited 2019 Nov 24];(7). Available from: http://doi.wiley.com/10.1002/14651858.CD006375.pub4.
11. Giusto LL, Zahner PM, Goldman HB. Management of the exposed or perforated midurethral sling. Urol Clin North Am [Internet]. 2019;46(1):31–40. Available from: https://doi.org/10.1016/j.ucl.2018.08.003.
12. Linder BJ, El-Nashar SA, Carranza Leon DA, Trabuco EC. Predictors of vaginal mesh exposure after midurethral sling placement: a case–control study. Int Urogynecol J. 2016;27(9):1321–6.
13. Cohen SA, Goldman HB. Mesh perforation into a viscus in the setting of pelvic floor surgery—presentation and management. Curr Urol Rep [Internet]. 2016;17(9):1–7. Available from: https://doi.org/10.1007/s11934-016-0621-3.
14. Krause M, Wheeler TL, Snyder TE, Richter HE. Local effects of vaginally administered estrogen therapy: a review. J Pelvic Med Surg. 2009;15(3):105–14.
15. Rahn DD, Ward RM, Sanses TV, Carberry C, Mamik MM, Meriwether KV, et al. Vaginal estrogen use in postmenopausal women with pelvic floor disorders: systematic review and practice guidelines. Int Urogynecol J Pelvic Floor Dysfunct. 2014;26(1):3–13.
16. Gaines N, Gupta P, Sirls LT. Synthetic midurethral slings: exposure and perforation. In: Goldman HB, editor. Complications of female incontinence and pelvic reconstructive surgery. Cham: Humana Press; 2017. p. 177–91.
17. Deffieux X, Thubert T, De Tayrac R, Fernandez H, Letouzey V. Long-term follow-up of persistent vaginal polypropylene mesh exposure for transvaginally placed mesh procedures. Int Urogynecol J. 2012;23(10):1387–90.
18. Abbott S, Unger CA, Evans JM, Jallad K, Mishra K, Karram MM, et al. Evaluation and management of complications from synthetic mesh after pelvic reconstructive surgery: a multicenter study. Am J Obstet Gynecol. 2014;210(2):163.e1–8.
19. Giri SK, Sil D, Narasimhulu G, Flood HD, Skehan M, Drumm J. Management of vaginal extrusion after tension-free vaginal tape procedure for urodynamic stress incontinence. Urology. 2007;69(6):1077–80.
20. Bartley J, Han E, Gupta P, Gaines N, Killinger KA, Broura J, et al. Transvaginal trigger point injections improve pain scores in women with pelvic floor hypertonicity and pelvic pain conditions. Female Pelvic Med Reconstr Surg. 2019;25(5):392–6.
21. Murphy AM, Goldman HB. Thigh exploration for excision of a transobturator sling. Int Urogynecol J. 2017;28(5):793–4.
22. King AB, Tenggardjaja C, Goldman HB. Prospective evaluation of the effect of thigh dissection for removal of transobturator mid urethral slings on refractory thigh pain. J Urol. 2016;196(4):1207–12.
23. Kowalik CG, Cohn JA, Kakos A, Lang P, Reynolds WS, Kaufman MR, et al. Road to recovery after transvaginal surgery for urethral mesh perforation: evaluation of outcomes and subsequent procedures. Int Urogynecol J. 2018;29(6):887–92.
24. Rac G, Greiman A, Rabley A, Tipton TJ, Chiles LR, Freilich DA, et al. Analysis of complications of pelvic mesh excision surgery using the Clavien-Dindo classification system. J Urol. 2017;198(3):638–43.
25. Duckett J, Bodner-Adler B, Rachaneni S, Latthe P. Management of complications arising from the use of mesh for stress urinary incontinence-International Urogynecology Association Research and Development Committee opinion. Int Urogynecol J. 2019;30(9):1413–7.

Severe Urethral Stenosis/Complete Urethral Obliteration

21

Rachel C. Barratt and Tamsin J. Greenwell

Introduction

Complete urethral obliteration occurs, in the main, as the result of trauma to the urethra, causing extensive urethral strictures or urethral loss. Traumatic injuries to the urethra are commonly iatrogenic with vaginal/urethral surgery (in particular following urethral diverticulectomy and mid-urethral tape insertion) and pelvic radiotherapy as causative agents in the majority of cases [1–3]. Pelvic fracture urethral injury is also a cause of traumatic urethral obliteration, although it is more likely to cause a longitudinal tear of the urethra with resulting incontinence than obliteration [4, 5]. In developing countries, obstetric trauma is still the most common cause with cases of prolonged or obstructed labour, causing severe pressure necrosis and tissue damage to the urethra [6, 7]. Rarer indications include severe genitourinary infection, rare skin conditions (e.g. lichen sclerosus/planus) and malignancy (primary urethral or vaginal/cervical) [8–10].

Pre-operative diagnostics include (where possible) examination of peri-urethral and vaginal tissues (Fig. 21.1) to assess for underlying skin condition such as lichen planus, cystoscopic assessment and bougie calibration of the urethra (Fig. 21.2), voiding cystourethrography, video cystometrogram (Fig. 21.3) to characterise proximal site of obliteration/stricture and magnetic resonance imaging of the urethra (Fig. 21.4) to exclude sinister pathology. If the aetiology of urethral obliteration is unknown, then a biopsy of the diseased urethral segment may be performed.

Case Scenario 1

A 50-year-old women (Ms. A) presented with an episode of acute urinary retention 4 weeks following excision of a large circumferential urethral diverticulum (Fig. 21.5) and 1-week routine post-operative removal of catheter following satisfactory peri-catheter urethrogram. Attempts by both emergency and urology department staff to catheterise her urethrally failed. A 14F supra-pubic catheter (SPC) was inserted under local anaesthetic. Following this, she elected to pursue minimally invasive management and had cystoscopy and urethral dilation. At cystoscopy, she was

Commentary by Jaspreet S. Sandhu, Memorial Sloan-Kettering Cancer Center, Department of Surgery, Urology Service, New York, NY, USA

R. C. Barratt · T. J. Greenwell (✉)
University College London Hospitals and University College London, Department of Urology, UCLH@ Westmoreland Street Hospital, London, UK
e-mail: Tamsin.greenwell2@nhs.net

K. C. Kobashi, S. D. Wexner (eds.), *Female Pelvic Medicine*,
https://doi.org/10.1007/978-3-030-54839-1_21

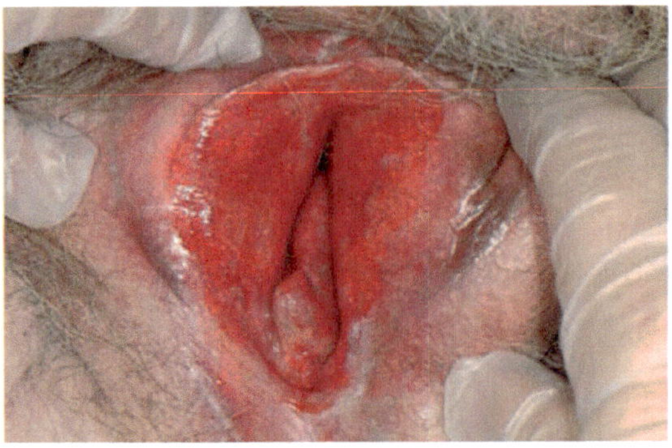

Fig. 21.1 Vaginal lichen planus. (Reused with permission. Copyright John Wiley and Sons [68])

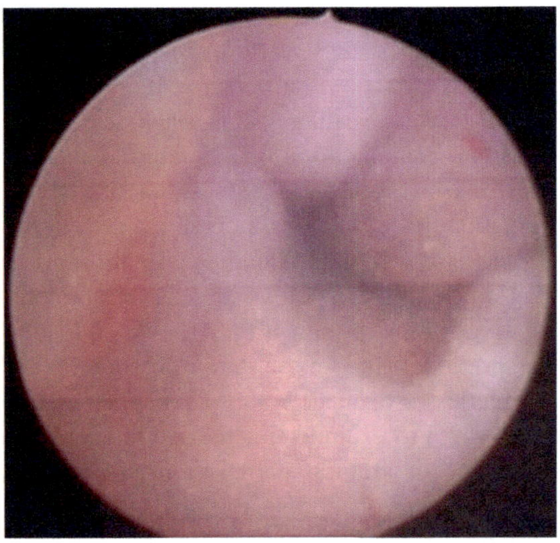

Fig. 21.2 Cystoscopic appearance of female stricture. (Courtesy of Tamsin Greenwell, MD)

found to have near-obliteration of her urethral meatus with exuberant granulation tissue (Fig. 21.6). Following treatment of her granulation with a combination of excision biopsy and silver nitrate stick application, her meatus was accessed and her urethra dilated to 30F and her SPC was removed.

Unfortunately, she suffered a recurrent episode of acute urinary retention after a further 3 weeks. Again, she opted to pursue minimally invasive treatment. She was returned to theatre for further urethral dilation. The findings were very much as at her initial cystoscopy – with an occluded urethral meatus and significant granulation tissue. Her urethra was dilated to 30F, and a new 16F SPC and 16F urethral catheter sited. Her urethral

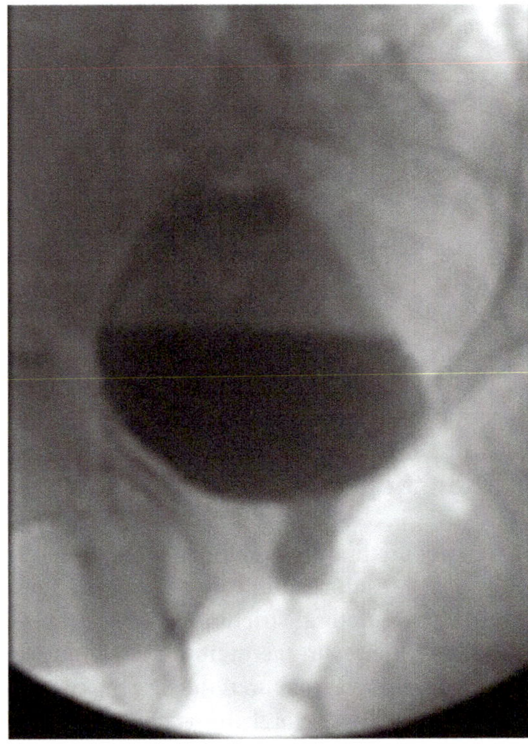

Fig. 21.3 VCMG of female stricture/obliteration. (Courtesy of Tamsin Greenwell, MD)

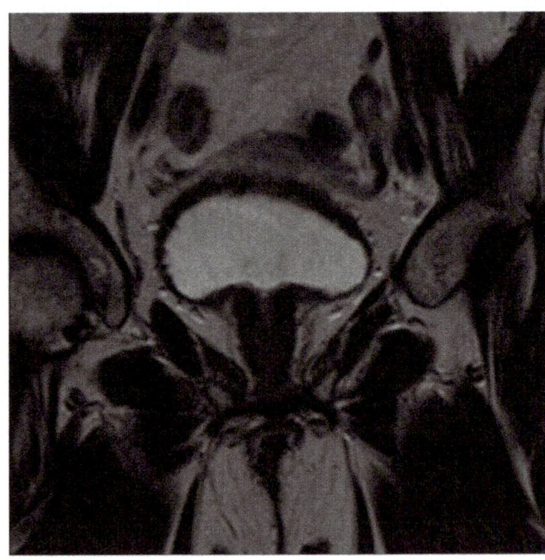

Fig. 21.4 MRI female stricture. (Courtesy of Tamsin Greenwell, MD)

catheter was removed after 2 days, and she was taught intermittent self-catheterisation (ISC) by a Continence Nurse Specialist. On discharge, she was performing ISC daily with a 16F catheter

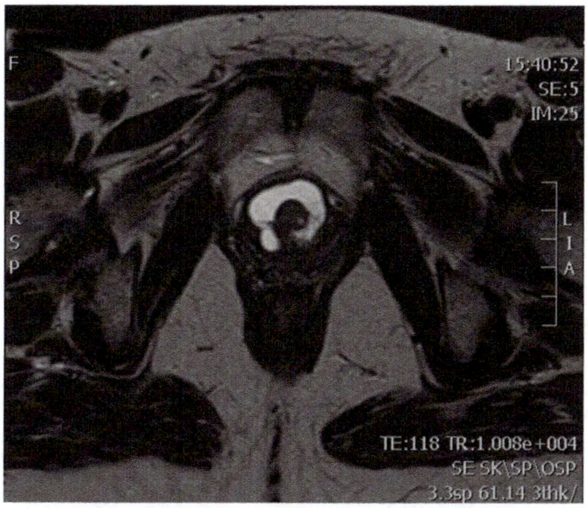

Fig. 21.5 MRI large circumferential urethral diverticulum. (Courtesy of Tamsin Greenwell, MD)

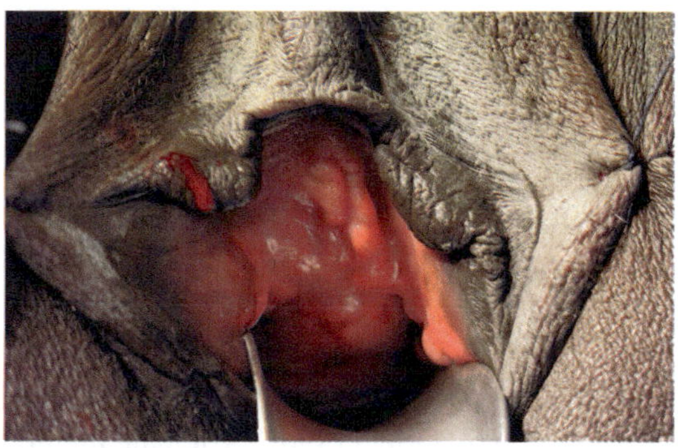

Fig. 21.6 Picture of distal obliteration with granulation tissue. (Courtesy of Tamsin Greenwell, MD)

and had her SPC on a catheter valve left in situ as a 'safcty valvc'.

Minimally Invasive Treatments: Urethrotomy, Urethral Dilation and Intermittent Self Catheterisation

Indications

Urethral dilation +/− urethrotomy or "cut-to-the-light" procedures are often attempted for patients with severe urethral stenosis/urethral obliteration as a primary intervention. This is not an unreasonable first step; however, although the evidence is limited, success rates are poor, with large studies quoting a maximum of 49% of patients being recurrence-free over 4 years follow-up and patients often required intermittent self-catheterisation to maintain urethral patency [11–13]. There is no consensus regarding type and size of catheter or frequency and duration for successful ISC [14, 15].

Following discharge, Ms. A had increasing difficulty performing her daily ISC and presented at 3 months post initial episode of retention having been completely unable to pass her ISC catheter for the preceding 7 days.

As outlined, minimally invasive techniques are rarely useful, particularly for complete urethral obliteration. The mainstay of management therefore is either urinary diversion (with Mitrofanoff supravesical channel formation or ileal conduit [16, 17]) or urethral reconstruction using urethroplasty techniques [18–20].

Urethroplasty

There are different options for urethroplasty in female severe urethral stenosis/urethral obliteration. Certain procedures may be more suitable for select patient groups, but, in general, evidence for reconstructive options in this setting is limited to small case series and expert opinion [21–25]. Techniques used in general depend on the skills and experience of individual surgeons and stricture/diseased urethral segment characteristics.

Advancement Meatoplasty

In cases of short distal severe urethral stenosis/urethral obliteration, a relatively simple advancement meatoplasty may be all that is required [26]. Circumferential, interrupted, non-absorbable sutures are placed at least 2 mm proximal to the diseased distal urethra in healthy tissue. A distal urethrectomy is subsequently performed and the healthy proximal urethra advanced forward and anastomosed to healthy vaginal epithelium using a fine absorbable suture. The non-absorbable sutures are then removed. Topical oestrogen is often helpful in promoting healing in these cases post-operatively, particularly in post-menopausal women [27]. Side effects are recurrent stenosis in up to 16.5%, spraying of urethral stream and vaginal reflux on voiding [26, 28, 29].

Ms. A elected to have an advancement meatoplasty. This was performed without event

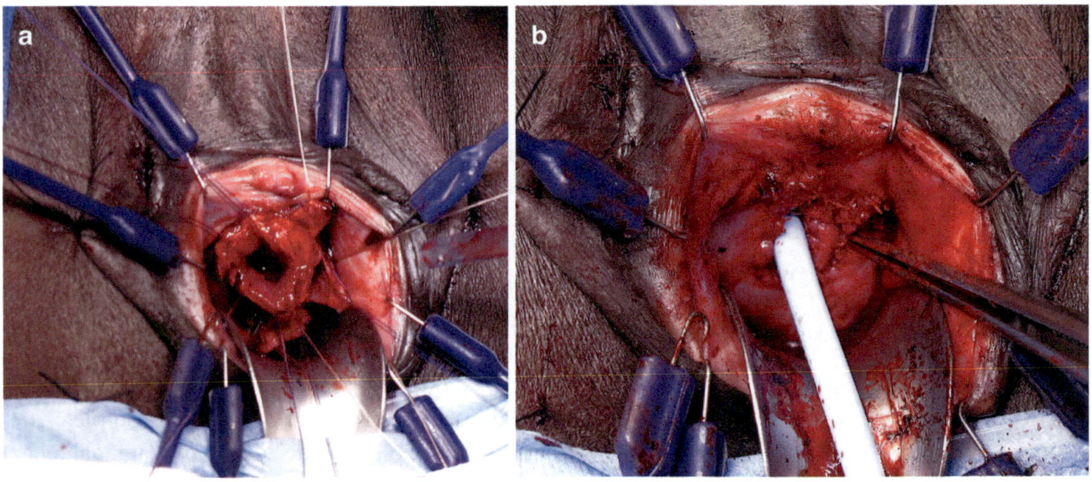

Fig. 21.7 (**a**, **b**) Vaginal flap distal urethroplasty. (Courtesy of Tamsin Greenwell, MD)

5 months following excision of her urethral diverticulum (4 months following her initial episode of urinary retention). She was discharged home, voiding urethrally following removal of her post-meatoplasty indwelling urethral catheter with her SPC spigotted in situ as a 'temporary' safety valve. She failed to return for routine follow-up but returned 10 weeks later having suffered a further episode of acute urinary retention. After further counselling, she progressed to having a vaginal flap distal urethroplasty (Fig. 21.7a, b).

Grafts and Flaps for Reconstruction

Indications Graft Versus Flap

Graft or flap-based urethroplasty may be necessary for cases of severe urethral stenosis or complete urethral obliteration. Grafts are more commonly used to augment shorter segments of diseased urethra [30, 31] but may be utilised to augment the whole length of the female urethra [32–34]. More commonly in cases of full-length severe urethral stenosis or urethral obliteration, a flap-based tubularised neo-urethra is required as there is no functional urethral plate on which to graft [35, 36]. The choice of graft or flap depends on patient and surgeon preference, the condition of local vaginal and putative graft or flap tissues and the extent of the urethral disease. In the case of fibrotic, poorly vascularised urethral stricture disease (as in this case), a flap-based urethroplasty may be more suitable as this is already well vascularised and not dependent upon local ingrowth of vessels.

Flap Options for Urethral Reconstruction

Vaginal Flap Urethroplasty

The vaginal flap urethroplasty was first described by Blaivas and Heritz (1996) for female urethral reconstruction [35]. An inverted U-shaped incision is made in the anterior vaginal wall with the apex of the incision level with the inferior border of the urethral meatus. In general, this flap is 1–1.5-cm wide, but it may be modified according to the degree of enlargement in urethral calibre required and can be utilised to completely replace an absent or completely obliterated un-reconstructable urethra. The urethra is incised at 6 o'clock ventrally through the stenotic part, extending 0.5 cm into proximal healthy mucosa. The apex of the vaginal flap is sutured into the proximal apex of the urethral incision (with the vaginal epithelium facing in towards the urethral lumen) (Fig. 21.8). Subsequently, the edges of the flap are apposed to the lateral sides of the urethral incision around a 16Ch urethral catheter to re-tubularise the urethra using interrupted or continuous (as per surgeon preference) absorbable sutures [35, 36].

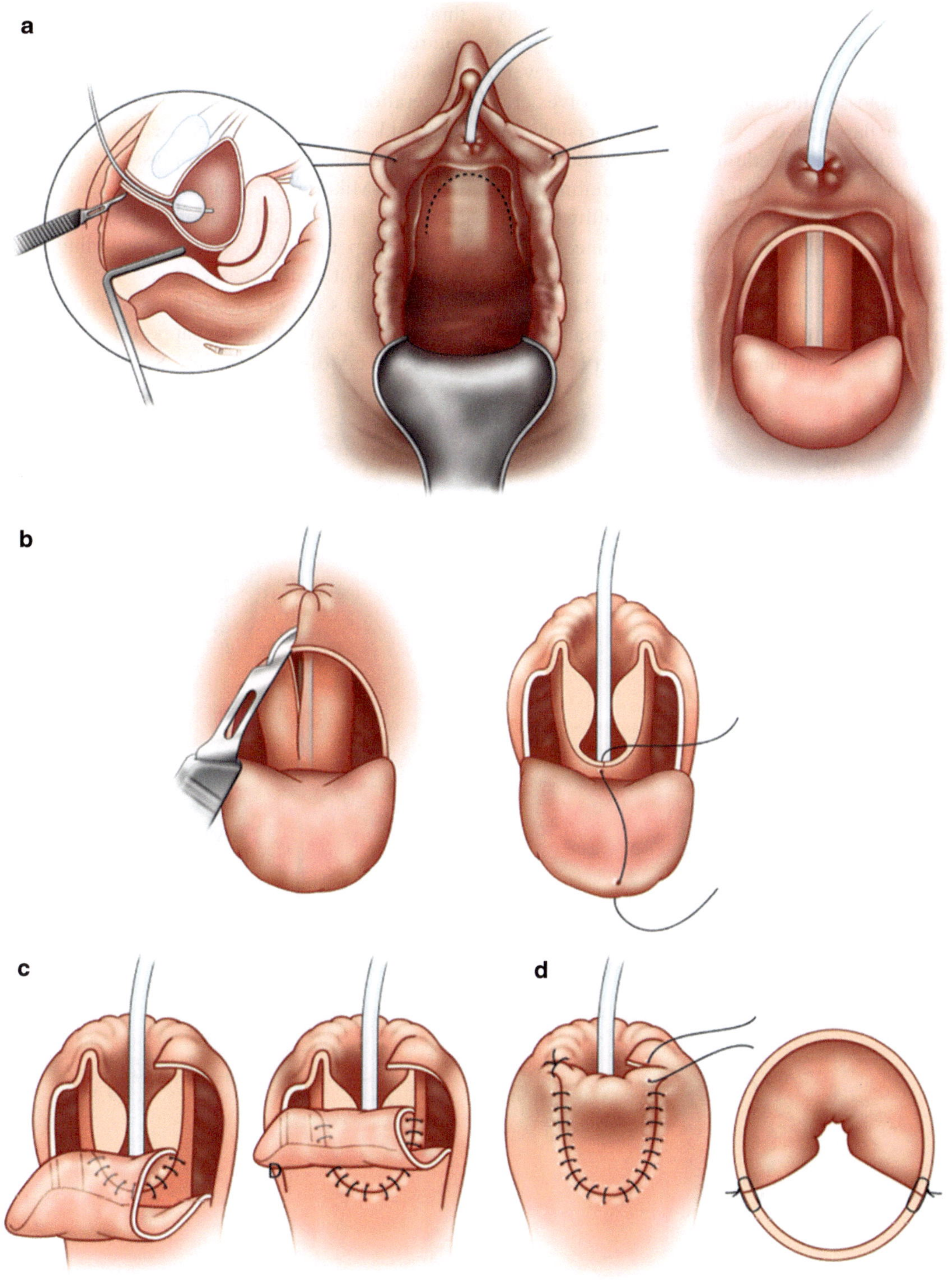

Fig. 21.8 Inverted-U vaginal urethroplasty. (Reused with permission. Copyright Springer Nature [69]). (**a**) Inverted U vaginal incision to raise flap. (**b**) Ventral urethral sticturotomy with suture of apex of inverted U flap to proximal apex of stricturotomy. (**c**) Bilateral suture of inverted U flap to both edges of stricturotomy to complete urethroplasty

A modification of the vaginal flap urethroplasty (the lateral vaginal flap urethroplasty) has been reported as an alternative for cases of severe urethral loss/obliteration [37]. This involves creating a flap between two parallel incisions on either side of the urethral stump or bladder neck in a urethral obliteration case (a urethrectomy would be performed first to reach healthy tissue). These two incisions can either be joined with a distal or proximal (to the meatus) transverse incision to free the flap on a pedicle. This flap is then sutured to the distal end of the urethral stump/bladder neck and tubularised around a 16Ch urethral catheter using interrupted absorbable sutures to form a neo-urethra (Fig. 21.9) [37, 38].

Alternately, as in Case Scenario 1, if the obliteration is limited to the distal urethra/meatus, a lateral U-shaped flap can be used to form a V-Y advancement distal urethroplasty using the Heinieke-Mikulicz principle (Fig. 21.10) [39]. Ms. A had a successful trial of void 3 weeks post vaginal flap urethroplasty and is voiding well 6 months post urethroplasty 4.

Most cases require a modified Martius labial fat pad interposition flap for support (Fig. 21.11a–f) unless very distal as in Case Scenario 1. If the

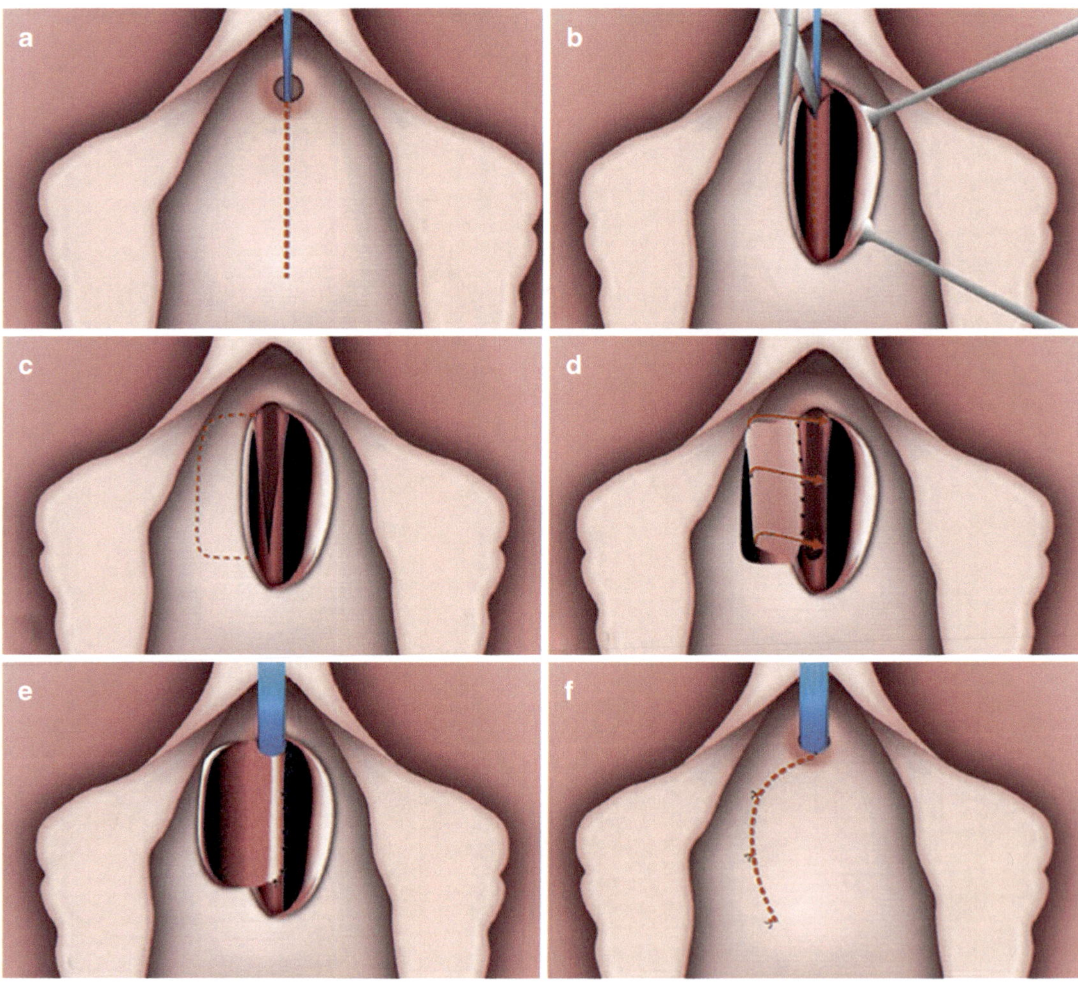

Fig. 21.9 Lateral vaginal urethroplasty. (Reused with permission. Copyright Elsevier [33]). (**a**) Midline ventral vaginal incision. (**b**) Midline ventral urethral stricturotomy. (**c**) Lateral vaginal flap outlined. (**d**) Medial side of lateral vaginal flap sutured to right edge of stricturotomy. (**e**) Lateral side of flap sutured to left edge of stricturotomy to complete the urethroplasty - with complete inversion of vaginal epithelium. (**f**) Vaginal incision closed

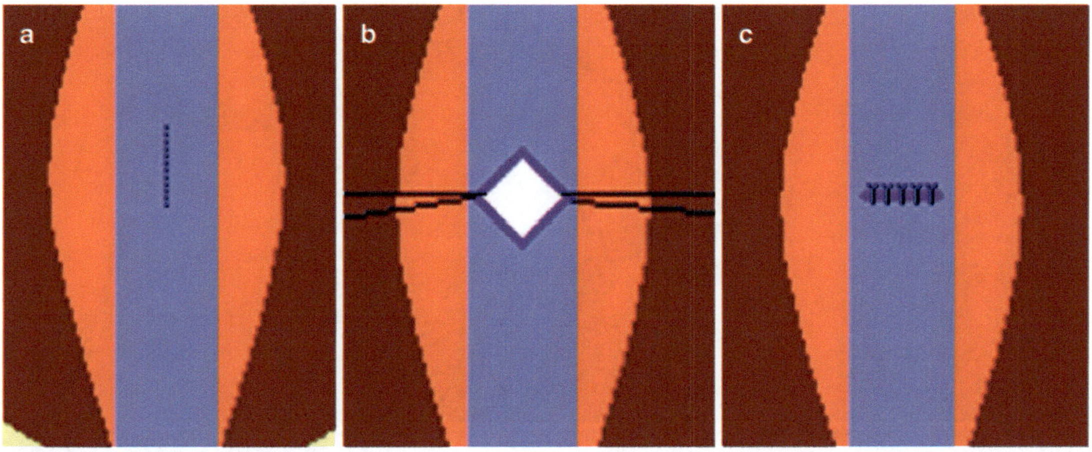

Fig. 21.10 Heineke-Mikulicz urethroplasty. (Reused with permission. Copyright Elsevier [70]). (**a**) Midline longitudinal urethral incision through stricture. (**b**) Lateral stay suture traction to pull urethral incision horizontally. (**c**) Horizontal closure of stricturotomy

disease/obliteration affects the proximal/mid-urethra (the sphincter active area), the possibility of post-reconstruction stress urinary incontinence must be discussed. Some surgeons advocate a concurrent autologous pubo-vaginal sling [40]. We prefer to reconstruct and assess and treat any consequent stress urinary incontinence at a later date, as we have been surprised to find post-operative continence, even in women with full urethral replacement.

Rosenblum and Nitti (2011) also described the use of labia minora (Fig. 21.12) and thigh flaps (Fig. 21.13) in female urethroplasty for cases where the anterior vaginal wall is scarred or of poor quality [41]. However, as both these structures are less elastic, with a higher associated morbidity, due to the increased distance from the sight of reconstruction, they are best kept in reserve for very challenging cases. Thigh flaps have the additional disadvantage of being hair bearing [42–44].

Case Scenario 2

A 46-year-old woman, (Ms. B), presented with recurrent UTIs, poor flow and urgency incontinence. She had been diagnosed with urethral stricture 10 years previously and had been managed with urethral dilation and ISC. She was unable to perform ISC for 6 months secondary to pain and had required increasingly frequent urethral dilations – most recently 3 monthly. She was voiding urethrally, albeit with a very slow flow rate (Fig. 21.14), her MRI revealed enlarged and thickened peri-urethral tissue – a combination of sphincter and peri-stricture inflammation (Fig. 21.4), and she was unable to void during video-urodynamics which otherwise revealed normal capacity bladder with end-fill overactivity (Fig. 21.3). She elected to have an urethroplasty and was consented for buccal mucosal graft urethroplasty or vaginal flap urethroplasty +/− Martius labial fat pad interposition.

At time of surgery, the urethra was found to be completely inaccessible to all attempts at passage of a cystoscope (adult and paediatric, rigid and flexible) and it was impossible to pass even a guidewire per urethral meatus. A suprapubic cystostomy and an attempt to pass a guidewire from above also failed due to 'near'-complete obstruction of the urethra. Obstruction was termed 'near'-complete, because she was still managing to pass urine urethrally. A formal small Pfannenstiel incision was performed, and her bladder opened to access the bladder neck. A Clutton's sound was placed in the bladder neck and the proximal urethra/bladder neck area accessed from the vagina by cutting down onto the sound. An alternative approach taken in a

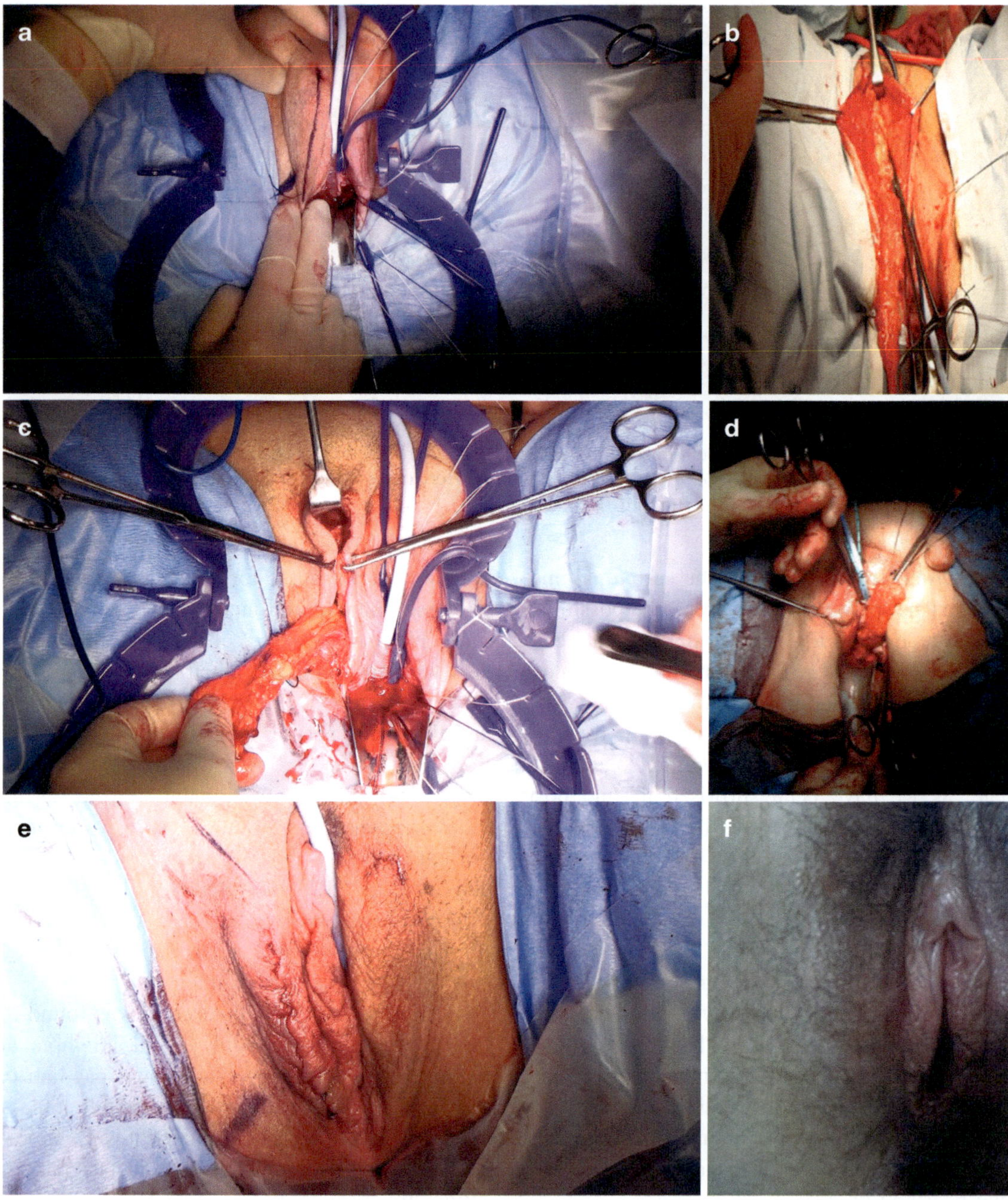

Fig. 21.11 (**a–f**) Martius fat pad. (Courtesy of Tamsin Greenwell, MD) (**a**) Labial skin incision outlined. (**b**) Fat pad flap harvest in process with fat pad mobilised off medial, lateral and posterior aspects. (**c**) Fat pad flap harvest on posterior pedicle completed. (**d**) Transposition of fat pad flap from labia into the vaginal incision by tunnelling under the side wall of the vagina. (**e**) Appearance of labial harvest site immediately post operatively. (**f**) Appearance of labial harvest site 6 weeks post operatively

similar case was to pass a needle into the bladder under guidance of supra-pubic cystoscopy. A widely spatulated opening was formed between the vagina and bladder neck using absorbable sutures (Fig. 21.15). Options then considered for urethral reconstruction included vaginal flap urethroplasty or bladder flap urethroplasty. A vaginal flap urethroplasty was performed using the classical Blaivas technique, with the apex of a wide inverted U flap centred

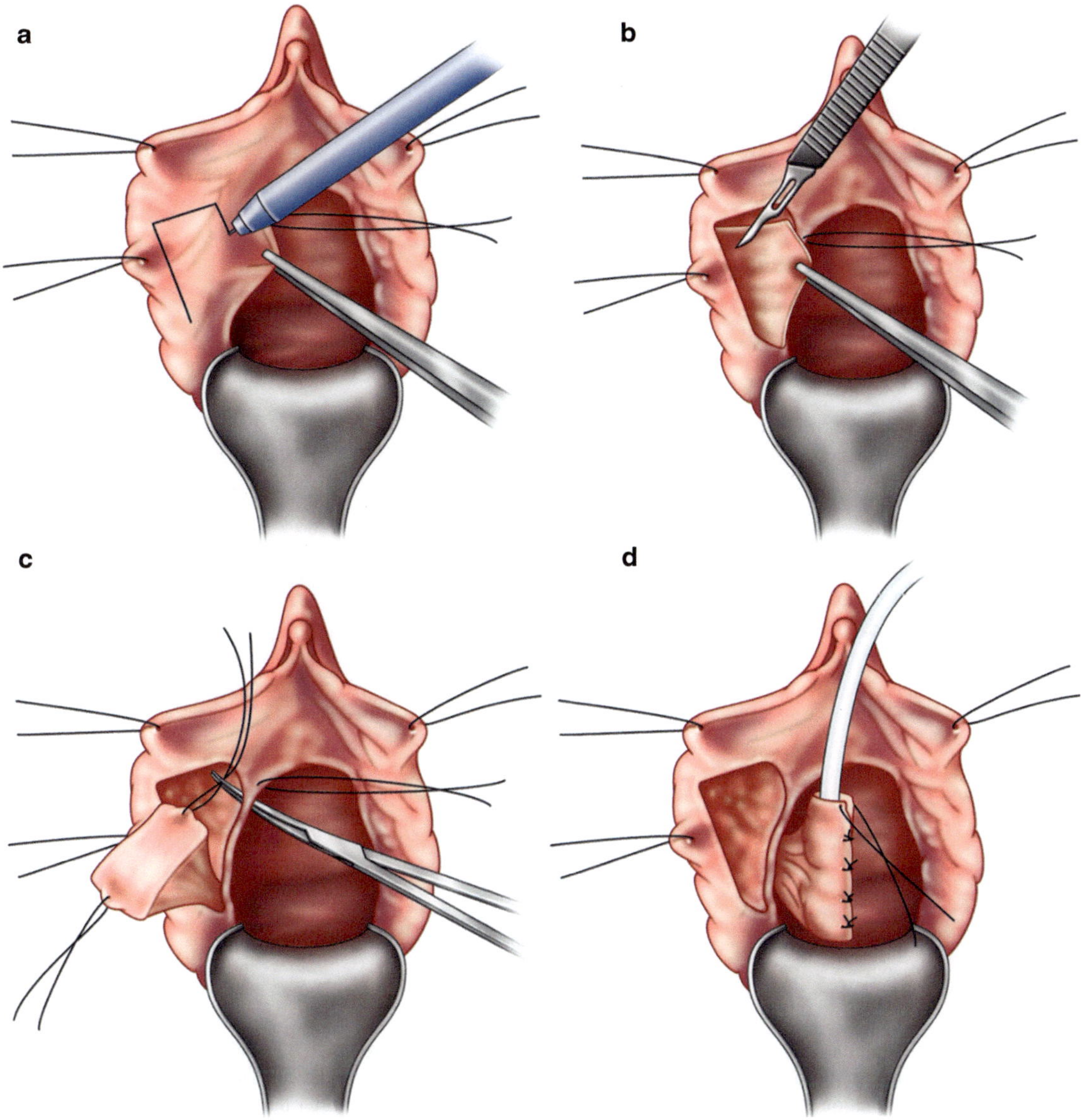

Fig. 21.12 Labia minora flap. (Reused with permission. Copyright Springer Nature [69])

at and sutured to the bladder neck opening (Fig. 21.8). The flap was then sutured to itself over a 16F catheter using continuous absorbable suture. A modified Martius labial fat pad flap was raised bilaterally and sutured over the flap neo-urethral to support it. It was decided not to perform a simultaneous pubo-vaginal sling but to allow all to settle post-surgery and assess whether further intervention was required. She had a successful trial of void after healing was confirmed at her 3-week post-surgery urethrocystogram. She was reviewed in outpatients at 3 and 6 months post-surgery – and is voiding well with no urinary incontinence.

Bladder-Flap Urethroplasty

In very proximal cases of urethral obliteration, complete urethral obliteration or complete urethral loss, bladder flap urethroplasty may be the flap of choice as it is adapted for many of the same conditions as the urethra and has alpha-adrenergic and circular smooth muscle fibres,

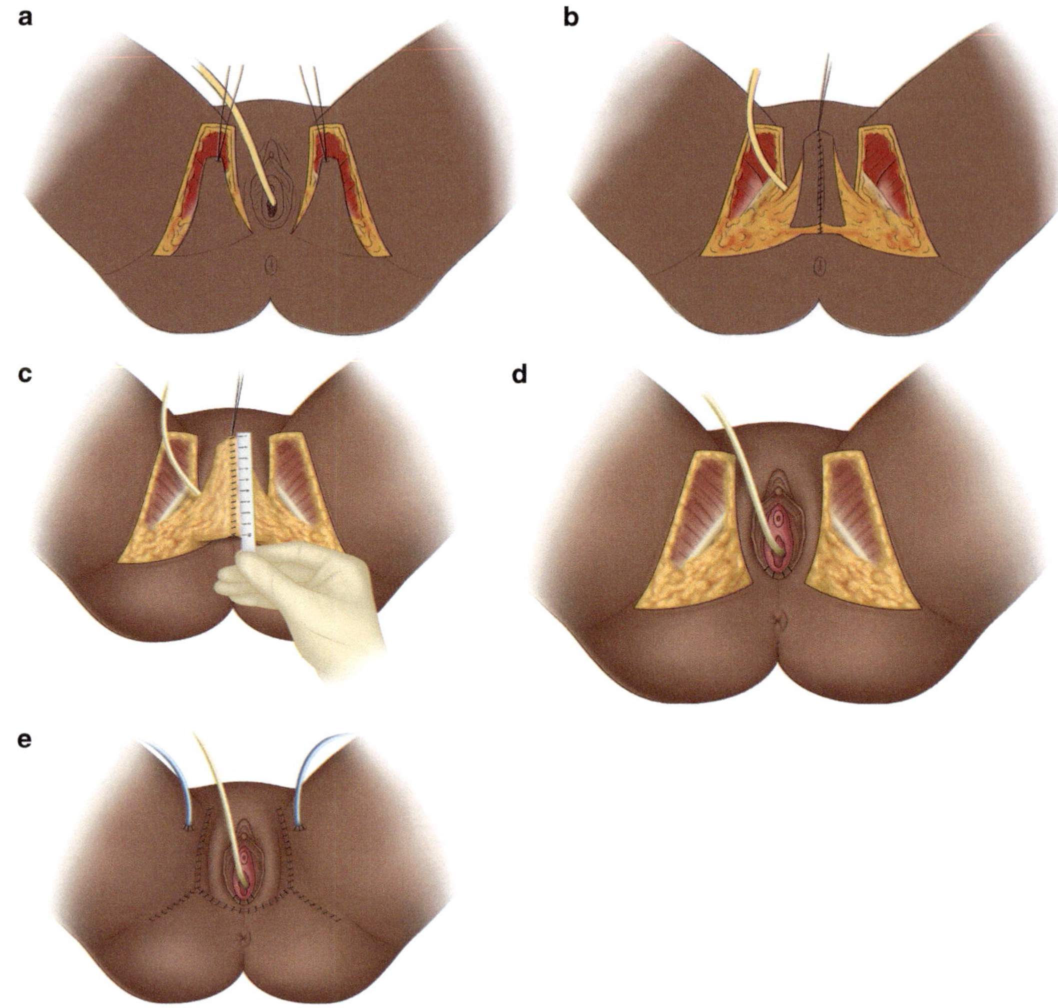

Fig. 21.13 (**a**–**e**) Thigh flap (Singapore) (**a**) Mobilisation of medial thigh flap(s) lateral to the labia majora on a posterior pedicle. (**b**) Formation of the posterior (dorsal) wall of the neourethra. (**c**) Formation of the anterior (ventral) wall of the neourethra. (**d**) Inversion of the neourethra into the vagina, deep to the anterior vaginal wall. (**e**) Final external appearance after harvest site closure

both of which can contribute to improving continence outcomes. Most bladder flap techniques rely on the vascular pedicle supply coming supero-laterally from the dome of the bladder. The two most common procedures described in the literature are outlined below although many authors have reported their own modifications to these techniques [45, 46].

Oblique flap bladder flap urethroplasty harvests a flap from the bladder neck obliquely towards the ureteric orifice. This is harvested and tubularised over a 16Ch catheter to form a neo-urethra. The advantage to this technique is that the suture line is not in the mid-line and therefore, the risk of fistulation between the neo-urethra and vagina is lower. However, the distance from the bladder neck to the ureteric orifice limits the length of the flap, and therefore, this technique is often not able to provide a sufficiently long neo-urethra [45].

A vertical anterior bladder flap urethroplasty, by contrast, involves creation of a flap from the posterior bladder wall. This can be extended up to the dome of the bladder if required to create a suitable length neo-urethra. The flap is tubularised over a 16Ch catheter (Fig. 21.16); however,

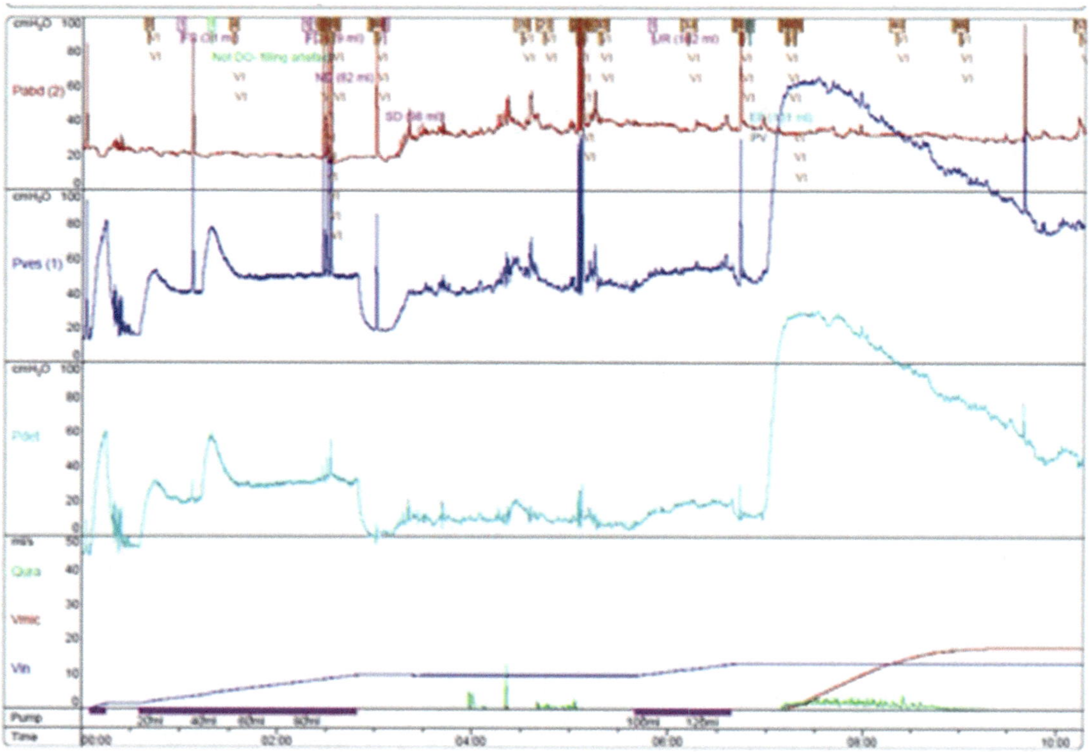

Fig. 21.14 Pressure flow trace for patient B showing severe bladder outflow obstruction. (Courtesy of Tamsin Greenwell, MD)

as the suture line is ventral and in the mid-line, it lies adjacent to the anterior vaginal wall with significant risk of fistulation and, therefore, a modified Martius fat pad interposition flap is essential [46].

Once a neo-urethra has been tubularised over a catheter, it is then routed through a space dissected between the anterior vaginal wall and pubic bone to form, where possible, an anatomical neo-meatus in the vaginal vestibule. Women may develop significant stress urinary incontinence following bladder flap urethral reconstruction. The possibility of either a concurrent or delayed anti-incontinence procedure, (which, for most, is an autologous pubo-vaginal sling although some authors report using bulking agents) must be discussed [47]. There is very little data to inform the timing of an anti-incontinence procedure – and this is best determined by patient and surgeon preference; again we prefer to wait and re-assess continence following recovery from reconstruction.

Success Rates and Complications

Evaluating all the available literature for vaginal flap urethroplasty procedures related to urethral damage reconstruction reveals 124 patients in 11 case series with variable follow-up. Mean success rates are 87% (range 80–100%) [19, 25, 33, 35–38, 40, 48–50] (although in one study, all patients performed CISC routinely post-op as part of their protocol). Failures appear to be able to be salvaged successfully in 86% with a second procedure – often, this is a buccal mucosal graft (BMG) urethroplasty [50]. Blaivas et al. (2012) found that stricture recurrence occurred following vaginal flap urethroplasty between 62 and 72 months post-surgery, echoing the finding in male stricture disease that recurrence happens most often in the medium- to long-term post-operative period [50]. Continence is not thoroughly reported but appears, from the available literature, to be excellent with 95–100% dry at last follow-up although some had concurrent autologous pubo-vaginal sling at time of repair [50, 51]. No significant post-operative

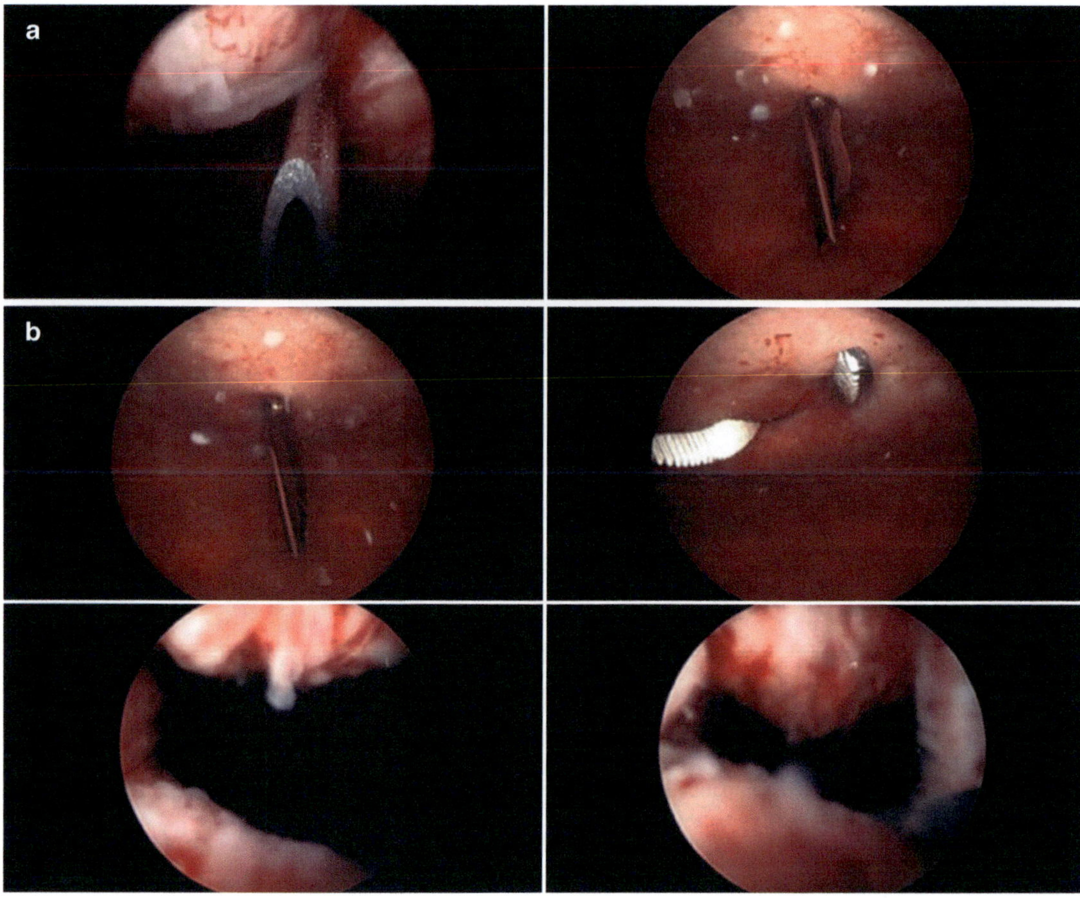

Fig. 21.15 Cut through to bladder neck. (Courtesy of Tamsin Greenwell, MD) (**a**) Suprapubic cystoscopic guided insertion of needle from the vaginal aspect through the occluded urethra into the occluded bladder neck with subsequent passage of scalpel blade along side it. (**b**) Suprapubic cystoscopy guided incision of the bladder neck with subsequent passage of clip to demonstrate newly reopened bladder neck. (**c**) Final suprapubic cystoscopy appearance of newly reopened bladder neck after placement of initial eversion sutures

complications are reported in the literature although bleeding with haematoma formation, infection, fistulation and stricture recurrence are all possible [19, 25, 33, 35–38, 40, 48–50]. Some authors have reported de novo irritative lower urinary tract symptoms post-operatively, but these did not appear to be significant [19, 25, 33, 35–38, 40, 48–50].

There is a single case series of 2 patients with labial minora flap urethroplasty performed via a ventral approach. Success was quoted at 100% for both patients at 24 months follow-up. No significant complications were reported [42]. Tubularised labia minor and/or major flap replacement urethroplasty has been reported in 8 females with obliterative urethral stricture associated with urethrovaginal fistula [43]. Success was reported in 87.5% at a mean follow-up of 48.25 months after the procedure. No complications other than transient stress urinary incontinence in 1 patient were reported.

Finally, for tubularised bladder flap urethroplasty, data is, as expected, limited. It is reported as a technique for urethral reconstruction (urethral loss/obliteration) in 4 case series with a cumulative total of 5 patients undergoing this technique. No recurrent strictures were reported, but continence is an issue. Hemal et al. (2000) report continence at 2–4 hourly intervals in their 3 patients, and this relatively poor continence outcome is reflected in the other series [45–47, 52].

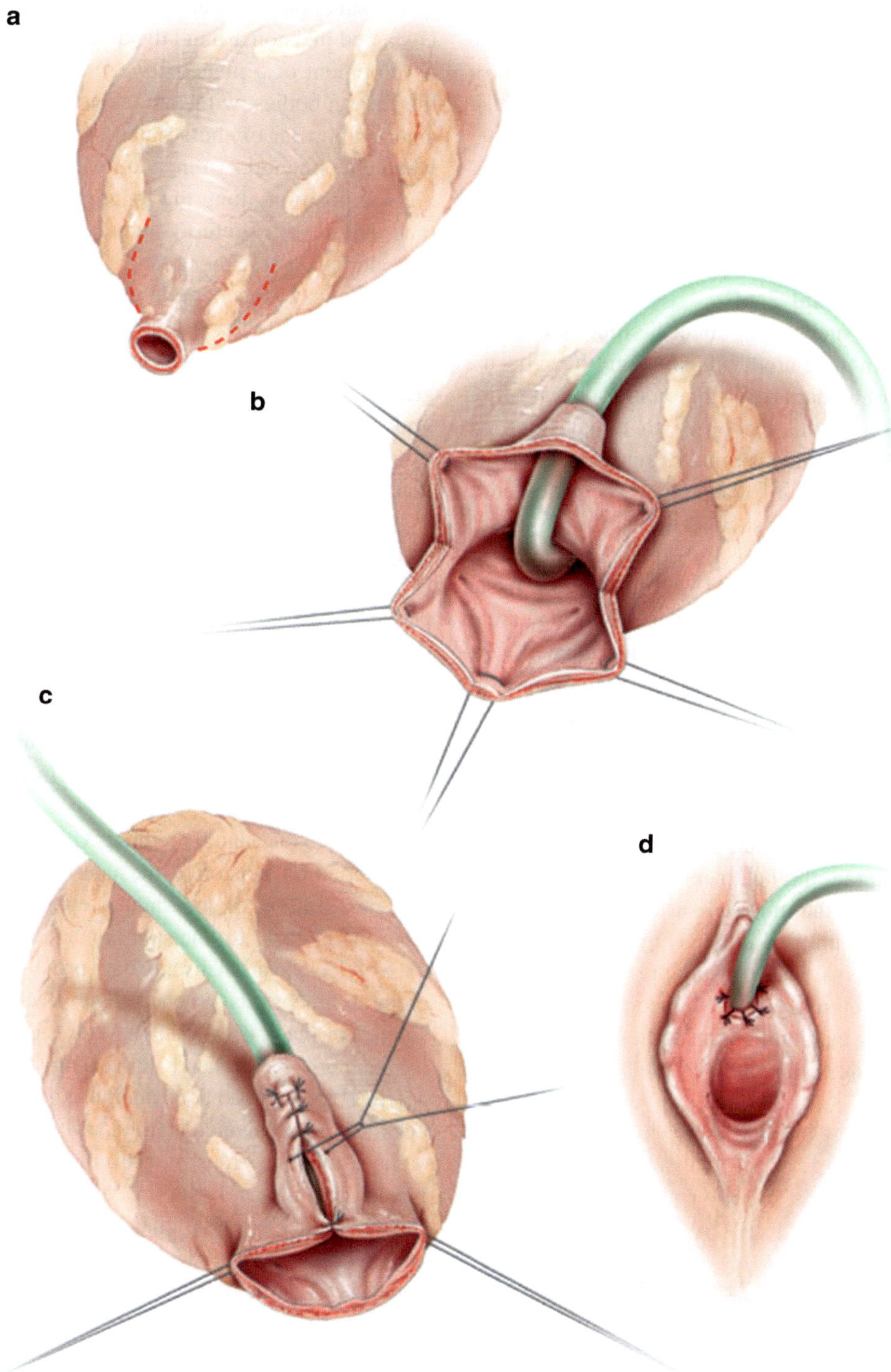

Fig. 21.16 Bladder wall flap. (Reused with permission. Copyright John Wiley and Sons [71]). (**a**) Outline of U flap on anterior bladder wall with apex on posterior wall of bladder immediately below trigone. (**b**) Anterior bladder wall flap incised with temporary displacement of pre-existing bladder opening superiorly onto anterior bladder wall. (**c**)Longitudinal closure of sides of anterior bladder wall flap to form neourethra. (**d**) After full closure the neourethra has been transposed deep to the anterior vaginal wall and a neomeatus has been created

Case Scenario 2

If a guidewire had passed, then a graft urethroplasty may also have been an option.

Graft Options: Buccal, Lingual, Tissue Engineering

Buccal Mucosal Graft

After the success of buccal mucosal grafts (BMGs) in male urethroplasty, there have been a number of authors reporting on the success of the translation of this technique to female urethroplasty. Buccal mucosa makes an excellent graft for the urethra as it is hairless and accustomed to moist environments such as the urethra.

BMG harvest has been previously described and involves removing a graft of buccal tissue from the inner surface of one cheek taking care to avoid Stenson's duct (parotid duct, located adjacent to the upper 2nd molar). The size of the graft depends on the length of urethra requiring reconstruction but in complete obliteration often needs to be 2–3-cm wide and normally at least 3–4-cm long [53]. The graft once harvested should be thinned and then sutured into place over a 16 Fr indwelling urethral catheter with non-absorbable sutures with the mucosal surface facing inwards towards the urethral lumen (Fig. 21.17).

Both dorsal and ventral approaches for BMG female urethroplasty have been described, but due to the small number in studies, comment cannot be made with regards to the best approach.

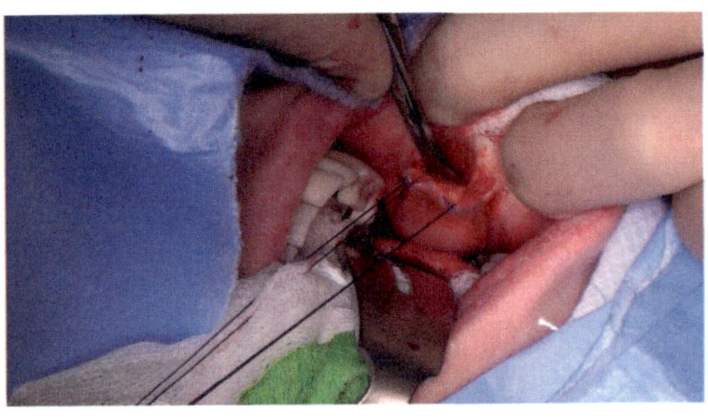

Fig. 21.17 BMG harvest. (Reused with permission. Copyright John Wiley and Sons [32]). Stay sutures are in distal buccal mucosa to hold old to length and allow manipulation as the graft is harvested off the underling buccinator

Dorsal approaches are performed via a reverse U-shaped incision around the urethral meatus and development of a plane between the urethra and the clitoral bodies, with care taken to preserve the anterior portion of the striated sphincter muscle when encountered. An incision is made in the 12 o'clock position along the length of the stricture (and into healthy urethra), and the graft is anastomosed in place to either side of the incision. If the graft extends to the external urethral meatus, then it is fashioned to form a slit-like meatus. Some authors recommend quilting of the augmented graft to the clitoral bodies to aid maturation of the graft (Fig. 21.18). Dorsal approaches are favoured by some authors due to the postulated reduction in sacculation of the graft and better voiding stream as well as providing a well-vascularised and well-supported plate for the graft to establish upon [32]. This technique may be almost essential for patients with poor vaginal epithelium and high risk of urethrovaginal fistula formation and reconstruction failure with a ventral approach. Its disadvantages are that the dorsal incision is bisecting the omega-shaped female urethral sphincter at its thickest part if the incision extends into the middle 2/3 of the urethra [54].

Access to the ventral urethra is via a longitudinal (or inverted U) incision on the anterior vaginal wall and mobilisation of the vaginal epithelium away from the urethra. An incision is made this time in the 6 o'clock position distally until proximal healthy urethral mucosa is reached. The BMG is then sutured in place (Fig. 21.19). With this approach, the authors recommend harvesting a modified Martius labial fat pad flap and transposing this to lie between the augmented urethral BMG graft and the vaginal wall in order to prevent fistulation and breakdown of the repair. A ventral approach is thought to decrease the chances of post-operative urinary incontinence due to the female urethral sphincter's ventral deficiency [32, 54].

In the main onlay, graft approaches have been described. There is a single case reported of a ventral inlay technique with patency of the repair at 10 months follow-up, but this is unlikely to be suitable for extensive cases of urethral obliteration (Fig. 21.20) [55].

Morbidity related to buccal mucosa is low. Reduction in sensation in the area of graft harvest

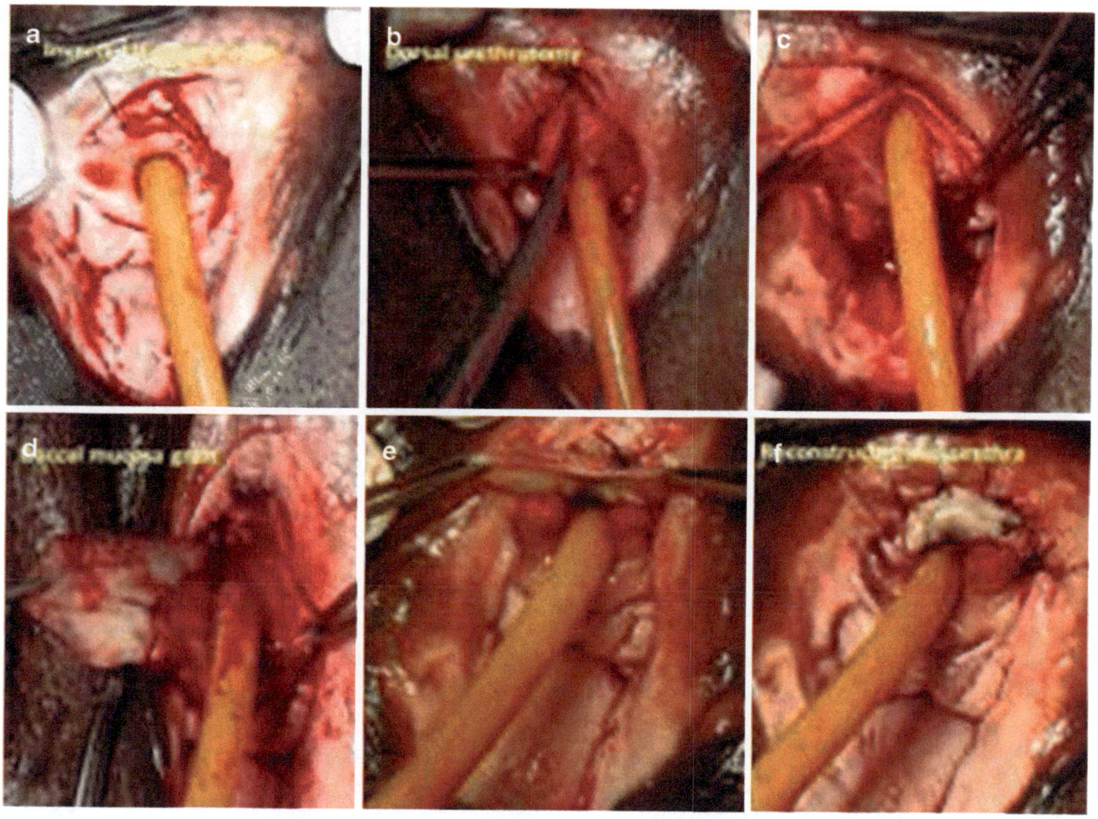

Fig. 21.18 Dorsal BMG urethroplasty. (Reused with permission. Copyright Springer Nature [69]). (**a**) Inverted U incision around dorsum of meatus. (**b**) Dorsal mobilisation of urethral with dorsal stricturotomy. (**c**) Further dorsal mobilisation of urethra with advancement of stricturotomy. (**d**) Suture of BMG to apex of stricturotomy. (**e**) BMG sutured at apex and bilaterally onto either side proximally. (**f**) Final appearance

has been reported in 29%, change is saliva production in 11%, and reduction in maximal mouth opening in 9% [56].

Lingual Mucosal Grafts

In cases of suboptimal buccal mucosa, success has also been reported with the use of lingual mucosa (Fig. 21.21). Sharma et al. (2009) have published on the use of this graft in women, and previously in males, and have shown it to be well tolerated with minimal morbidity when compared to BMG [57]. In larger male series, graft-related morbidity is slurring of speech in 8%, parageusia in 5% and ventral tongue numbness in 17% [58]. However, due to the lack of further evidence, the authors would currently recommend utilising this only in cases in which BMG mucosa is not available (e.g. patient choice and previous graft site).

Vaginal/Labial Graft

Vaginal grafts are not widely reported in the literature as common sense would dictate that if the vagina is to be used, then a vaginal flap would be more suitable as it is better vascularised and does not require the maturation process of a graft. However, a small series of 11 patients has been reported by Petrou et al. (2012) of dorsal vaginal graft urethroplasty [59]. This follows a similar approach to the dorsal BMG urethroplasty but utilises a graft harvested from the anterior vaginal wall or medial aspect of the labia minora. The vaginal wall/labial defect is then subsequently closed prior to proceeding to either a dorsal or ventral approach urethroplasty after careful haemostasis as bleeding is an obvious risk. Success rates are discussed below.

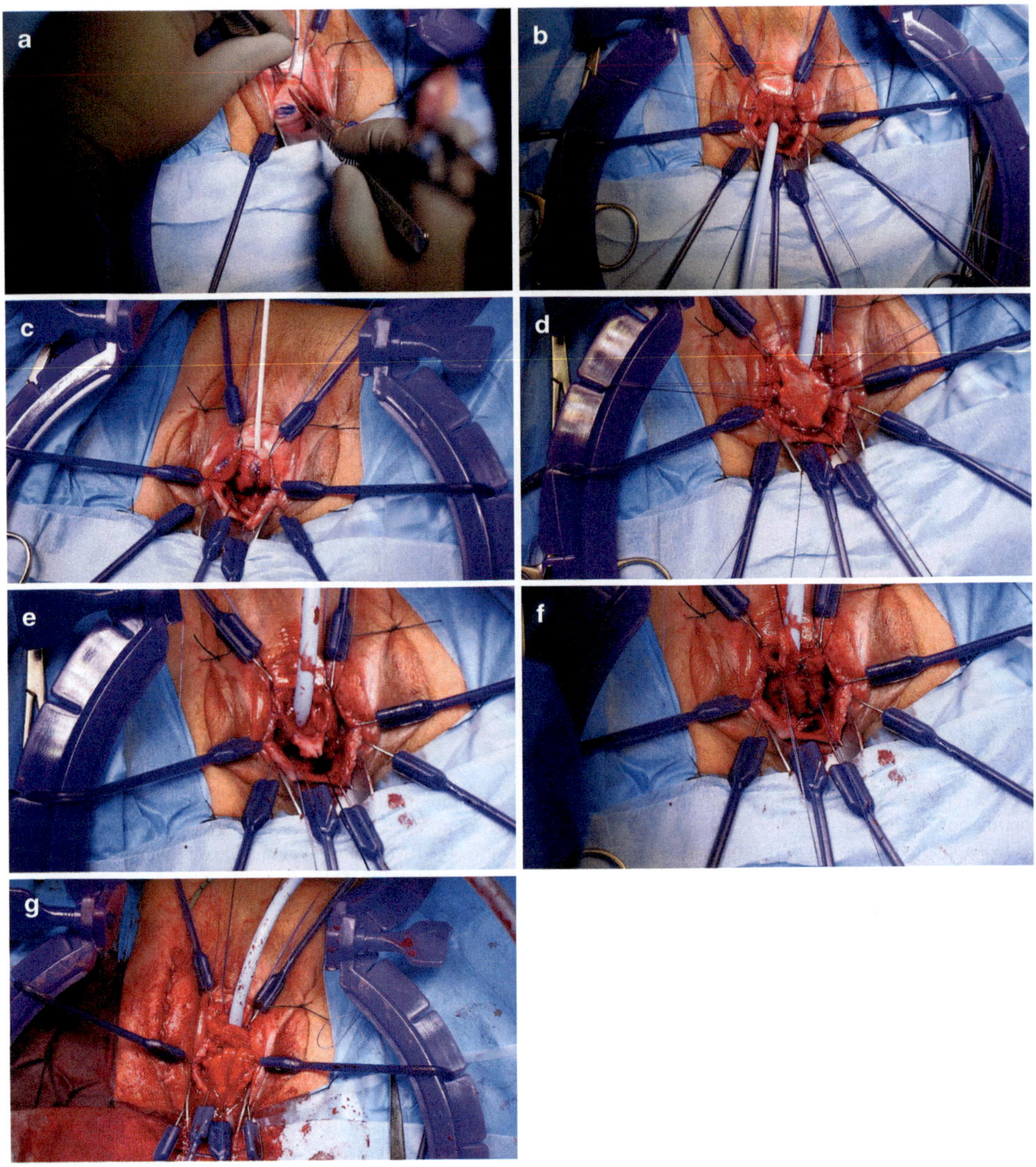

Fig. 21.19 (**a**–**g**) Ventral BMG urethroplasty. (Reused with permission. Copyright John Wiley and Sons [32]). (**a**) Proximal end of stricture marked on vagina after determination using embolectomy catheter. Midline vaginal incision about to commence. (**b**) Anterior vagina mobilised off anterior and lateral urethra. (**c**) Proximal end of stricture and midline longitudinal urethral incision site marked. (**d**) BMG harvested, sutured to apex of midline ventral stricturotomy and held in place laterally with stay sutures. (**e**) BMG sutured bilaterally to stricturotomy to level of meatus. Excess distal BMG is to allow creation of a neomeatus. (**f**) Overlying periurethral tissue is closed without tension. (**g**) Martius fat pad flap is transposed into the vaginal wound and sutured over the completed urethroplasty - with quilting especially distally to support the graft

Tissue Engineering: Acellular Porcine Urinary Bladder Matrix

The ideal graft would avoid having to borrow from another part of the body, which obviously incurs morbidity at another site distant from the repair and therefore, there is active research in development of acellular biological grafts. El-Kassaby et al. (2008) previously showed the

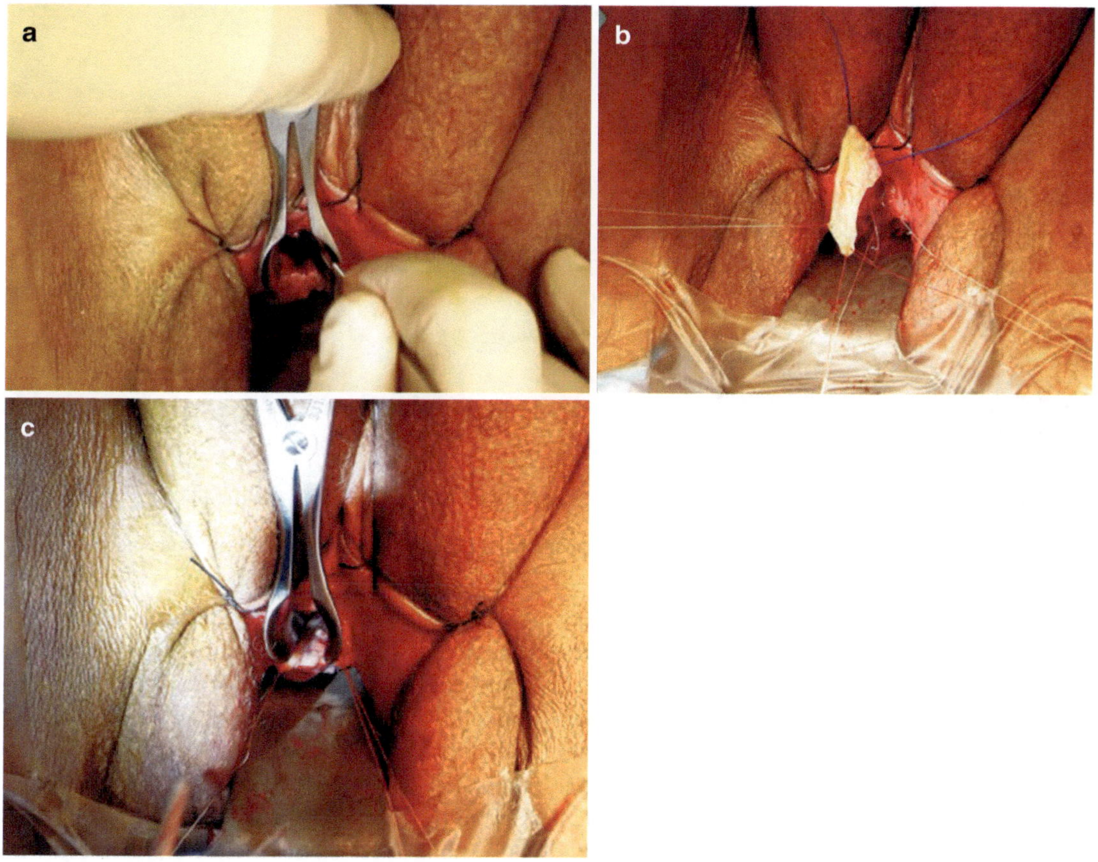

Fig. 21.20 Vaginal sparing ventral inlay (**a**) Inverted u incision to dorsum of meatus to allow dorsal mobilisation to distal edge of stricture. (**b**) Suprapubic cystoscopy to level of proximal aspect of stricture. (**c**) and (**d**) Suprapubic cystoscopic guidance of sutures passed from vaginal aspect of stricture to proximal aspect of stricture and back to distal aspect - to allow subsequent division of scar tissue and anastomotic urethroplasty

feasibility of acellular bladder matrix grafts in male urethroplasty but noted that it appeared that a healthy graft bed was required to ensure success of the acellular graft, whereas BMG could survive even in difficult, poorly vascularised graft beds [60].

Ansari and Karram (2017) have subsequently reported on 2 patients who underwent female urethral reconstruction using acellular porcine urinary bladder matrix, Martius fat pad interposition and insertion of an autologous pubo-vaginal sling [61]. Both patients had improved continence and appeared to have developed subjectively 'normal' urethral mucosa at the site of grafting. The authors recognise that further work is required to prove histologically that this acellular matrix can transform to urethral mucosa, but this has previously been shown to be possible in the El-Kassaby et al. series [60]. Work in this area is ongoing but promising.

Success Rates and Functional Outcomes

As expected, there is a paucity of evidence for each specific graft-based urethroplasty technique. A systematic review of surgical techniques for female urethral stricture disease by Osman et al. (2013) found a total of 32 cases of oral mucosal graft urethroplasty reported by 7 studies [62]. Mean success rates were 94% over an average follow-up of 15 months. Reported complications included graft site haematoma and temporary storage lower urinary tract symptoms. No incontinence was reported in any study. However, it should be acknowledged that, save for one large series by Mukhtar et al. of 22 patients, these are generally small series with

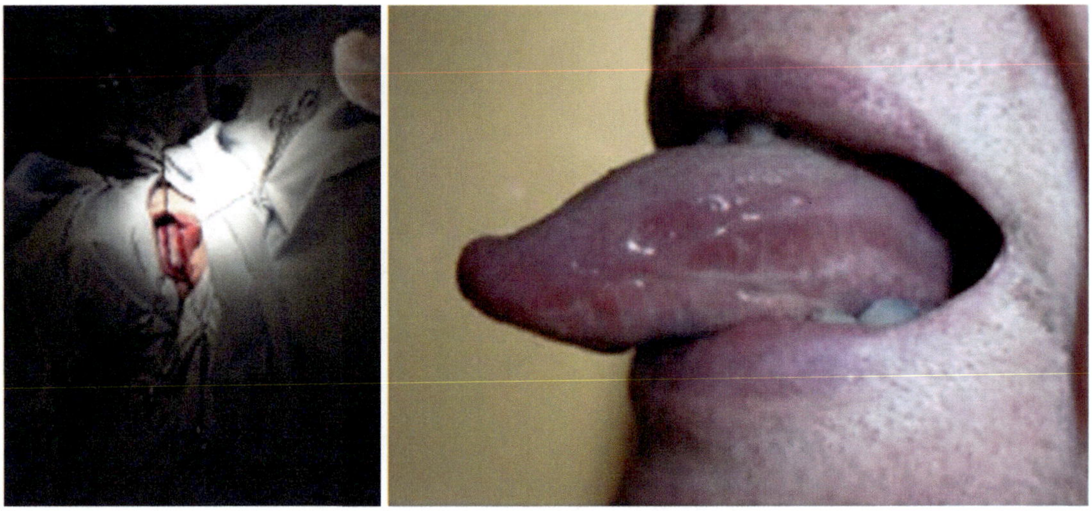

Fig. 21.21 Lingual mucosal graft harvest and final appearance of harvest site. (Courtesy of Mr. Paul Anderson)

short follow-up (it is worth noting that male series of BMG urethroplasty note recurrent strictures over 10 years after the primary operation) [32].

For vaginal/labial graft urethroplasty, Osman et al. found 4 studies with a total of 25 patients and mean follow-up of 22 months and mean success rates were 80% [62]. Petrou et al. (2012) showed no post-operative stress urinary incontinence but did report one case of de novo urge urinary incontinence. No other significant complications were noted [59].

Excision and Re-anastomosis Urethroplasty

Due to the short length of the female urethra, traditional excision and re-anastomosis techniques result in increased morbidity. Dorsal mobilisation of the urethra can cause significant bleeding and proximal dissection risks stress urinary incontinence. Extensive mobilisation of the urethra, particularly distal to the stricture, must also be avoided as this can cause devascularisation of the urethra. Due to the shorter female urethral length, this technique is only suitable for short segments of urethral obliteration. As a result, it is not widely used/described in the literature, with Patil et al. reporting on one case [63] and Rovner and Wein (2003) describing success with this technique in the context of urethral diverticulectomy (Fig. 21.22) [1].

Lengthening Incision Techniques

Longitudinal ventral incision of the urethra and transverse re-anastomosis using the Heineke-Mikulicz principle has been described by Ackerman et al. [64]. However, there are no case reports or series on this procedure's success rates. Certainly, it is acknowledged that this procedure is only suitable for short strictures, preferably with less extensive dorsal scarring (as this will risk stricture recurrence) and therefore may be less suitable for cases of complete urethral obliteration. Recurrence rates and complications are not currently published.

Graft or Flap-Based Urethroplasty

Graft or flap-based procedures are the mainstay of treatment for urethral obliteration, as a significant increase in urethral calibre needs to be achieved. This involves either dorsal or ventral incisions in the urethra at the diseased segment (with healthy margins at either end) and anastomosis of an augmentation graft or flap to widen the urethral lumen. In some cases where there are long segments of urethral obliteration or loss of a full substitution graft/flap, urethroplasty has to be performed to create a neo-urethra. Indications for grafts versus flap-based procedures and choice of graft/flap are described in the next section.

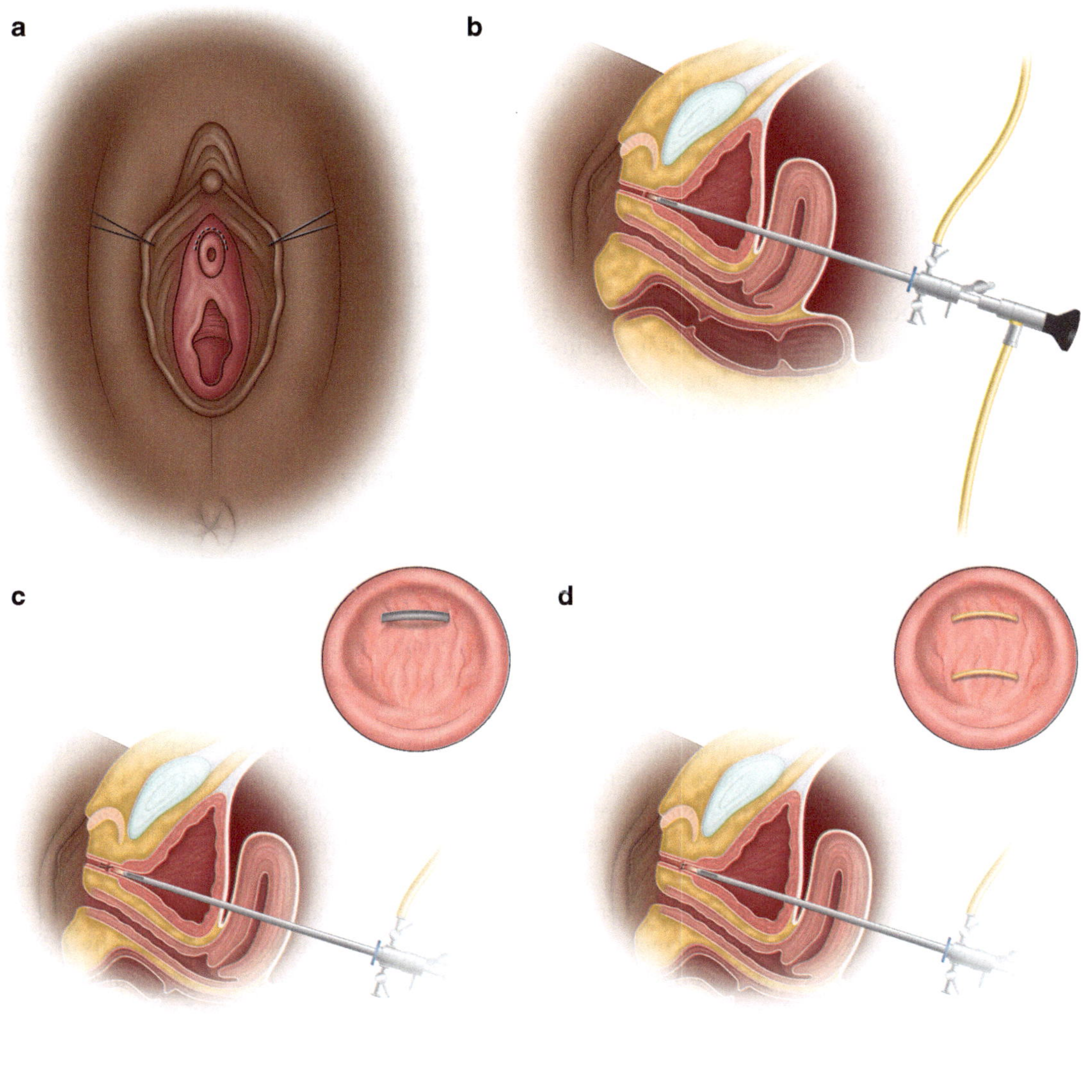

Fig. 21.22 (**a–d**) Anastomotic urethroplasty

Technical Considerations

Use of Martius Fat Pad

One of the key principles of urethral reconstruction is ensuring adequate cover of urethral sutures with peri-urethral tissue in order to prevent fistulation in ventral repairs. Often the peri-urethral tissue is poor due to extensive fibrosis and alternative tissue must be found to cover the urethral repair suture line. A modified Martius labial fat pad flap interposition has proved to be a durable and safe graft and protects the urethral repair with minimal morbidity for the patient (<2% complication rate) [32, 65]. It is also readily accessible and easy to move into position to quilt onto the urethral repair (Fig. 21.11).

Concomitant Anti-incontinence Procedure

With any urethral reconstruction, there is a risk of post-operative stress urinary incontinence, even with careful dissection and a good understanding of the relevant anatomy. Some authors describe concurrent placement of an autologous fascial sling. Flisser and Blavias (2003) report concurrent use of autologous pubo-vaginal sling in 56 out of 74 patients undergoing vaginal flap urethroplasty for various pathologies, with 87% of patients reporting cure/significant improvement post-operatively [66]. They postulate that a concurrent anti-incontinence procedure should be considered in any patient with extensive proximal urethral dissection or who is judged to be at high risk of post-operative urinary incontinence. The timing (staged vs. concurrent) is still up for debate, however. There is no evidence in the literature for the use of synthetic slings in this setting and, given the known complications of urethral/vaginal erosion and fistula formation, should be avoided as they may increase the rate of reconstruction failure [67].

Summary

Severe urethral stenosis/complete urethral obliteration is a rare and difficult condition to treat with limited evidence for the multiple surgical reconstruction techniques described. Due to the complexity, variability and unpredictability of the condition, it is important to have a range of techniques in the armamentarium of a reconstructive urologist in order to adapt to the clinical scenario presented. Continence is a key issue, which can be maintained in many cases with careful dissection and a sound anatomical understanding of the urethra. However, in proximal urethral obliteration, it may not be possible to preserve continence and additional anti-incontinence procedures may be required either concomitantly or subsequently – the authors recommend autologous pubo-vaginal sling as the best solution.

Reconstruction can be performed using a ventral or dorsal approach with neither approach having superiority over the other. However, it is important to remember the risk of urethrovaginal fistulation if there are ventrally placed sutures and the authors recommend utilisation of a modified Martius labial fat pad flap interposition between the urethra and vagina in this scenario. For the majority of cases of complete urethral obliteration, formation of a neo-urethra is required, and therefore, tubularised flap-based urethroplasty techniques that create a neo-urethra are often the most useful for this scenario. Ultimately though, for urethral reconstruction to be successful, there must be a healthy graft bed or a healthy well-vascularised flap, this must be anastomosed to healthy tissue (i.e. proximal to the diseased segment) and the repair must be watertight. It is important to remember the lessons learnt in male urethroplasty that strictures may recur in repaired urethral segments up to 10 years after the initial reconstruction, and therefore, it is important to carry out extended follow-up for these patients on a regular basis.

Commentary

Jaspreet S. Sandhu

This chapter presents a case-based review of severe female urethral stricture disease including a detailed summary of available female urethral reconstructive techniques. These techniques range from endoscopic management such as internal urethrotomy or urethral dilation followed by intermittent self-catheterisation to flap or graft-based urethroplasty.

The authors correctly state that a common aetiology of female urethral strictures in the western world is iatrogenic, specifically following urethral surgery (e.g. urethral diverticulectomy or removal of mid-urethral sling). Pelvic radiation, such as that for gynaecological or colorectal malignancies, is another common cause for female strictures. It is also noted that, unlike in males, pelvic fractures are not a common aetiology of female urethral strictures.

The history and physical exam are extremely important in women presenting with symptoms of urethral stricture. Specifically, urethral cancer should be on the differential diagnosis in women with no obvious cause for urethral stricture based on history. A physical exam or pelvic imaging finding of a urethral mass or urethral thickening in this setting should prompt a urethral biopsy and if cancer is found, the patient should be managed by an oncologist. At our centre, we have diagnosed urethral cancers in multiple women who presented with recurrent urinary tract infections and/or difficulty voiding.

Treatment options for female stricture disease are varied and are reviewed nicely in this chapter. Minimally invasive methods such as urethral dilation or internal urethrotomy are often the first-line treatment and can sometimes be the only treatment needed, specifically if intermittent self-catheterisation is added [15]. Vaginal wall and other flaps have been described with reasonable efficacy. More recently, buccal mucosal grafts have been used with similar efficacy. The small number of patients in these series, however, limits our ability to conclude if one technique is better than another or even if flaps or graft are better than endoscopic management. The fact that the two meta-analyses referenced in this chapter were compilations of studies that average 5–7 patients each is concerning. Furthermore, a recent report on the experience of 6 surgeons with dorsal buccal graft urethroplasty in female urethral stricture disease included approximately 6 cases per surgeon over a 9-year period [72]. Not only is the number of patients in these series low, follow-up remains limited. As more surgeons gain experience and offer these techniques, more robust reporting is expected and perhaps, one technique will prove better than others.

Female urethral strictures associated with previous pelvic radiation are a uniquely difficult problem to treat. It appears that more women are presenting with urethral strictures after radiotherapy; yet, there is very little reported in literature on this topic. In our experience, urethral strictures post-radiotherapy are best managed with minimally invasive methods. These patients tend to have severely ischaemic tissue resulting in diminished wound healing and complications after surgery are difficult to treat and can potentially be devastating. Specifically, urinary incontinence or vesicovaginal fistula rates are likely higher after urethroplasty in radiated patients. If these are subsequently treated, the surgeon is dealing with a radiated and previously operated field and sometimes, these patients are left with a urinary diversion as their only option.

Finally, a urinary diversion or a suprapubic-tube placement are important techniques to use as a 'back-up' for patients with severe female urethral stricture disease. Permanent supra-pubic tubes are not ideal, but some patients prefer the simplicity of this method and are comfortable with frequent scheduled replacements of these catheters.

A simple cystectomy may be performed with a urinary diversion regardless of whether it is a continent cutaneous diversion or an ileal conduit urinary diversion. While a cystectomy with urinary diversion is technically straightforward, it is important to note that these patients have a high rate of subsequent complications particularly if the cystectomy is for benign disease [73] as in the setting of severe female urethral strictures. Cutaneous continence mechanisms, such as those based on the Mitrofanoff principle, can be added to an existing bladder in the setting of complete urethral occlusion. However, it should be noted that women that presented with urinary incontinence also need a bladder neck closure. A previous history of radiation can cause a bladder neck closure to subsequently fail; in which case, these women either need a tight pubo-vaginal sling or a cystectomy with urinary diversion.

Female urethral stricture disease is being recognised as an important malady that needs treatment. This chapter provides an excellent review of the surgical techniques currently available for treating this disease. Because of the limited evidence base, it is extremely important to take into account patient preference and goals of care and discuss the risks and possible complications of treatment with patients in a shared decision-making model.

References

1. Rovner ES, Wein AJ. Diagnosis and reconstruction of the dorsal or circumferential urethral diverticulum. J Urol. 2003;170:82–6; discussion 86.
2. Angulo JC, Mateo E, Lista F, Andrés G. Reconstructive treatment of female urethral stenosis secondary to erosion by suburethral tape. Actas Urol Esp. 2011;35:240–5.
3. Rubio SM, Casado JS, Chamorro MV, Martín PG, Fuertes ME, Sierra JM. Other radiological lesions of the lower urinary tract in patients after isolated pelvic radiotherapy and combined with surgery. Arch Esp Urol. 2016;69:59–66.

4. Carter CT, Schafer N. Incidence of urethral disruption in females with traumatic pelvic fractures. Am J Emerg Med. 1993;11:218–20.
5. Latini JM, McAninch JW, Brandes SB, Chung JY, Rosenstein D. SIU/ICUD consultation on urethral strictures: epidemiology, etiology, anatomy, and nomenclature of urethral stenoses, strictures, and pelvic fracture urethral disruption injuries. Urology. 2014;83(3 Suppl):S1–7.
6. Hamlin RH, Nicholson EC. Reconstruction of urethra totally destroyed in labour. Br Med J. 1969;2(5650):147–50.
7. Monseur J. Reconstruction of the female urethra using the roots of the clitoris. Eleven cases. J Urol Nephrol (Paris). 1976;82:581–91.
8. Hussain M, Askari H, Lal M, Naqvi SA, Rizvi SA. Experience at a stricture clinic in a developing country. J Pak Med Assoc. 2013;63:234–8.
9. Pérez-López FR, Vieira-Baptista P. Lichen sclerosus in women: a review. Climacteric. 2017;20:339–47.
10. Kang M, Jeong CW, Kwak C, Kim HH, Ku JH. Survival outcomes and predictive factors for female urethral cancer: long-term experience with Korean patients. J Korean Med Sci. 2015;30: 1143–9.
11. Romman AN, Alhalabi F, Zimmern PE. Distal intramural urethral pathology in women. J Urol. 2012;188(4):1218–23.
12. Takao M, Asano T, Nakamura H. Urodynamic studies before and after gradual dilation with metal sounds for female urethral stricture. Hinyokika Kiyo. 1992;38:15–7.
13. Popat S, Zimmern PE. Long-term management of luminal urethral stricture in women. Int Urogynecol J. 2016;27:1735–41.
14. Parsons BA, Narshi A, Drake MJ. Success rates for learning intermittent self-catheterisation according to age and gender. Int Urol Nephrol. 2012;44:1127–31.
15. Smith AL, Ferlise VJ, Rovner ES. Female urethral strictures: successful management with long-term clean intermittent catheterization after urethral dilatation. BJU Int. 2006;98:96–9.
16. Ahmed S, Kardar AH. Construction of a neourethra in girls: follow-up results. Pediatr Surg Int. 2000;16:584–5.
17. Faure A, Cooksey R, Bouty A, Woodward A, Hutson J, O'Brien M, Heloury Y. Bladder continent catheterizable conduit (the Mitrofanoff procedure): long-term issues that should not be underestimated. J Pediatr Surg. 2017;52(3):469–72.
18. West C, Lawrence A. Female urethroplasty: contemporary thinking. World J Urol. 2018. https://doi.org/10.1007/s00345-018-2564-4.
19. Spilotros M, Malde S, Solomon E, Grewal M, Mukhtar BM, Pakzad M, Hamid R, Ockrim JL, Greenwell TJ. Female urethral stricture: a contemporary series. World J Urol. 2017;35:991–5.
20. Tsivian A, Sidi AA. Dorsal graft urethroplasty for female urethral stricture. J Urol. 2006;176:611–3.
21. Goel A, Paul S, Dalela D, Sankhwar P, Sankhwar SN, Singh V. Dorsal onlay buccal mucosal graft urethroplasty in female urethral stricture disease: a single-center experience. Int Urogynecol J. 2014;25:525–30.
22. Osman NI, Mangera A, Chapple CR. A systematic review of surgical techniques used in the treatment of female urethral stricture. Eur Urol. 2013;64:965–73.
23. Rehder P, Glodny B, Pichler R, Exeli L, Kerschbaumer A, Mitterberger MJ. Dorsal urethroplasty with labia minora skin graft for female urethral strictures. BJU Int. 2010;106:1211–4.
24. Gozzi C, Roosen A, Bastian PJ, Karl A, Stief C, Tritschler S. Volar onlay urethroplasty for reconstruction of female urethra in recurrent stricture disease. BJU Int. 2011;107:1964–6.
25. Önol FF, Antar B, Köse O, Erdem MR, Önol ŞY. Techniques and results of urethroplasty for female urethral strictures: our experience with 17 patients. Urology. 2011;77(6):1318–24.
26. Okur H, Küçĭkaydin M, Kazez A, Turan C, Bozkurt A. Genitourinary tract injuries in girls. Br J Urol. 1996;78:446–9.
27. Gilliver SC, Ashcroft GS. Sex steroids and cutaneous wound healing: the contrasting influences of estrogens and androgens. Climacteric. 2007;10:276–88.
28. McAninch LN. External meatotomy in the female. Can J Surg. 1965;8:382–8.
29. Biedwald W, Duda SH. Surgical therapy of congenital distal urethral stenoses in girls by meatoplasty. Int Urol Nephrol. 1987;19:327–32.
30. Migliari R, Leone P, Berdondini E, De Angelis M, Barbagli G, Palminteri E. Dorsal buccal mucosa graft urethroplasty for female urethral strictures. J Urol. 2006;176:1473–6.
31. Berglund RK, Vasavada S, Angermeier K, Rackley R. Buccal mucosa graft urethroplasty for recurrent stricture of female urethra. Urology. 2006;67:1069–71.
32. Mukhtar BMB, Spilotros M, Malde S, Greenwell TJ. Ventral-onlay buccal mucosa graft substitution urethroplasty for urethral stricture in women. BJU Int. 2017;120:710–6.
33. Romero-Maroto J, Verdú-Verdú L, Gómez-Pérez L, Pérez-Tomás C, Pacheco-Bru JJ, López-López A. Lateral-based anterior vaginal wall flap in the treatment of female urethral stricture: efficacy and safety. Eur Urol. 2018;73:123–8.
34. Montorsi F, Salonia A, Centemero A, Guazzoni G, Nava L, Da Pozzo LF, Cestari A, Colombo R, Barbagli G, Rigatti P. Vestibular flap urethroplasty for strictures of the female urethra. Impact on symptoms and flow patterns. Urol Int. 2002;69:12–6.
35. Blaivas JG, Heritz DM. Vaginal flap reconstruction of the urethra and vesical neck in women: a report of 49 cases. J Urol. 1996;155:1014–7.
36. Gormley EA. Vaginal flap urethroplasty for female urethral stricture disease. NeurourolUrodyn. 2010;29(Suppl 1):S42–5.
37. Simonato A, Varca V, Esposito M, Carmignani G. Vaginal flap urethroplasty for wide female stricture disease. J Urol. 2010;184:1381–5.

38. Kowalik C, Stoffel JT, Zinman L, Vanni AJ, Buckley JC. Intermediate outcomes after female urethral reconstruction: graft vs flap. Urology. 2014;83:1181–5.
39. de Geeter P. Surgery of the female urethra: meatusplasty, operation of the urethral caruncle, urethral prolapse and urethral diverticulum. Aktuelle Urol. 2006;37:226–38.
40. Blaivas JG. Vaginal flap urethral reconstruction: an alternative to the bladder flap neourethra. J Urol. 1989;141:542–5.
41. Rosenblum N, Nitti VW. Female urethral reconstruction. Urol Clin N Am. 2011;38:55–64.
42. Tannello M, Frego E, Simeone C, Cunico SC. Use of pedicle flap from the labia minora for the repair of female urethral strictures. Urol Int. 2002;69:95–8.
43. Xu YM, Sa YL, Fu Q, Zhang J, Xie H, Jin SB. Transpubic access using pedicle tubularized labial urethroplasty for the treatment of female urethral strictures associated with urethrovaginal fistulas secondary to pelvic fracture. Eur Urol. 2009;56:193–200.
44. Zorn KC, Bzrezinski A, St-Denis B, Corcos J. Female neo-urethral reconstruction with a modified neurovascular pudendal thigh flap (Singapore flap): initial experience. Can J Urol. 2007;14(1):3449–54.
45. Radwan MH, Abou Farha MO, Soliman MG, El Refai M, Ragab MM, Shaaban AM, Abou Farha OM. Outcome of female urethral reconstruction: a 12-year experience. World J Urol. 2013;31:991–5.
46. Mitsui T, Tanaka H, Moriya K, Suzuki H, Mouri G, Hashimoto A, Nonomura K. Construction of neourethra using flipped anterior bladder wall tube in a prepubertal girl with complete disruption of urethra. Urology. 2010;76:112–4.
47. Elkins TE, Ghosh TS, Tagoe GA, Stocker R. Transvaginal mobilization and utilization of the anterior bladder wall to repair vesicovaginal fistulas involving the urethra. Obstet Gynecol. 1992;79:455–60.
48. Sawant A, Kasant GV, Kumar V, Pawar P, Tamnankar A, Bansal S, Kapadnis L, Savalea A. Reconstruction of female urethra with tubularized anterior vaginal wall flap. J Clin Diagn Res. 2016;10:PC01–3. (49 vaginal flap urethroplasties).
49. Hajebrahimi S, Maroufi H, Mostafaei H, Salehi-Pourmehr H. Reconstruction of the urtehra with an anterior vaginal mucosal flap in female urethral stricture. Int Urogynecol J. 2019. https://doi.org/10.1007/s00192-019-03910-3.
50. Blaivas JG, Santos JA, Tsui JF, Deibert CM, Rutman MP, Purohit RS, Weiss JF. Management of urethral stricture in women. J Urol. 2012;188:1778–82.
51. Angulo JC, Mateo E, Lista F, Andres G. Reconstructive treatment of female urethral estenosis secondary to erosion by suburethral tape. Actas Urol Esp. 2011;35:240–5.
52. Hemal AK, Dorairajan LN, Gupta NP. Posttraumatic complete and partial loss of urethra with pelvic fracture in girls: an appraisal of management. J Urol. 2000;163:282–7.
53. Morey AF, McAninch JW. When and how to use buccal mucosal grafts in adult bulbar urethroplasty. Urology. 1996;48:194–8.
54. Delancey JO. Functional anatomy of the female lower urinary tract and pelvic floor. Ciba Found Symp. 1990;151:57–69.
55. Hoag N, Gani J, Chee J. Vaginal-sparing ventral buccal mucosal graft urethroplasty for female urethral stricture: a novel modification of surgical technique. Investig Clin Urol. 2016;57:298–302.
56. Wood DN, Allen SE, Andrich DE, Greenwell TJ, Mundy AR. The morbidity of buccal mucosal graft harvest for urethroplasty and the effect of nonclosure of the graft harvest site on postoperative pain. J Urol. 2004;172:580–3.
57. Sharma GK, Pandey A, Bansal H, Swain S, Das SK, Trivedi S, Dwivedi US, Singh PS. Dorsal only lingual mucosal graft urethroplasty for urethral strictures in women. BJUI. 2009;105:1309–12.
58. Kumar A, Goyal NK, Das SK, Trivedi S, Dwivedi US, Singh PB. Oral complications after lingual mucosal graft harvest for urethroplasty. ANZ J Surg. 2007;77:970 3.
59. Petrou SP, Rogers AE, Parker AS, Green KM, McRoberts JW. Dorsal vaginal graft urethroplasty for female urethral stricture disease. BJUI. 2012;110:E1090–5.
60. El-Kassaby A, AbouShwareb T, Atala A. Randomized comparative study between buccal mucosal and acellular bladder matrix grafts in complex anterior urethral strictures. J Urol. 2008;179(4):1432–6.
61. Answari S, Karram M. Two cases of female urethral reconstruction with acellular porcine urinary bladder matrix. Int Urogynecol J. 2017;28(8):1257–60.
62. Osman NI, Chapple CR. Contemporary surgical management of female urethral stricture disease. Curr Opin Urol. 2015;25(4):341–5.
63. Patil S, Dalela D, Dalela D, Goel A, Snakhwar P, Sankhwar SN. Anastomotic urethroplasty in female urethral stricture guided by cystoscopy – a point of technique. J Surg Tech Case Rep. 2013;5:113–5.
64. Ackerman AL, Blaivas J, Anger JT. Female urethral reconstruction. Curr Bladder Dysfunct Rep. 2010;5:225 32.
65. Malde S, Spilotros M, Wilson A, Pakzad M, Hamid R, Ockrim J, Shah PJ, Greenwell T. The uses and outcomes of the Martius fat pad in female urology. World J Urol. 2017;35(3):473–8.
66. Flisser AJ, Blaivas JG. Outcome of urethral reconstructive surgery in a series of 74 women. J Urol. 2003;169:2246.
67. Blaivas JG, Sandhu J. Urethral reconstruction after erosion of slings in women. Curr Opin Urol. 2004;14(6):335–8.
68. Tanbo T, Kirschner R, Jebsen P, et al. Vaginal involvement in genital erosive lichen planus. Acta Obstet Gynecol Scand. 2010;89(7):966–70.
69. Baxter ZC. Urethroplasty for female urethral stricture disease. In: Firoozi F, editor. Female pelvic surgery. Cham: Springer; 2020.

70. Lumen N, Monstrey S, Goessaert A-S, Oosterlinck W, Hoebeke P. The Heineke-Mikulicz principle. Urethroplasty for strictures after phallic reconstruction: a single-institution experience. Eur Urol. 2011;60(1):150–8.
71. Tanagho EA. Surgical atlas anterior detrusor flap in urogenital sinus repair. BJU Int. 2008;107:647–61.
72. Hampson LA, Myers JB, Vanni AJ, et al. Dorsal buccal graft urethroplasty in female urethral stricture disease: a multi-center experience. Transl Androl Urol. 2019;8(suppl 1):S6–S12.
73. Zillioux J, Rapp D, Smith-Harrison L, et al. Assessment of complications following urinary diversion for benign indications. Can J Urol. 2019;26:9720–5.

Index

K. C. Kobashi, S. D. Wexner (eds.), *Female Pelvic Medicine*,
https://doi.org/10.1007/978-3-030-54839-1

GPSR Compliance

The European Union's (EU) General Product Safety Regulation (GPSR) is a set of rules that requires consumer products to be safe and our obligations to ensure this.

If you have any concerns about our products, you can contact us on ProductSafety@springernature.com

In case Publisher is established outside the EU, the EU authorized representative is:

Springer Nature Customer Service Center GmbH
Europaplatz 3
69115 Heidelberg, Germany

Batch number: 10166143

Printed by Printforce, the Netherlands